SENSORY PROCESSES

SENSORY
PROCESSES

David R. Soderquist
University of North Carolina at Greensboro

Sage Publications
International Educational and Professional Publisher
Thousand Oaks ▪ London ▪ New Delhi

For information:

Sage Publications, Inc.
2455 Teller Road
Thousand Oaks, California 91320
E-mail: order@sagepub.com

Sage Publications Ltd.
6 Bonhill Street
London EC2A 4PU
United Kingdom

Sage Publications India Pvt. Ltd.
M-32 Market
Greater Kailash I
New Delhi 110 048 India

Printed in the United States of America

Library of Congress Cataloging-in-Publication Data

Soderquist, David R.
 Sensory processes / by David R. Soderquist.
    p. cm.
Includes bibliographical references.
 ISBN 0-7619-2333-0
 1. Senses and sensation. I. Title.
 QP431 .S575 2002
 612.8—dc21   2001004335

01 02 03 04 05 06 10 9 8 7 6 5 4 3 2 1

Acquiring Editor:	Jim Brace-Thompson
Editorial Assistant:	Karen Ehrmann
Production Editor:	Diana E. Axelsen
Typesetter/Designer:	Marion Warren
Indexer:	Jeanne Busemeyer
Cover Designer:	Sandra J. Ng

Contents

Preface

For over three decades I have taught graduate and undergraduate courses in psychology. Although the courses have varied in their depth of presentation, content, and titles (Introductory Psychology, Perception, Sensation and Perception, Sensory Processes, Biological Psychology, Auditory Perception, Animal Psychophysics), they all focused on or emphasized particular perceptual aspects of human and animal existence. Because perception is one of the major intellectual pursuits of psychologists, it is well recognized that "There is nothing that is in the intellect that is not first in the senses" (Blaise Pascal).

This statement underscores the aim of this book; namely, to provide an introductory text that emphasizes all the sensory systems from a neuroscience perspective. The text is designed to meet a new and relatively unique niche in the neurosciences. The first two chapters provide the basic neural and physiological foundations for the remaining chapters. The text then continues by focusing on the neurological processes associated with each sensory modality. Although the emphasis is on the neurological aspects of each sensory system, perception is not disregarded. Perceptual processes are introduced and discussed from a neurological perspective. A unique aspect of the text is the inclusion of anomalies and dysfunctions for each sensory modality. In addition, a Glossary provides definitions for each highlighted term or concept discussed in the chapters. Given this approach, the content of the book is most likely to attract individuals interested in neuroscience, psychology, and biology. The text, however, also recommends itself to those in other disciplines (anthropology, premedicine, predentistry, preveterinarian).

Acknowledgments

I would like to thank the senior editor at Sage Publications, Jim Brace-Thompson, for his continual support and enthusiastic endorsement of this project. There were, as every author knows, times when I became weary and even cynical that the text would not come to fruition. Jim urged me on with good humor and skill. I would like to acknowledge Karen Ehrmann for her on-the-spot and on-the-job efforts with an apprentice author. Her personal approach to publishing makes her a true pleasure to work with. My skilled and dedicated copy editor, Denise McIntyre, is high on my list for praise. I thank her sincerely for being so polite in repairing an author's spelling and misstatements.

I would also like to acknowledge the great amount of labor and artistic skill displayed by Melissa Ball and Jason Rickards. They interpreted my hand drawings and produced the final published figures. I appreciate their dedication. I would also like to thank the following reviewers for their comments: Michael Sloane, Paul Dassonville, Rickye Heffner, Henry Heffner, Rick Jenison, Ellen Covey, Steven J. Haase, and Bruce Halpern. Their insights and thoughtful comments were much appreciated.

I would also be negligent if I did not acknowledge the continual support and encouragement of my students over the years. They urged me on with simple comments and sometimes with raw and occasional comical suggestions. I have probably surprised many of you by taking your comments seriously. I thank you for reading so closely and making your notes available. Finally, and with great devotion, I would like to thank my significant other, Aloha E. Bryson. She told me I should and knew I could. Thank you love, I needed that.

CHAPTER 1

Introduction to the Nervous System

The world is mostly unknown. This statement immediately emphasizes the point that we are not conscious of most of the environmental events that occur around us. The world consists of stimuli of which we may or may not be aware. These stimuli are pressure variations, chemicals, electromagnetic radiation, temperature, and even gravity. Figure 1.1 emphasizes this situation. This world of ours contains many events we do not focus on but also some we simply cannot perceive. We process the sensory information we interpret automatically each moment. However, we overlook many interesting aspects of our existence. For example, there are different types of pain. If you pause and think about it, you can recognize this. Remember the day you bumped your head. The immediate pain, sharp and crisp, was followed by a duller but still acutely painful ache and throb. You may even recall being told to "rub it, it'll feel better." The light rubbing usually does reduce the pain, but what happens if you rub too hard? It does not feel better. Pain is a confusing sensation when examined closely. Another example is to stare at a waterfall for a minute and then look at the grass. You would see the grass grow upward right in front of you. This illusion is the response of an active and normal visual system.

In this chapter, we examine the human nervous system and some principles that govern its operation. The nervous system can be understood more easily by first partitioning it in smaller components. Even when the nervous system is partitioned, however, it is cumbersome when first encountered. The goal of this chapter, and the one that follows, is to provide the knowledge

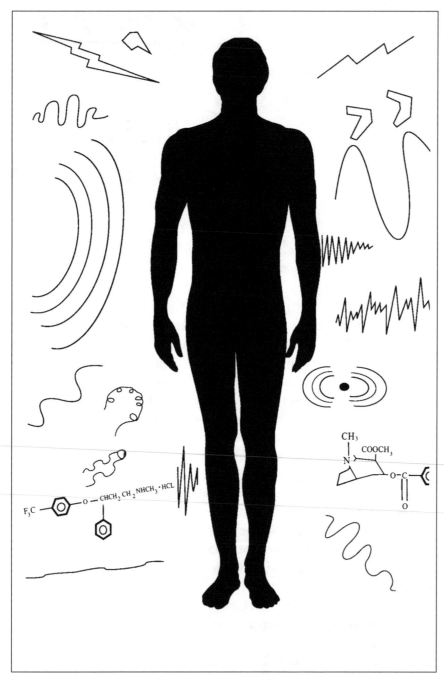

Figure 1.1. The Physical Energy in Our Surrounding Environment

necessary to appreciate the sensory systems discussed in later chapters. This chapter concludes with a discussion of some nervous system dysfunctions.

The Nervous System

The old adage that says "You are what you eat" can be more correctly stated, from a neurological perspective, as "You are what your nervous system permits." This simply means, in an emphatic way, that your thoughts, feelings, emotions, sensations, desires, dreams, ideas, creative urges, language, and life itself are under the control of the most complex structure in the world—your brain. This, of course, does not mean that there are no other physical structures or systems having important roles in your life—for example, digestive processes, internal organs, glands, and hormones. However, the nervous system is undoubtedly in control. It is no overstatement to say that the function of 100 to 120 billion neurons composing the nervous system is one of the most elusive mysteries of science today. The task of understanding the brain has been difficult but rewarding. The study of the nervous system is one of the most intellectually stimulating fields of study. Indeed, it is intriguing to realize that the nervous system investigates the nervous system. This is a simple matter of one brain investigating itself—a unique situation.

The immense magnitude of the nervous system requires, or demands, that investigators limit themselves to the study of relatively small and restricted features. Even by investigating small regions at a time, however, investigators are continually amazed at the bewildering complexity. The intricacy occurs in the realms of functions—what the nervous system does, and structure—how the nervous system is put together. It is our goal to examine the operation of the nervous system from only one of the multitude of different perspectives, namely, how does the nervous system receive information from the environment and, once the information is received, how does it process the information? In other words, how do we "sense" the stimuli in our environment? Because our lives depend on well-functioning sensory systems, we seek to understand what the nervous system does to provide us with a "real" world. The real-world environment also includes internal bodily activities such as stomachaches and joint movements. The nervous system monitors, reacts to, and interprets the world external to the body while continually monitoring the shifting environment within.

The nervous system is commonly partitioned in two parts: the **peripheral nervous system (PNS)** and the **central nervous system (CNS)**. These two interacting and communicating systems are in actuality a continuous entity.

The peripheral nervous system effectively merges into the central nervous system so dividing the nervous system in two separate parts is, in fact, an artificial partition. For the sake of description, however, it is a necessity. Furthermore, the central nervous system is usually partitioned in two additional sections: the brain and the spinal cord. The sectioning of the central nervous system is a useful procedure that is adhered to for our purpose of exposition. Figure 1.2 shows, diagrammatically, the division of the human nervous system into the peripheral nervous system and the central nervous system. We discuss each in turn.

The Peripheral Nervous System

The peripheral nervous system in Figure 1.2 shows the 31 pairs of **spinal nerves.** They are called "spinal" because they carry information to and from the spinal cord (Heimer, 1983). There are also 12 **cranial nerves** that conduct information to and from the brain more directly; that is, they do not involve the spinal cord. We discuss the cranial nerves associated with sensory systems as we examine each sensory modality. We focus here on the spinal and peripheral nerves and their organization.

Before we discuss the plan of the peripheral nervous system, it is important at the outset to briefly examine the idea of a nerve. All **nerves** are composed of thousands of small strands of fibers called **axons.** The axon is the conducting portion of a neuron. The peripheral nervous system and central nervous system process the neural impulses conducted by each axon. Many of these axons are individually wrapped with a covering called **myelin.** The axons are often gathered together to make a nerve. An analogy may be useful. We can compare a nerve with a telephone cable. A telephone cable (the nerve) consists of thousands of individually insulated wires (the axons). Each wire (axon) is capable of carrying a separate message. The insulation around each wire is the myelin. In addition, the insulation for each wire in the cable is often color coded, as is the myelin; it appears white when viewed with a microscope. The white appearance indicates to investigators that they are viewing a pathway of the nervous system. Neurons themselves appear gray.

The spinal nerves emerge from both sides of the spinal cord in a very specific manner. They emerge from the **dorsal** and **ventral horns.** The words *dorsal* and *ventral* refer to the back and belly of the spinal cord, respectively. The ventral portion of the spinal nerve sends information to muscles and glands and thus has an **efferent** function. *Efferent* refers to the conveying of information away from the central nervous system. The ventral portion of the nerve is also referred to as a "motor" nerve because it is often concerned with the

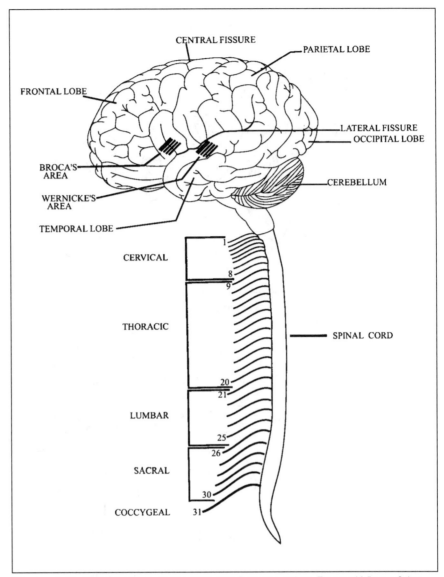

Figure 1.2. The Divisions of the Nervous System and an External View of the Brain and Spinal Cord

movement of the skeletal muscles. The dorsal portion of the spinal nerve is **afferent** in nature and carries information toward the central nervous system. The afferent portion of the spinal nerve provides the sensory information while the efferent axons allow the central nervous system to send messages to muscles, internal organs, and glands. Figure 1.3 shows a simplified diagram of this arrangement.

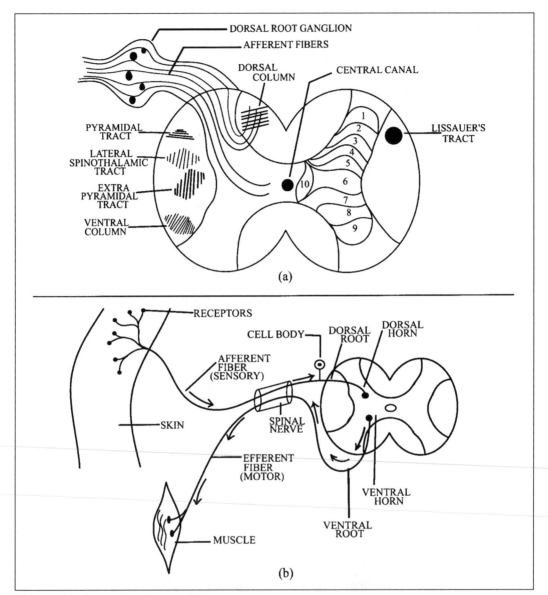

Figure 1.3. The Spinal Cord and Pathways

NOTE: (a) Cross-section of the spinal cord showing pathways and laminae within the cord and (b) Overview of the afferent and efferent paths.

Some of the spinal nerves are referred to as mixed nerves because they contain a mix of sensory (afferent) and motor (efferent) fibers. The classical division of the spinal nerve in two parts, shown in Figure 1.3(b) as the **dorsal** and **ventral roots**, is known as the **Bell-Magendie law**—the dorsal root is sensory and the ventral root is motor. Recent evidence has shown, however, that some afferent fibers enter the ventral horn, so the Bell-Magendie "law" may be more of a rule of thumb than a law.

Figure 1.3(a) shows the dorsal root ganglion as an enlargement of the sensory nerve. The axon fibers that compose the nerve require a **cell body** or **perikaryon** as a means of life support. The cell body is the main protoplasmic mass of a cell. The cell body produces an internal constituent called **axoplasm.** The axoplasm provides the axon with the metabolic means of existence. The dorsal root ganglion is a gathering together of the cell bodies associated with each sensory fiber in the spinal nerve. Because the cell bodies are not covered with myelin, visual inspection yields the gray appearance. Thus, to repeat, one of the first general rules of the nervous system is that pathways are white and cell bodies are gray. There is no ganglion for the efferent fibers. The cell bodies for the efferent fibers are located within the spinal cord itself.

Examination of Figure 1.3(b) shows that the distal end of axons, the end farthest from the central nervous system, often have special **arborizations** or treelike branching near their terminals. In the case of the sensory or afferent fibers, the arborizations enable the neural element to receive stimulation simultaneously from several sources in the environment. In addition, the axon often has additional arborizations that permit a single axon to send impulses to and communicate with many other cells. At the distal end of the neural element, there is often a specialized modification. The modification is a receptor (discussed in the next chapter). The rule to remember at this point is simple: No receptor = no sensation.

Peripheral and Spinal Nerves

Until now, we have not differentiated between the spinal nerves and the peripheral nerves. The situation is, at first glance, somewhat confusing. It can be readily understood, however, by noting that the spinal nerves come directly from the spinal cord and combine to form a peripheral nerve, see Figure 1.4. As the spinal nerve begins its journey toward the periphery of the body, a number of **plexuses** occur. *Plexus* is Latin for "braid." This means that the sensory portions of the spinal nerves are composed of individual fibers that diverge to different peripheral nerves. Each peripheral nerve, as a result, is made up of fibers from several spinal nerves. The peripheral nerves then continue to specific areas of the body. It is this very organization of the peripheral nervous system that causes differences in sensitivity as a function of different types of physiological insult—that is, an injury or surgical procedure. If a peripheral nerve is severed, the sensations are eliminated from a fixed and relatively small, circumscribed area of the body. Each peripheral nerve serves a

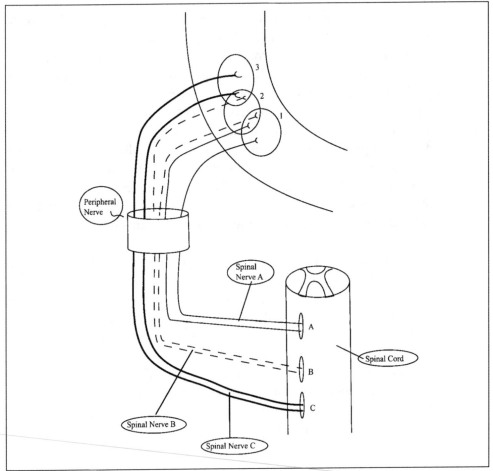

Figure 1.4. An Example of the Spinal and Peripheral Nerve Configuration

NOTE: Spinal nerves A, B, and C form a peripheral nerve and synapse on dermatomes 1, 2, and 3.

restricted portion of the body surface. If, on the other hand, a spinal nerve is cut there may be very little loss in feeling because fibers from other spinal nerves innervate the same surface area of the body. Figure 1.4 shows, diagrammatically, how this can occur. If spinal nerve A were severed, there would be little loss of sensitivity at the body surface labeled 1. This is because the innervations provided by spinal nerve B overlaps with the body surface previously served by spinal nerve A. In short, the loss of the fibers due to the severing of spinal nerve A is offset by the innervations provided by spinal nerve B. If, however, you were to cut the peripheral nerve, then all three body surfaces shown in Figure 1.4 would be devoid of innervations. The entire body area served by the peripheral nerve would be numb.

Each circular area of the body surface shown in Figure 1.4 is innervated by a spinal nerve. Specifically, spinal nerves A, B, and C innervate body surfaces 1, 2, and 3, respectively. The body surface innervated by the dorsal root of a spinal nerve is called a **dermatome**. Although each dorsal root (recall that there are 31 pairs) innervates its own specific dermatome (body surface) the dermatomes overlap to a large degree.

What this means, most simply, is that the entire surface of the body is partitioned and subdivided into specific areas served by spinal nerves. Figure 1.5 shows the dermatomes of the body associated with the spinal nerves. The dermatomes shown in Figure 1.5 do not overlap as indicated by the previous discussion. Figure 1.5 examines the spinal innervations and the spinal nerves of the arm. The cervical spinal nerve, labeled C6, innervates the area associated with the thumb. If you were to cut this spinal nerve, the area associated with the thumb and associated forearm would be incapable of sending information to the central nervous system. Because the peripheral radial nerve, composed of several spinal nerves, also innervates the thumb, it should be clear that there still would be some feeling in the thumb. In other words, cutting spinal nerve C6 does not eliminate all feeling and sensations from the thumb because there are other spinal nerves serving the thumb area via the radial nerve. There is a decrease in sensitivity, but not a complete loss of sensation.

The Central Nervous System

As mentioned previously, the central nervous system is composed of two parts: the spinal cord and the brain. We begin by describing the afferent and efferent portions of the spinal cord and some of the intricate interactions within the cord.

We can assume that every pain you perceive depends on information within your brain. The maxim to remember here is a simple one: No brain, no pain. There are pathways within the spinal cord that transmit pain information from the extremities of the body. If the spinal cord were severed (a transection), you could obtain an idea of how the pathways within the spinal cord are organized. Figure 1.3(a) shows such a cross section with the incoming fibers arriving at the dorsal horn. The interior of the cord is shaped like a butterfly and is gray in appearance. This grayness is a clear cue that one is viewing millions of unmyelinated cell bodies. The cell bodies, and the myelinated pathways, have been extensively studied and labeled. The diagram shown in Figure 1.3(a) briefly introduces the terminology necessary to discuss the conduction and function within the spinal cord. Once we have this overview, we can continue our discovery within the brain itself.

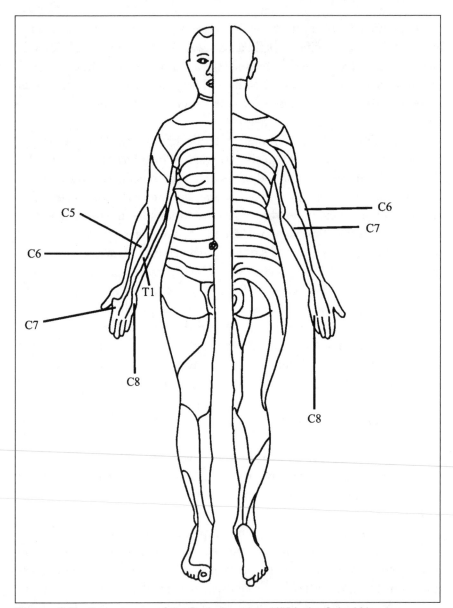

C5

C6

C7

T1

C8

C6

C7

C8

Figure 1.5. Dermatomes of the Body Associated With the Spinal Nerves

Spinal Gray Matter

The butterfly shape within the spinal cord is divided into three areas. Two of the classifications have already been discussed: the dorsal and ventral horns. The third is the intermediate area lying between the two extremes. The intermediate zone consists of a dense grouping of cells known as **interneurons.** Interneurons are small neurons that interact with each other within the layers of the spinal cord. The dorsal horn, intermediate area, and ventral horn have been further divided in 10 separate layers (see Figure 1.3[a]). There are five **laminae** or layers within the dorsal horn, three laminae within the intermediate zone, and two laminae in the ventral horn. There are only about 5 of the 10 that are directly concerned with the transmission and integration of sensory information. These five are the laminae located in the dorsal horns. For clarity, the laminae are only shown on the right half of the spinal cord in Figure 1.3(a). For the time being, we label them from 1 to 5. When we discuss pain in a later chapter, more details of the function and interaction of these cellular layers will be apparent. Our goal at this point is to be aware of the fact that the cellular center of the spinal cord is fairly well defined and has distinctive structural and functional layers.

Spinal Pathways

The pathways that surround the central gray matter conduct information to the brain—the afferent pathways—and away from the brain—efferent pathways. Figure 1.3(a) shows, in the white area surrounding the central butterfly, the two major afferent pathways: the **dorsal column** and the **lateral spinothalamic tract.** The afferent pathways are only shown on the left of the diagram. The pathways in reality, of course, ascend and descend throughout the area surrounding the butterfly central core. In addition to the afferent pathways, there are three major descending paths coming from higher centers in the brain: the **pyramidal tract,** the **extrapyramidal tract,** and the **ventral column.** At first glance, these paths may appear difficult to remember. However, once you get a feel for how these paths got their names , you can recall more easily their destination and location. The fibers in the dorsal column travel throughout the spinal cord and are named according to their dorsal location, near the back. Likewise, the fibers in the lateral spinothalamic tract are located laterally, to the side, of the spinal cord and conduct information from the spinal cord to an area within the brain called the thalamus. The lateral spinothalamic tract has also been called the anterolateral funiculus, the neospinothalamic tract, paleospinothalamic tract, and the spinoreticular tract. For our purposes of discussion, we retain the more descriptive nomenclature of the lateral spinothalamic tract.

The pyramidal tract is actually triangular or pyramidal in shape when viewed in cross section. The extrapyramidal tract is, therefore, just another pyramidal tract when viewed in cross section. Hence, it is an "extra" pyramidal pathway. The ventral column conducts information down the spinal cord in the ventral horn, near the belly. Finally, Figure 1.3(a) shows a small pathway called **Lissauer's tract,** named after the individual who first described it. Many functional aspects of the nervous system got their names from their discoverers. Lissauer's tract is relatively short in comparison with the other pathways. It is located dorsal and lateral to the dorsal horn. The fibers that enter this tract travel a short distance, both up and down, and then reenter the spinal cord. Thus, information that comes in at one level of the spinal cord makes contact with other levels of the spinal cord by way of Lissauer's tract.

Although Figure 1.3 is instructive in terms of providing structural labels and an overall view of the organization of the spinal cord, it is far from complete. If we move on to Figure 1.6, we see a larger perspective of the sensory path from skin to brain.

Figure 1.6 shows a fiber entering the spinal cord via the dorsal root. Once the fiber has entered the cord, it joins other fibers already ascending in the dorsal column. For clarity, the other fibers are not shown. These first-order fibers (first in the sequence) travel upward, enter the brain stem, and make a connection within an area known as the **medulla.** Once the first-order fiber has made this connection the second-order axons leave the medulla and cross the midline to the opposite side of the body. The ascent then continues toward the **thalamus** through the pathway called the **medial lemniscus** (band or ribbon of fibers). The second-order fibers that enter the thalamus make a connection with the third and last group of fibers in the sequence. These third-order fibers then ascend to the cortex and terminate within the primary somatosensory cortex on the **postcentral gyrus** of the **parietal lobe.** A **gyrus** is a convolution or bump in contrast with a **sulcus** that is a groove or fissure. The entire pathway consists of just three sequences: first-, second-, and third-order neurons, and two connections. An important aspect of the dorsal column pathway is that the fibers enter the spinal cord and ascend **ipsilaterally** (on the same side). The fibers do not cross the midline until they have ascended to the brain stem in the medulla. Once they arrive at the brain stem, they cross the midline and continue their journey to the cortex. The right hemisphere receives the sensory activity from the left side, and the left hemisphere receives sensory input from the right side.

The course traveled by the fibers within the lateral spinothalamic tract differs from that in the dorsal column. Figure 1.6 also shows the lateral

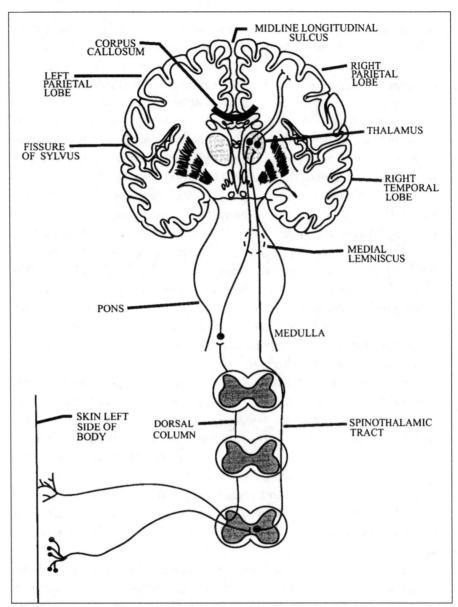

Figure 1.6. Dorsal Column and Lateral Spinothalamic Tract

NOTE: The dorsal column travels ipsilaterally to the medulla and then crosses the midline. The spinothalamic tract synapses in the spinal cord and crosses the midline before ascending to the cortex.

spinothalamic path. The first-order sensory fibers that make up the lateral spinothalamic tract connect with the second-order fibers in the ipsilateral dorsal horn of the spinal cord. Following this first connection, the second-order fibers immediately cross the midline in the spinal cord to the contralateral side of the body. The second-order fibers then ascend, via the lateral spino-thalamic tract, to the thalamus. Once in the thalamus, the third-order fibers are contacted to continue the ascent to the postcentral gyrus of the cortex.

Referring back to Figure 1.2, you can see additional information about the brain structure itself. This view shows the four lobes in the left hemisphere of the brain: the **frontal lobe** is behind the forehead, the **temporal lobe** is on the side near the temple, the **occipital lobe** is at the back of the head, and the parietal lobe is anterior to the occipital lobe and behind the frontal lobe. The fissure of Rolando, also called the **central fissure,** separates the frontal and parietal lobe. The central fissure is, from the side view shown in Figure 1.2, located near the central part or center of the brain. The area immediately behind or posterior to the central fissure, postcentral, is the parietal lobe. The postcentral gyrus is the final destination of afferent sensory information regarding bodily sensations such as touch or pressure on the skin. These portions of the parietal lobe are, therefore, directly associated with the somesthetic experiences. The particulars of this portion of the cortex are discussed in more detail in a later chapter.

Immediately in front, anterior, of the central fissure is the motor cortex that initiates the commands for movement. The occipital lobe is the final destination for visual sensations. The temporal lobe has functions for auditory sensations as well as the capacity to process visual information. In summary, the pathways for somesthesis terminate at the highest level in the postcentral gyrus of the parietal lobe. The primary visual processes terminate within the occipital lobe, and auditory and visual sensations reside within the temporal lobe. The fissure that runs laterally and divides the temporal lobe from the frontal and parietal lobes is the fissure of Sylvus. The fissure of Sylvus is also known as the **lateral fissure.**

Referring back to Figure 1.2, you can see two functional areas of the brain known as **Broca's area** and **Wernicke's area.** These two portions of the brain are discussed in detail in later chapters. For the moment, it is only necessary to note that Broca's area has motor-speech functions and is located in the frontal lobe adjacent to the motor cortex. Broca's area is directly associated with phonation, articulation, and facial expression. Speech is directly under the neural control of a specific area of the brain—namely, Broca's area. Wernicke's area, on the other hand, appears to be responsible for the comprehension and understanding of language. The two areas have connecting pathways. Actually, the complete linguistic dominance of Broca's and Wernicke's areas within the left hemisphere is not entirely correct. The language functions are within the left hemisphere for about 90% of right-handed individuals. Left-handed people, however, have their linguistic dominance, speech production, and comprehension, in the left hemisphere only about 60% of the time. As usual, the brain and nervous system have shown their typical complexity.

The description of the nervous system to this point is exceptionally sketchy. Because there are more than 120 billion cells in the nervous system, perhaps many more, this is surely an understatement. In addition, there have been deliberate omissions of specific nuclei, cell groups, and pathways. This was done to simplify the discussion and still introduce structures, functions, and nomenclature needed in future chapters. As we proceed, the basic structures of the nervous system are expanded and modified for each sensory system. The meticulous details and the elegant organization of the nervous system are, unfortunately, beyond the scope of a single introductory text. Nevertheless, the goal is to entice you to examine and wonder about the most complex and intricate mechanism on earth: your brain.

The Neuron

Thoughts, memories, and all sensations are based on the same brain process. They all operate and depend on the transmission of neural impulses. As a straightforward analogy, consider the nervous system to be like a giant telephone system. What makes memories, thoughts, vision, speech, hearing, and pain different is that each system has a different area code and telephone number. Some of the memories have toll-free "800" numbers. Some of the numbers are occasionally busy, and some are misdialed. The numbers are all different but they all work on the same principle—the conductance of electrical impulses along neural pathways. The telephone system has calls going everywhere simultaneously. Some are routed through the local exchange, some through an intermediate system, some through communication satellites. The brain uses this same basic idea. The brain has pathways (axons), local exchanges (interneurons), intermediate substations (thalamus), and higher-level communication satellites (cortex). The points of exchange in the brain, however, are vastly more complex than any telephone or computer system. Facilitation of transmitted information, inhibition of information, and modulation or changes in the information occur at billions and billions of points along the brain's communication lines. In addition, the neural paths are monitored by literally millions of other neural paths. Shifts in the information can and do occur because of such monitoring. The bottom line is that the brain, pathways, and neurons, all operate on the same principle: electrical-chemical impulses.

A Brief Overview

In this section, we extend our view by focusing on the small neural elements that comprise the central nervous system. These individual parts, the neurons, provide the foundation for the construction of perceptions. The uniqueness of the neuron has some similarities with the common digital computer. Both the computer and the neuron operate on a binary system. Our brain and the individual cells are, however, several magnitudes more versatile than any computer. No computer, in existence now or even planned for the future, can ever match the processing abilities of our brain. After describing the distinctive characteristics of neurons, we consider some methods of recording and measuring their activity.

Neurons, remember, are both the paths to the brain and the centers used to produce sensory perceptions of the world. Knowledge of their operation is critical to understanding sensory processes and daily interactions with the environment. Any error or misfortune in their normal activity affects our perceptions, thoughts, and memories. It is important that we have this background. All sensory systems are based on these cells operating smoothly. When neurons fail, we fail.

The Anatomy of a Neuron

The nervous system is based on the electrical-chemical conductance of impulses over a multitude of paths. The neuron, the basic element of the nervous system, is a physiological structure and a unique entity in itself. Each neuron or cell is alive and independent, to some degree, of all other cells. It processes information that impinges on it by integrating (summing) all the messages it receives and then makes a "decision" whether to send the message on to other neurons. Even though all the cells operate on the same basic principle, they differ in size, shape, number of arborizations, number of receptive fibers (dendrites), and chemical messengers (neurotransmitters). In addition, we need to clarify an important element of the analogy. The neuron does operate on electrical charges and the conduction of impulses; however, the impulses are dependent on the chemical environment internal and external to the cell. The role of chemistry is examined more fully in a later section when we examine the origin of the electrical impulses.

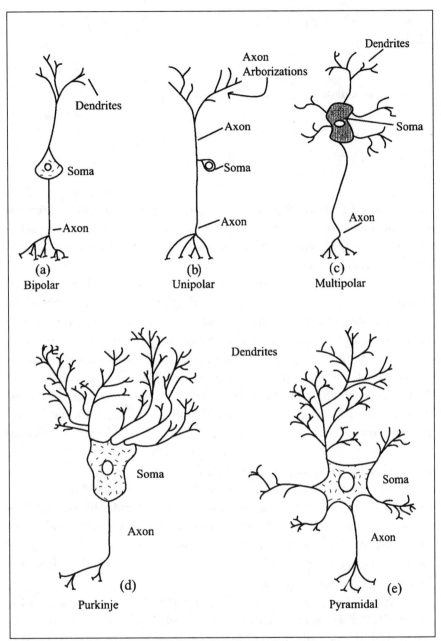

Figure 1.7. Example of Neurons in the Nervous System

NOTE: (a) bipolar cell, (b) unipolar cell, (c) multipolar cell, (d) Purkinje cell, (e) a pyramidal cell.

Figure 1.7 is a schematic drawing of neurons found in different parts of the nervous system. The cells, although they differ radically in shape, have several important features in common. Each neuron generally has four morphological regions:

1.   The cell body (also called the soma or perikaryon)
2.   Dendrites
3.   Axon
4.   The terminal end bouton

The end bouton is also referred to as the "presynaptic terminal" at the end of the axon arborizations. Each part of the neuron has a function of its own. Before we examine the common features, it is useful to examine the neurons shown in Figure 1.7 more closely.

Figure 1.7(a) shows a **bipolar neuron.** The name, as you may suspect, comes from the two fibers that originate from the cell body. One of the fibers is the dendrite and the other the axon. Based on the classical neuron theory, the dendrite and axon have two distinctively different functions. The function of the dendrite is to receive information from other cells whereas the axon conducts the information to the next cell in the sequence. The information flows in a unidirectional path from dendrite to axon. In respect to the bipolar cell shown in Figure 1.7(a), the dendrite receives the information and the axon sends it on. The bipolar cell can, for example, be found in the visual system at the back of the eye within the retina. More is said about this type of neural element when we discuss the visual system.

Figure 1.7(b) shows a neuron that we have discussed, although not specifically by name. This neuron is unipolar and has no dendrites; rather, it has a single axon emerging from the perikaryon that receives information at one end and sends it to the other end. This neuron is the common element in the conductance of information from the skin to the spinal cord. The cell body is located in the dorsal root ganglion.

A much more common neuron found within the nervous system is the multipolar cell shown in Figures 1.7(c), 1.7(d), and 1.7(e). Figure 1.7(c) shows a multipolar cell typical of the interneuron found in the central gray matter of the spinal cord and brain. The view of the multipolar neuron is much more complex than the previous two types of cells. There are several dendrites leaving the cell body. Each dendrite, in turn, has several branches and collaterals extending from its trunk. The branches also have small dendritic spines to which other neurons make functional contact. The multipolar cell, then, has most of its function devoted to the dendritic reception of inputs from other cells.

When you consider the fact that a neuron's soma also receives information in a manner similar to that of the dendrites, the function of the multipolar cell immediately appears to be primarily for reception and integration. Once the information is integrated, the cell makes a decision. The cell either forwards the message to the next cell or does not. Figure 1.7(d) and 1.7(e) show different multipolar neurons. These are the Purkinje cell from the cerebellum and the pyramidal cell from the cortex.

When you think about these cells, particularly the multipolar cells with their vast number of inputs, the complexity of the brain and nervous system becomes almost overwhelming. For example, we have already pointed out that the central nervous system contains an estimated 100 to 120 billion neurons, or more.

When you consider the fact that each multipolar cell probably makes about 1,000 connections with other cells (the axon has its collaterals and arborizations) and in turn receives literally thousands of inputs from other cells, the total number of possible functional connections within a human brain becomes truly astonishing. Scientists estimate the number of connections is as large as 10,000,000,000,000,000—ten quadrillion, and it is probably an underestimate. This estimate is larger than the estimated number of stars in our galaxy.

The neurons shown in Figure 1.7 are representative of the diversity found within the nervous system. Just as in the case of snowflakes, no two neurons are alike. This single fact makes the nervous system utterly unknowable in minute detail. Fortunately, the differences among neurons lie primarily in their morphology, not their basic functional operation. Because of this functional similarity, the telephone cable analogy is quite correct when it comes to the basic principle that all neurons conduct impulses along predetermined paths. This principle has allowed scientists to discover the neurological functions that permit an individual to sense the environment, think, have emotions, learn, remember, and be alive.

Our discussion has thus far touched on the function of three of the four features of a neuron. These are the dendrite, soma, and axon. What remains to be discussed is the presynaptic terminal or end bouton found at the end of the axon arborizations. This portion of the neuron is, perhaps, the most important because communication occurs at this point.

The presynaptic terminal, by its very name, suggests that it is only a part of a more complex structure. This is exactly the case. The functional connection between neurons is called a **synapse.** The synapse consists of three parts. The initial part is the structural **end bouton** found at the end of the axon. The second part of the synapse is in reality not a physical structure at all; rather, it is the gap between the axon end terminal and the neural structure on which the end bouton is functionally attached. The gap is known as the **synaptic cleft.** The post side of the synaptic cleft (the end bouton is the presynaptic side) is referred to as the postsynaptic portion of the functional connection. Thus, when a synapse is discussed it is in terms of the presynaptic terminal, the cleft, and the postsynaptic portion of the connection.

You should keep in mind several aspects of the synapse. The vast majority of synapses occur when an axon connects with a dendrite, **axodendritic,** or a soma **axosomatic.** Often there is a dendritic spine formed on a dendrite for the synaptic formation. Two other synaptic designations are the **axoaxonic,** synapse of one axon on another, and the axoaxonic and axodendritic combination, respectively.

A closer view of a representative neuron is provided in Figure 1.8 that shows a schematic of a multipolar neuron with several synaptic connections from other neurons. The synapses are axodendritic and axosomatic. Surrounding the single long axon is a myelin sheath. There are separations or interruptions in the myelin called nodes. These nodes, named after the individual who first observed them, are the **nodes of Ranvier.** The myelin sheath, as noted previously, is not found on every axon. However, when myelin is present it is the result of a specialized supporting cell. Within the central nervous system, myelin is formed by a glial cell known as an **oligodendrocyte.** This cell wraps itself around the axon in a tight spiral. In the peripheral nervous system, the myelin sheath is the result of a different glial cell called the **Schwann** cell. The general effect of having an axon wrapped in the myelin is to improve the speed of conduction of neural impulses. Unmyelinated fibers conduct their messages at a much slower rate. The swiftness of conduction in the myelinated fibers is the result of a process called **saltatory conduction.** When an axon is myelinated, the electrical impulses functionally leap from node to node along the axon.

This "leapfrogging," from one node of Ranvier to the next, increases the speed of conduction by a factor of six. At the end of the axon, which in humans may be over a meter in length, are the arborizations and synapses. One need exert very little intellectual effort to imagine the length of some of the axons in giraffes or pachyderms.

The shaded area of Figure 1.8, the point at which the axon leaves the soma, is known as the **axon hillock** or the **initial segment.** This particular sec-

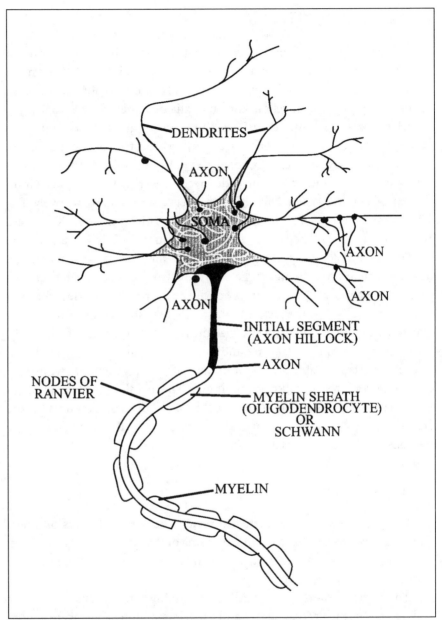

Figure 1.8. A Myelinated Multipolar Neuron With the Nodes of Ranvier and Multiple Axodendritic and Axosomatic Synapses

tion of the neuron plays a key role in determining whether the cell initiates an impulse within the axon. This section of the neuron is examined more closely in a following section of this chapter.

The Supporting Glia Cells

The nervous system is not an entity that consists entirely of neurons. In fact, the nervous system has another group of cells that is 9 to 10 times more numerous than neurons. (Can you imagine 900 to 1,000 billion more cells in the brain?) This group of cells is known as **glia** or sometimes **neuroglia.**

There are several different subclassifications of glia cells. For our purposes, we need only be concerned with astrocytes, oligodendrocytes, microglia, and Schwann cells. As noted previously, the oligodendrocytes and Schwann cells act primarily to provide myelin covering to the axons within the central nervous system and peripheral nervous system, respectively. The astrocytes, on the other hand, apparently have nutritive functions (Kimelberg & Norenberg, 1989). They make contact with neurons while simultaneously in contact with blood capillaries. In addition, when an injury occurs in the nervous system both the microglia and the astrocytes become actively engaged in the removal of the debris produced by the trauma and degeneration of the nerve cells. It is the glia cells, primarily the astrocytes and microglia, which react to the trauma and energize the recovery process. Unfortunately, the proliferation of the astrocytes and microglia can also lead to a **glial scar.** The glial scar is a possible reason for the lack of axon regeneration within the central nervous system following an injury. The fact that most central nervous system neurons are no longer capable of cell division accounts for the lack of new neurons. Some recent evidence suggests that the formation of new neurons in adult mammals is possible.

A Little History

Let us to take a few moments to review the past endeavors of scientists who have given us the current panorama of the synapse and the neuron. The synapse is perhaps one of the most interesting aspects of the nervous system.

The history of the discovery and understanding of the synapse covers several decades of intellectual debate and experimentation. There were, before the advent of the electron microscope and direct observation, differences of opinion regarding the manner in which electrical impulses crossed from one neuron to the next. According to the classical neural theory espoused earlier, there is a one-way path from the transmitting axon to a receptive dendrite or cell body. In the view of one group of investigators, a chemical diffuses across a synaptic cleft, a gap that was yet to be observed, to accomplish transmission from cell to cell. The chemical hypothesis said that the presynaptic end bouton released a chemical that, when it reached the postsynaptic side, initiated activity in the receiving neuron. Many individuals supported this view. If there is to be a controversy, however, it is important to have colleagues who support your theory and a group of colleagues who believe otherwise. Thus, the opposing camp reported strong and convincing arguments that the synapse is not chemically mediated; rather, they contended that information was passed from neuron to neuron by the electrical impulse simply being passed on by a physically present conductor among cells.

The debate continued until the weight of the evidence began to suggest that the chemical hypothesis was correct. One bit of evidence, for example, to support the latter position was that the time required for an impulse to cross a synapse was too long to support the electrical hypothesis. The time required to cross the synapse was measured to be in the neighborhood of 0.3 to 0.5 milliseconds (0.0003 to .0005 of a second). Although this appears to be a very short time, it is about the amount of time that is necessary for chemical release, diffusion, and the postsynaptic contact. This and other types of evidence continued to act as instigators for scientists to find a chemical that permits the transmission of an impulse from one neuron to the next. The search has yielded several chemical mediators. These chemical transmitters, discussed later, are critically important in the functioning of the nervous system and the sensory processes we take for granted every day.

The story, however, does not end here. The recognition of chemical transmitter substances and the direct observation of a synaptic gap between the neurons have secured the chemical mediation hypothesis. This conclusion does not eliminate the possibility of an electrical conductance by a direct structural connection between the neurons. The electron microscopist not only provided evidence to support the chemical mediation but also discovered the evidence for the electrical conductance. There are, in fact, physical connections called **gap junctions** between some neurons. These gap junctions provide the necessary conduit for the flow of electrical impulses. The gap junctions act like a pipeline between neurons. Thus, as is often the case in science, both of the synaptic hypotheses are correct. The electrical synapse is in the minority, however. The chemically mediated synapse is far more abundant within the nervous system. The electrical synapse, also called **electrotonic** transmission, has been known to exist in invertebrates and more recently was found in vertebrates. However, their occurrence is rare in humans.

A final bit of history important in the study of the nervous system is one that concerns many people. How do scientists determine what neurons, glia, synapses, and pathways look like and how did they discover the brain's organization and function?

The answer, which seems so obvious, is more complex than you might suspect. The obvious conclusion is that they looked with a microscope and drew pictures of what we saw. However, about 150 years ago anatomy was done painstakingly by dissection and macroscopic study of the parts. It was not until the 1800s that the appearance of the microscope and methods to stain tissue with dyes such as silver nitrate were found, and great strides were made in the morphological study of the nervous system. The microscope greatly enhanced the anatomist's ability to trace and follow pathways within the animals examined. It was well-known at that time that when central nervous system tissues were injured they degenerated. The degeneration of injured tissue provided, then as now, a built-in method of learning about nervous structure and function. When an axon is cut, an **axotomy,** it begins to degenerate distally and proximally from the site of the lesion. The initial degeneration is in the direction of impulse flow, away from the cell body and toward the axon terminal. This is known as anterograde degeneration, also called **Wallerian degeneration** and **orthograde degeneration. Retrograde degeneration** refers to the degeneration proximal from the zone of trauma, toward the cell body and dendrite. The loss of myelin, axon, dendrite, and soma can be mapped by the use of stains and dyes that differentially mark the degenerating parts of the cell. In this way, the origin and destination of the cut fiber can be determined.

Advances in cell study in the 1970s have used enzymes and radioactive markers to trace the fibers and reveal the morphological details of neurons. These substances are taken up by the metabolic activity of the neuron. Two important substances used to delineate the neural elements of a cell are the enzyme **horseradish peroxidase (HRP),** and radioactive 14C-deoxyglucose. The dendrites, soma, and axon are then identified and inspected. Tracing techniques have yielded the line drawings and photographs published in scientific journals. Knowledge concerning neural structure and pathways continues to grow in quantum leaps.

Single-Cell Recording

You already know by the heading of this section that the study of individual neuronal activity is possible. What is described here is a brief overview of endeavors that have led to Nobel prizes for scientists, cures for diseases, and intellectual pursuits for hundreds of people, including you.

When we speak of single-cell recording, or unit response, it is important to keep in mind that there are two basic procedures used to study the activity of living neurons. Both procedures detect and measure electrical voltage or current and variations in voltage or current. The variations may occur because of normal spontaneous activity or because of deliberate external stimulation under experimenter control. In either case, the objective is to record neural activity.

The first procedure entails recording electrical activity from outside the cell. The placement of a small microelectrode, approximately 10 microns in diameter at the tip, is placed near a living and active cell. This is the extracellular procedure because the electrode does not enter the cell from which it is recording. When the electrode is placed close to a cell, it is possible to record the electrical activity of the cell as the response flows by the electrode. Extracellular recordings do not reveal the small voltage variations within the neuron; rather, they reveal the relatively large impulses, about 100 millivolts (mv), that are conducted past the electrode. These impulses are formally known as the **action potentials** and are based on the transmission of information from one neuron to another. The action potentials are a large part of the secret to the nervous system, sensation, movement, thought, memories, and life itself (Hodgkin, 1964, 1992; Peters, Palay, & Webster, 1991).

The second method of examining the neural activity is intracellular recording. In this procedure, an electrode 1.0 micron or less in diameter is inserted directly into a cell. The electrode may be placed in the soma or within an axon. When the microelectrode tip is inside the cell, without damaging the cell, you can examine not only the larger action potentials that are recordable by the extracellular electrode but also the low-level electrical activity that leads to action potential generation. These small electrical changes are of different types and are known by various labels, but for the time being we call these smaller voltage variations, approximately 20 to 25 mv, **generator potentials.** This label is, in many ways, quite descriptive of these small electrical changes. These intracellular recordings are more difficult to obtain and reveal different types of information than does the extracellular procedure. Both techniques, however, are extremely important in the investigation of the nervous system and sensory processes.

Electrical Potentials of the Neuron

The stage is set now for the details of neural activity. The morphology has been explained, and the electrodes are waiting for our attention. So let us begin by examining Figure 1.9(a).

This schematic diagram shows an axon with an intracellular electrode within an axon. The electrode is attached to a meter to indicate changes in voltage. There must be, as any physics major knows, another electrode placed

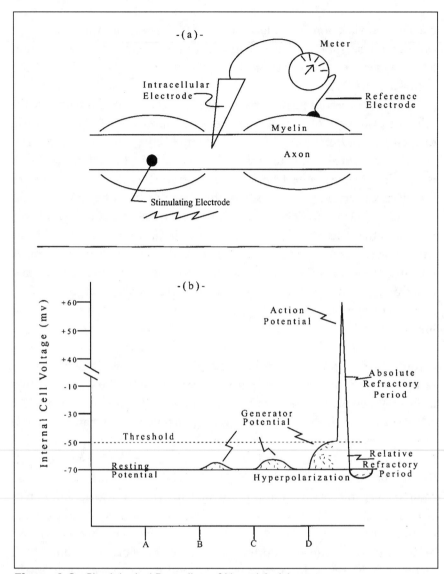

Figure 1.9. Physiological Recording of Neural Activity

NOTE: (a) example of intracellular recording electrodes and (b) results of four experiments that depolarize the cell.

somewhere if an electrical circuit is to be completed. This latter electrode, the reference electrode, is placed outside the cell membrane. This recording system, if it is sensitive enough, should measure the voltage difference across the cell membrane. Specifically, the two electrodes provide a quantitative difference, in millivolts, between the inside of the cell where the intracellular electrode is placed, and the outside of the cell where the reference electrode is located.

Figure 1.9(b) shows the results of a set of four experiments. Each experiment is an independent study with a different stimulus intensity. The four stimuli are applied to the neuron at four different times. The stimuli vary in their strength. Let us assume that the investigator has chosen four values of increasing magnitude. They are Stimulus A (no stimulus), Stimulus B (weak intensity), Stimulus C (moderate intensity), and Stimulus D (high intensity).

The experiment is discussed in four stages. Each stage is associated with one of the four stimulus intensities. We record the voltage across the membrane starting at the point when the stimulus is turned on (a brief electrical impulse) and stopping when the voltage returns to the starting value. The astute observer notes that there are actually two questions being asked by the investigator in this experiment. First, how does the voltage in millivolts change as stimulus intensity changes? Second, how does the voltage in millivolts change as time passes?

Stage I. The initial recording is done with Stimulus A. In this condition, we prepare the neural fiber for an electrical shock in the usual manner. However, the intensity of the stimulus is set to 0.0. In this condition, it is assumed that the voltage measured across the cell membrane is representative of the cell when it is in an unstimulated or resting state. It is important to emphasize that the procedures used to record the activity of a neuron with a stimulus intensity equal to 0.0 must be the same procedures as those used when a nonzero stimulus intensity is applied. If valid conclusions are to be drawn from the experiment, all stimulus conditions must be the same except for stimulus intensity.

The results of the experiment using Stimulus A is shown in Figure 1.9(b). The voltage is recorded at a constant –70 mv. The –70 mv is interpreted to mean that the inside of the cell is negative relative to the outside of the cell. The neuron, regardless of how you measure it, has a value of –70 mv when it is inactive and at rest. This voltage is called, not surprisingly, the neuron's **resting potential** when it is nonconducting, and unstimulated. This resting potential is the baseline you use when examining the effects of other stimulus values.

Because the inside of the cell is negative and the outside is positive, the cell is considered to be **polarized** in its resting condition. In other words, the cell has two poles, one negative inside and one positive outside. If you were to

depolarize the cell, you need to move the −70 mv potential toward 0.0. If a stimulus event occurred that caused the voltage difference across the membrane to move toward zero, you could say that the cell was in the process of depolarizing. Any event that depolarizes a cell moves the voltage more positive—that is, toward 0.0 from a −70 mv. Any event that caused the resting potential to become more negative could make the cell more polarized. The cell, in this latter case, is **hyperpolarized.**

You should keep this terminology firmly in mind as you progress through the book. A neuron's momentary state is always considered relative to its normal resting state. Thus, the terminology of hyperpolarization and depolarization should become second nature as you proceed. If a cell is depolarized, the internal potential is more positive than the resting value; if the cell is hyperpolarized it has become more negative within the cell.

Stage II. Stage II of our experiment proceeds exactly as before. However, in this case a weak stimulus, Stimulus B, is applied. The results are shown in Figure 1.9(b) as a depolarization of the cell. The application of the stimulus caused the voltage to move from −70 mv toward 0.0. The magnitude of the depolarization is small. In a period of approximately 10 milliseconds (msec), the cell changed from the resting state of −70 mv to −67 mv and back again to −70 mv. This is the first appearance of the generator potential. Let us try a more intense stimulus.

Stage III. The experiment is repeated exactly as before. This time the stimulus to activate the cell is increased to a moderate value, Stimulus C. Figure 1.9(b) shows the results for this condition. These data are very similar to those in Stage II with the weak stimulus. The exception is in the magnitude of the depolarization. The depolarization is 7 mv in Stage III (from −70 mv to −63 mv). If a conclusion were to be drawn from the data collected thus far it could run along the following lines: The size of the generator potential is a direct function of the stimulus intensity. The more intense the stimulus, the greater the depolarization.

Stage IV. The last stage of the experiment is conducted using Stimulus D, the most intense of the four levels. The recording begins, as before, when the stimulus impulse is turned on. The data are collected continuously until the cell has returned to its resting level of −70 mv. What do the data look like now?

Figure 1.9(b) shows the variation in voltage across the cell membrane as a function of time after stimulus onset. Figure 1.9(b) shows an initial depolarization when Stimulus D is turned on. It is similar to that seen in Stages II and III. That is, there is a relatively slow depolarization from –70 mv to –50 mv during the first few milliseconds following the stimulus onset. This portion of the data is the generator potential. Following this relatively slow depolarization, a unique feature of the data begins. At –50 mv the internal voltage of the cell makes a brief and rapid positive-going spike. This rapid depolarization, and its immediate return to a polarized state, lasts about a millisecond and is, as previously noted, the action potential. *Spike, impulse,* or *neural impulse* are used interchangeably with action potential. The action potential begins at –50 mv as indicated by the label *threshold.* The spike is considered complete after it has returned to the threshold value. The period of time required for an action potential to occur, 1 msec, is the **absolute refractory period.** The portion of the curve immediately following the spike is the **relative refractory period.** A portion of this latter interval consists of a period of hyperpolarization.

The experiment is now complete and the results can be interpreted. The first thing to note is the difference in voltage for the first three stages of the experiment in contrast with the change in voltage in Stage IV with Stimulus D. In the latter situation, when the most intense stimulus was used, an action potential occurred. The spike was nonexistent in the first three stages of the investigation. If we were to repeat the final stage of the experiment, we could find the same result every time. Each time Stimulus D, or a stimulus more intense than D, was presented a spike could occur. The interesting aspect of the replications is that the spike could be initiated at the same voltage level every time, –50 mv. A fixed amount of depolarization is required to generate a neural impulse. If a spike is to be produced, the cell must be depolarized to a threshold value. This threshold is –50 mv. If the slow depolarization, the generator potential, does not reach this threshold value, no impulse is produced. The action potential, then, either occurs or it does not; it is an all-or-none phenomenon. When the depolarization reaches the threshold value, the impulse is initiated. It completes the cycle from threshold-to-maximum depolarization and back to threshold in a millisecond. The size of the action potential is always the same for any one neuron.

The conclusions of the experiment may be summarized by noting that action potentials fire (are generated) on an all-or-none basis and are initiated when the generator potential reaches the threshold value. The magnitude of the generator potential is dependent on the stimulus intensity. A weak stimulus produces a small generator potential, also referred to as an electronic depolarization; a stronger stimulus produces a larger generator potential. The intensity of the stimulus does not affect the size of the action potential. Every action potential produced by any one neuron is the same magnitude.

Excitation and Inhibition

Thus far, the experiment has worked out well. The results are clear-cut. The conclusions are straightforward and easily interpreted. The stimulus that was used to generate the potential variations across the cell membrane was, however, somewhat loosely defined in the previous paragraphs. The stimuli were simply defined as electrical shocks with different intensities. The fact of the matter is, however, that the parameters of the stimulus are critically important in obtaining the observed results. It should come as no surprise that there are several ways in which the stimulus is applied. We used just one of them; namely, we applied a brief electrical shock so that the cell depolarized. The stimuli could be presented in such a way that they increase the negativity of the cell. If these latter stimuli were used, the results would have been remarkably different. Figure 1.10(a) demonstrates the results of the experiment we just completed, depolarization and action potential generation, and shows a new outcome in Figure 1.10(b). This experiment assumes that the stimulus was reversed in its effect. The internal portion of the cell became more negative. The stimuli are labeled E, F, and G and represent negative stimulus intensities in an increasing order of magnitude. The results of such an experiment are clear: The cell becomes increasingly hyperpolarized and action potentials never occur.

The results of the entire experiment, including the negative stimulus condition, show that the internal voltage can vary both above and below the resting value of –70 mv. When a stimulus depolarizes the cell, it is possible to generate a spike. When a stimulus causes the cell to become hyperpolarized, there is no spike generation. It may have occurred to you that if a cell happens to be hyperpolarized when confronted with a depolarizing stimulus, the cell is less likely to generate an impulse. This is indeed the case. The further removed from the critical threshold potential (–50 mv) the cell is, the less likely it is that the cell becomes depolarized enough to initiate an impulse. If, for example, a cell is hyperpolarized to –75 mv, the amount of depolarization required to initiate a spike is 25 mv (from –75 to –50 mv). If the cell is at resting potential, it requires just 20 mv of depolarization to initiate the spike (–70 to –50 mv). A cell that is hyperpolarized is in a state of **inhibition,** and the inhibition must

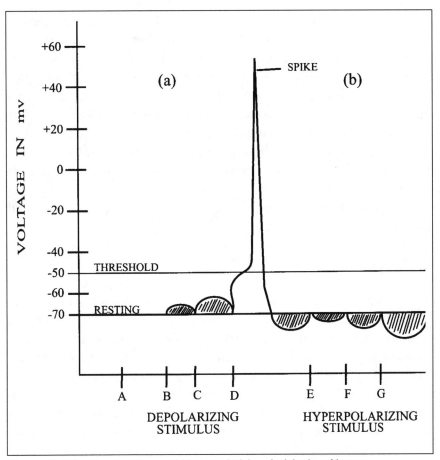

Figure 1.10. Depolarizing and Hyperpolarizing Activity in a Neuron

be overcome if a spike is to be initiated. In contrast with inhibition is the idea of **excitation.** As you have already guessed, excitation is associated with the depolarization of the cell. A stimulus, then, can lead to depolarization (excitation) or hyperpolarization (inhibition).

The ideas of inhibition and excitation are extremely important in understanding the nervous system and sensory processes. The complexity of the system is almost overwhelming when you consider the fact that each neuron is at any moment in time in a continuous state of agitation. Furthermore, as you already know, there are literally thousands of synapses attached to each neuron. Each one of these synapses is shouting at the top of its "chemical" voice. Some synapses are excitatory and urgently request that the postsynaptic cell depolarize to immediate activity (excitation). Other synapses are inhibitory in nature and request an urgent message of inhibition and hyperpolarization. You might think that the cacophony of such a situation, repeated billions of times, would be utter chaos. This, fortunately, is not the case. Each neuron makes a calm and rational decision. The decision is made at the initial segment or axon hillock of the neuron (see Figure 1.8) through a process similar to algebraic summation. That is, excitation (depolarization) and inhibition (hyperpolarization) are "added up" by the cell with depolarization considered as positive and hyperpolarization as negative. If the result of the summation is a depolarization to threshold (–50 mv), at the axon hillock, then an action potential is initiated. This summation is a continuous algebraic integration of all synaptic inputs. An action potential is generated only when the generator potential reaches the threshold value at the initial segment.

Intensity Coding

It may have occurred to you that the generation of a single action potential, as discussed in the previous experiment, is not sufficient to produce a sensation, movement, or thought. This is certainly the case. A single impulse from a single neuron is an insignificant event in the operation of the entire brain. There are literally billions of action potentials being generated in your brain and nervous system at this very moment. This occurs even while you sleep. There is a continuous bombardment of activity from one neuron to the next, via the synapses, which gives rise to life and active organisms—humans, cats, dogs, insects, frogs, and so on.

The interesting aspect concerning the brain activity and the sensations that occur is that everything is done by action potentials. However, the end result of neural activity is clearly not the same. Vision is not the same as touch. Hearing is certainly different from taste. Yet, all these sensations are based on the same brain process: the neural impulse and the associated synaptic activity. The reason for the different sensations is, to a large degree, the result of where the impulses originate and where they are sent. Impulses that originate from the skin and end up in the somesthetic area of the brain do not produce a visual perception. Impulses from the auditory nerve do not end up in the visual cortex. Thus, the telephone analogy is accurate in many respects. This "direct line" concept of neural operation is often referred to as the **specificity theory**. This theory is encountered repeatedly as we progress through the book.

Although the specificity theory can help account for intermodality differences, differences between different sensory systems, a question still exits concerning intramodality differences, differences within the same sensory system. We all acknowledge that sounds are seldom of equal loudness. The difference in loudness, an intramodality difference, raises the question: What is the neural cause for the variation of intramodality sensations? Neuroscientists, physicians, engineers, and sensory psychologists (among others) are interested in the processes that cause these various sensations.

The examination of sensory systems has resulted in a variety of procedures and techniques. One fruitful methodological attack was represented by our previous experiment: The direct neurological or physiological approach. A second very useful procedure is psychophysics (Kandel, Schwartz, & Jessel, 1995; Posner, 1989). Psychophysics, for the moment, may be briefly introduced by noting that it is a methodological procedure directed toward elucidating the relationship between a stimulus and a sensory response. The stimulus, for example, may be a light or sound of a certain magnitude. The response may be a simple button press, a verbal response, or an animal's behavior. Psychophysics finds its primary use in laboratories directed toward sensory questions using humans and intact organisms. Seldom are invasive procedures used—for example, no ablation, lesion, axotomy, or single-cell recording. Because you seldom find a human volunteer for a neurological ablation or single-cell recording investigation, the psychophysical procedure is extensively used with humans. Furthermore, ethical and moral obligations clearly take precedence with investigations using both human and animal participants.

Thus, much of the human and animal data come primarily from experiments that use psychophysical procedures. Although there are experiments that have used human participants with nonpsychophysical procedures, these latter investigations have occurred under strict ethical conditions, legal and medical. These latter experiments were accomplished during necessary brain operations. They are discussed in later chapters. Our aim now is to examine the relationship between the stimulus intensity and the organism's response, both psychophysically and physiologically.

Physiological Recording

Because we know that sensations are dependent on action potentials, stimulus intensity must somehow be encoded in the form of neural impulses. The impulses are dependent on stimulus intensity first because the stimulus must be intense enough to cause the generator potential to reach threshold and generate a spike. Thus, one of the goals of investigations in sensory processes is to break the neural code and discover how the nervous system generates the multiplicity of sensations from action potentials. A first step in this enterprise is to examine more thoroughly the relationship between neural impulses and stimulus intensity.

The procedure we use is the one we are familiar with from the previous single-cell experiment. The intracellular electrode is implanted within the cell, and the neutral electrode is placed outside the cell membrane. The independent variable is stimulus intensity. The dependent variable is the variation in voltage across the cell membrane recorded intracellularly in response to stimuli of different magnitudes. There is, however, a difference in the duration of the stimulus. In the previous experiment, we had a very brief stimulus shock. In the present experiment, the stimulus, a depolarizing one, is turned on and remains on for a longer period. The longer duration of the intracellular recording not only allows us to examine the voltage changes we saw before but also permits us to count the number of impulses that occur as a function of the stimulus intensity and duration.

The previous experiment was somewhat artificial because it was assumed that the stimulus generated only a single action potential. In practice, this is seldom the case. Any stimulus that evokes a spike, nearly always evokes more than one. Figure 1.11 shows, diagrammatically, the responses of a neuron to a stimulus that is long in duration at three different intensities. The stimulus is denoted by the rectangles below the data in Figure 1.11(a). The most obvious result is that the number of spikes increases as a function of stimulus intensity. This conclusion is further shown in Figure 1.11(b). The size of the action potential, as noted previously, does not increase as the stimulus intensity increases; rather, the intensity affects the number or frequency of spikes that occur during the interval. The stronger or more intense the stimulus, the more neural impulses there are. Part of the neural code, then, is that as the stimulus in the environment increases in strength, the nervous system increases the number of action potentials generated. This is the **frequency-intensity** principle.

Close inspection of Figure 1.11(a) reveals the manner in which the action potentials are increased in frequency. The spikes occur more often with more intense stimuli because each impulse is initiated earlier in the cycle. That is, after a spike has been generated, the action potential does not completely dissipate or return to resting level before the next impulse is generated. This means that the interval between spikes decreases as the stimulus intensity increases and, as a result, there are more spikes within the same interval of time. This results in the increase in the number of action potentials as the intensity of the stimulus increases. You should note, however, that there is a limit to the

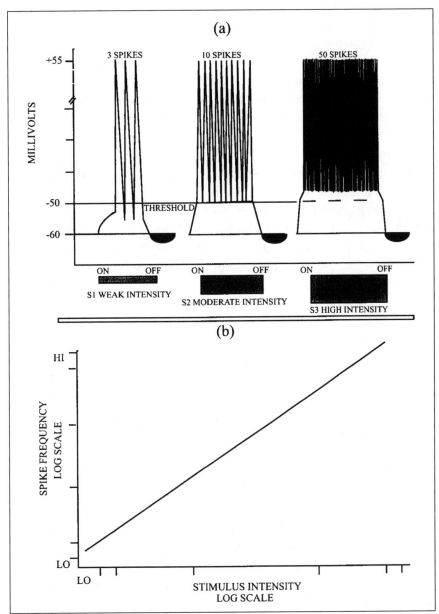

Figure 1.11. The Frequency of Impulses Increases as a Function of Increasing the Intensity

NOTE: (a) the effect of increasing stimulus level on neural activity and (b) a plot of the frequency-intensity principle.

number of action potentials a neuron can produce. At some point, as the stimulus intensity continues to intensify, the neuron will stop increasing its spike production. At this point, the neuron has reached its maximum activity or its saturation point.

Note, once again, that the axis for Figure 1.11(b) is logarithmic. These data are representative of a power function. There is a linear relationship when the data are plotted on the log-log scale within the neuron's dynamic range. A log-log scale refers to data plotted logarithmically on both the X and Y axis.

It may appear possible to infer from these data that sensations such as brightness and loudness are dependent on the frequency-intensity principle. That is, the sensation depends on the frequency of the neural impulses. For example, the number of impulses received by the brain within a second indicates the loudness of the sound. This is generally known as a strong inference, based on reasoned logic and suggestive data. It should be emphasized, however, that the data presented here do not, by themselves, support such an inference. You must be extremely careful in drawing conclusions from data. The task of finding relationships between sensory experience and neural activity requires data from several different experiments.

What then can be concluded from the data? What does the coding of intensity to frequency of neural firing show? The acknowledged relationship in sensory physiology is that a single neuron's activity is dependent on the stimulus intensity. When several neural fibers increase their activity, there is a perceptual increase in the experienced sensation. So, the frequency-intensity principle is clearly related to our perceptions.

Action Potentials

This section outlines how neurons process and conduct information. If environmental events are to be sensed and perceived it is important to understand how a neuron conducts its daily routine. The neuron's operation includes topics such as passive and active transport, sodium pumps, and action potentials. The activity that occurs between neurons, at synapses, is the topic of the next chapter.

The voltage variations across a cell membrane, from a resting potential near −70 mv to a positive potential near +55 mv has been introduced and discussed. The task now is to explain, as simply as possible, a complex system of electrical and chemical events. The events provide the basis for the observed changes across the neural membrane. To be more specific, the question we are going to address is: What occurs within a cell to maintain a polarized resting state (−70 mv) and how does depolarization occur during an action potential (+55 mv)?

The discovery of neural operation has followed a normal course of scientific investigation. Considerable curiosity, perseverance, skill, luck, and intellectual brilliance have led to the present state of knowledge. The breadth of this knowledge is, of course, still evolving. Experiments are currently underway in laboratories throughout the world that undoubtedly will suggest new directions and understanding.

Ions and Ionic Flow

The cellular examination of living matter, whether it is nervous tissues or oak trees, necessitates some knowledge of chemistry and electricity. For our purposes, the chemical and electrical ideas are relatively simple. For example, if we put common table salt, NaCl, (called a solute) into a glass of water (called a solvent) the result is not only a glass of salty tasting water but also the production of electrically charged substances called ions. The ionic theory states that, in particular circumstances, the salt molecules dissociate in two parts called ions. An **ion** is simply an atom that has gained or lost an extra electron (or two). When the molecule of salt breaks apart in water, the chloride ion retains an extra orbiting electron that was previously shared. Because electrons have a negative charge, the chlorine atom takes on a negative charge, Cl^-. The loss of the electron by the sodium results in a positive ion (Na^+). Furthermore, these positive and negative ions are attracted by electrical potentials with opposite charges because opposite charges attract and like valences repel. The movement of ions creates **ionic flow** and is the basis for *ion,* the Greek verb that means "to move."

The internal constituents of a neuron reveals that the cytoplasm or **axoplasm** of a neuron contains potassium (K^+), sodium (Na^+), chlorine (Cl^-), calcium (Ca^{2+} has lost two electrons), and large amino acids and proteins that have a negative charge, labeled A–, and called anions.

The concentration of these different ions within the cell, however, is not equal. There are fewer sodium (Na^+), chlorine (Cl^-) and calcium (Ca^{2+}) ions inside the cell than there are potassium (K^+) ions. The concentration of K^+ within the cell is approximately 20 times higher than outside it. The Na^+ distribution, moreover, is almost 9 times more concentrated outside of the cell. The Cl^- distribution across the cell membrane (inside relative to the outside) is nearly 5 times greater outside the cell. Finally, the Ca^{2+} ions have a greater concentration outside the cell than inside it. These unequal distributions of ions with their associated electrical charges are shown in Table 1.1. These charges and ion distributions are the basis of the negative resting potential and the action potential. The cell membrane contains "channels" or "pores"

TABLE 1.1   Distribution of Ions Across the Cell Membrane

Ion	Concentration Inside	Concentration Outside	Ratio
Na^+	50	440	1:9
K^+	400	20	20:1
Cl^-	40-150	560	1:6
Ca^{2+}	0.3×10^{-3}	10	—

through which ions can flow under certain conditions. This movement of ions is the aforementioned ionic flow. The flow can be either an **influx** of ions into the interior of the cell, or an **efflux** when ions exit the cell.

When ion channels are open, ionic flow occurs for two reasons—namely, concentration and electrical gradients. These two gradients form the basis for passive ion movement. The ions, in turn, determine the resting and action potentials in all neurons.

Concentration and Electrical Gradients

Concentration gradients begin with diffusion, a simple nonmetabolic process in which there is no expenditure of energy by the cell. Diffusion is the process by which ions tend to equalize themselves throughout a solution. If, for example, there were nine ions on the inside of a cell and only one ion on the outside, this difference could generate a concentration gradient and diffusion could occur provided they could cross the membrane. In an axon, the uneven distribution of K^+ ions on the inside relative to the outside of the cell leads to diffusion and an ionic flow. The ions attempt to diffuse and equalize the number of ions on each side of the membrane. When there is a difference in concentration, an inequality exists. The inequality in ion concentrations on each side of the membrane results in a **concentration gradient.** The diffusion of ions from an area of high concentration to an area of low concentration reduces the concentration gradient.

Another reason for ionic flow is electrical. As noted previously, like charges repel, and unlike charges attract. In terms of ions, a positive area repels positively charged ions such as K^+ and Na^+. A negatively charged area attracts the positively charged ions and repels ions like Cl^-. When differences in electrical charge exist between areas, for example, the inside and the outside of a cell, there is an electrical inequality known as an **electrical gradient.** For example, an electrical gradient causes the Na^+ ions to flow from an area with a positive valence or charge to an area with a negative valence. The Na^+ influxes from the outside of the cell to the inside.

The flow of ions may be viewed as analogous to the flow of electrons in a flashlight. A flashlight battery is a polarized cell, like a neuron. Indeed, the flashlight battery is called, for example, a "D cell," an "AA cell," or a "C cell." The voltage, as measured from one pole of the battery to the other, is like the electrical gradient across a neural membrane. The flow of electrons through a bulb in the flashlight is analogous to the ionic flow across the cell membrane. The flow in both cases is due to an electrical gradient.

Passive Transport

It is time to consider a neuron's charge when the ions are not distributed equally on both sides of the cell membrane. That is, when the cell is at rest near −70 mv, what keeps it there and how does it get negatively charged in the first place?

Similarly, what happens to the ions when an action potential occurs and the inside of the cell spikes to a value near +55 mv? To answer these questions, we need to consult Figure 1.12. The sketch is, of course, highly diagrammatic and inaccurate in terms of how an axon appears. Nevertheless, we can get a solid feeling for the processes and the general operation of **passive transport** by considering the simplified view. Passive transport refers to the movement of ions without metabolic cell involvement. The neuron does not actively move the ions across its membrane.

Figure 1.12(a) shows the membrane when there is an equal number of K^+, Na^+, Cl^-, Ca^{2+}, and anions inside and outside the cell. The voltage across the membrane is, in this case, balanced because both the concentration and electrical gradients are equal. If we were to arbitrarily remove the K^+ ions from the outside, as shown in Figure 1.12(b), an imbalance is apparent. The inside of the cell would become positive due to the abundance of the K^+. In addition, there would be both a concentration gradient and an electrical gradient across the membrane. These gradients tend to draw out the K^+ from the cell passively. This is shown by the arrows and the notation Ge and Gc in Figure 1.12(b). In other words, the concentration gradient, Gc, causes the K^+ ions to diffuse out through the membrane and the electrical gradient, Ge, repels the K^+ toward the outside. If nothing occurred to change this situation, the K^+

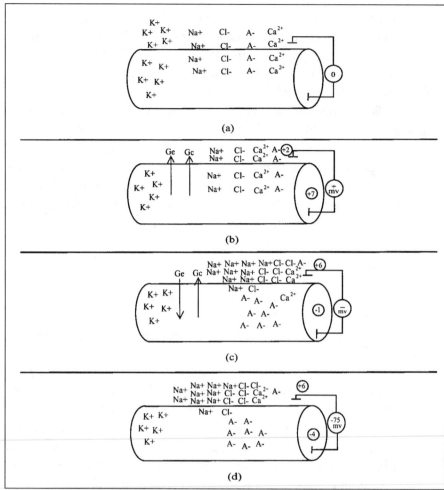

Figure 1.12. Ion Distribution Within an Axon and the Concept of Passive Conduction

NOTE: (a) Equal distribution of ions on each side of the membrane results in a zero membrane potential, (b) unequal distribution of K^+ produces an electrical and concentration gradient for K^+ efflux, (c) a more realistic ion configuration results in electrical influx and efflux gradients for different ions, and (d) ion concentrations leading to a –75 mv resting potential across the cell membrane.

ions eventually distribute themselves equally on each side of the membrane. The cell is then similar to the one shown in Figure 1.12(a).

If the Na^+, Cl^-, Ca^{2+}, and anion concentrations were distributed across the membrane as shown in Figure 1.12(c), the situation changes. In this case, the distribution of ions reflects a more realistic situation. It is based on the data given in Table 1.1.

So far in our discussion, we have assumed that the membrane is impervious to Na^+, Cl^-, Ca^{2+}, and anions and only K^+ could pass through. In this situation the inside of the cell is, as noted in Figure 1.12(c), slightly negative relative to the outside. This can be verified in the example by counting the positive and negative charges on each side of the membrane. The negativity and the high concentration of K^+ inside the cell produce an interesting milieu. The K^+ is, as expected, drawn out of the cell because of the concentration gradient, labeled G_c in Figure 1.12(c). As each K^+ ion leaves the cell, due to the diffusion, it takes with it a positive charge. The more the efflux of the K^+ ions continues, due to the concentration gradient "drawing" them out, the more electrically negative the inside of the cell becomes. Eventually there is an electrical gradient set up across the membrane that equals the concentration gradient, but in the opposite direction. The electrical gradient is labeled G_e in Figure 1.12(c). The negative valence within the cell draws the K^+ ions into the cell because the K^+ ions are positive; simultaneously, the concentration gradient forces the K^+ to leave the cell. The result is a stalemate. The concentration gradient draws K^+ out, but only to a certain point. The point of equilibrium is reached when the K^+ no longer diffuses outward because the negativity within the cell acts as a magnet to draw them back in. When a balance is reached between the concentration gradient and the electrical gradient, the voltage drop across the membrane is –75 mv, only 5 mv away from the neural resting potential.

Figure 1.12(d) shows the situation when the cell is near the resting potential. Ignoring the other ions for a moment, it is clear that the resting potential of –70 mv is primarily the result of a balance of two forces: the concentration gradient drawing the K^+ out and the electrical gradient, which draws the K^+ back in. The K^+ ionic flow yields a negative interior of –75 mv, a value very close to the resting potential. An important point concerning the K^+ flow is that the potential of –75 mv is done without any active help from the cell itself. The cell is, in this sense, passive. As noted earlier, the process of ionic flow without metabolic cell activity defines passive transport. Before we consider the flow of ions during an action potential, it is necessary to digress slightly and consider an important mechanism known as the sodium-potassium pump. Once this phenomenon is understood, we can more clearly understand the ionic flow that produces the maintenance of the –70 mv resting potential and the observed difference of 5 mv.

The Sodium-Potassium Pump

The situations depicted in Figure 1.12 are somewhat artificial. When a more realistic situation is examined in which the concentrations of Na^+, Ca^{2+}, and Cl^- are higher on the outside of the cell than within, it becomes apparent that there is a strong tendency for the Na^+ and Ca^{2+} to attempt to cross the membrane and enter the cell. The high concentration of Cl^- also sets up a concentration gradient for Cl^- to enter the cell. However, this Cl^- concentration gradient is offset by the opposite force of the electrical gradient; Cl^- is driven out of the cell due to the high negative charge in the cell (due to the A−). We focus, for the moment, on the Na^+ and Ca^{2+} ions.

Returning to Figure 1.12(d), we see the large number of Na^+ and Ca^{2+} ions concentrated outside the cell, and the interior of the cell has a negative resting potential. Both the concentration and electrical gradients for the Na^+ and Ca^{2+} are producing an influx force to move the Na^+ and Ca^{2+} inward. The electrical gradient produces an influx gradient because the negative resting potential within the cell attracts the positive sodium and calcium ions. The concentration gradient is an influx force because of the difference in ions inside and outside the cell. At this point it is time to acknowledge that the cell membrane is not completely impervious to Na^+ and Ca^{2+}. The strong influx gradients force a leakage of Na^+ and Ca^{2+} through the membrane. The consequence of the leakage is a decrease in the negativity of the cell interior. The continual leakage of positive ions into the cell makes the interior of the cell more positive and slowly depolarizes it. Furthermore, as the inside of the cell starts to become positively charged, the K^+ tend to efflux. The K^+ leaves because like charges repel and because there is a concentration gradient attracting the K^+ ions outward.

In summary, there is a constant influx of Na^+ and Ca^{2+} ions into the cell and an efflux of K^+. This constant leakage of ions moves the electrical potential of the cell interior from negative toward positive. If this leakage continues unabated, the negative resting potential dissipates and eventually becomes zero. The polarization is removed and the cell "runs down" analogous to a flashlight that has been turned on all night. If nothing is done by the cell to recharge and prevent the Na^+ and Ca^{2+} ions from leaking in and the K^+ ions from leaving, the negative potential within the cell continues to decrease and eventually becomes zero just as is shown in Figure 1.12(a).

The manner in which the leakage is counteracted entails the active participation of the neuron. The cell transports the Na^+ ions back to the outside of the cell while moving the K^+ back inside. This involvement of the cell in the transport of Na^+ and K^+ is called **active transport**. To be more specific, the active transport of Na^+ from the inside of the cell to the outside and the active transport of K^+ into the cell is accomplished by a metabolic process known as the **sodium-potassium pump.** The sodium-potassium pump not only removes the Na^+ from the inside of the cell but simultaneously ensures that the concentration of K^+ is maintained at the appropriate level by pumping K^+ into the cell. The sodium-potassium pump does not exchange ions equally, however. The ratio of exchange is near 3:2; three ions of Na^+ are removed for each insertion of two K^+. This inequality, however, causes no problem because the leakage of Na^+ and the outflow of K^+ is at the same rate. Three Na^+ ions leak in for every two K^+ ions that leave. Thus, the exchange ratio of the sodium-potassium pump matches the leakage. The sodium-potassium pump is shown diagrammatically in Figure 1.13. The figure shows the clockwise movement of the pump as it removes Na^+ from the cell and brings K^+ into the cell.

Calcium Removal

You have probably noted by now that the active transport system of the sodium-potassium pump has not handled the infusion of the Ca^{2+} ions. The removal of the Ca^{2+} is done by a different method. Briefly, the Ca^{2+} removal is a by-product of the influx of the Na^+. That is, as the Na^+ leaks into the cell there is an automatic and continual removal of Ca^{2+}. An analogy may help to simplify the concept. The in-pouring of the Na^+ ions may be viewed as a continuous stream of water that turns a waterwheel. The waterwheel is mechanically coupled to a large millstone in a flour mill. As the waterwheel is turned, the millstone grinds the grain to flour. In this analogy, the Na^+ ions represent the water that turns the waterwheel. The mechanical linkage to the millstone is analogous to an automatic linkage in the cell membrane. The influx of Na^+ ions is the "power" that "mechanically" removes the Ca^{2+} ions. There is no special active transport system for the Ca^{2+} removal. Figure 1.13 shows a situation in which the Na^+ and Ca^{2+} leak into the cell and the sodium-potassium pump transports the Na^+ back out. The sodium-potassium pump also replaces the K^+ that has "escaped" to the outside. The mechanical removal of the Ca^{2+} occurs when the Na^+ leaks into the cell.

Chlorine Distribution

The concentration of Cl^- is predominantly outside the cell relative to the inside. This, at first glance, tends to cause some concern about their effect on the potential of the cell. Surprisingly, the effect of Cl^- is relatively small. The primary reason for such a state of affairs is that the membrane of the cell is

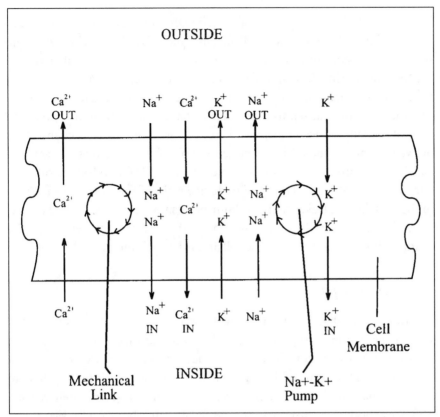

OUTSIDE

INSIDE

Mechanical
Link

Na+-K+
Pump

Cell
Membrane

Figure 1.13. Diagram of the Active Transport System Using the Sodium-Potassium Pump to Remove the Na⁺ and Return the K⁺

NOTE: The mechanical removal of Ca²⁺ by Na⁺ influx and K⁺ and Ca²⁺ leakage is also shown.

"open" to the free movement of the Cl⁻ ions. This freedom of movement allows the Cl⁻ ions to arrange themselves in such a manner that they balance, and the concentration and electrical gradients are equalized at the value of the resting potential. Said differently, the sodium-potassium pump maintains a fixed ionic concentration for Na⁺ and K⁺ but the Cl⁻ ions are free to "settle" at an equilibrium across the membrane that is at the value set by the sodium-potassium pump.

The 5 mv Difference

To visualize why the resting potential of the cell is –70 mv rather than –75 mv requires that we acknowledge the actual permeability of the cell membrane and the activity of the sodium-potassium pump. Let us review the situation briefly.

When the membrane is permeable only to K^+, then the potential across the membrane is −75 mv. The assumption is that the membrane is permeable only to K^+. The assumption is incorrect. There is a tendency for Na^+ to leak into the cell because of the concentration and electrical gradients. Like most biological systems, the neural membrane is imperfect, it leaks. Consequently, the membrane is not likely to remain at −75 mv. The influx of Na^+ and the leakage of K^+ across the membrane results in a decrease in the internal potential of the cell from the −75 mv. The sodium-potassium pump, of course, operates to offset the leakage of Na^+ and K^+, but the pump can only do so if it has been activated. When the sodium-potassium pump begins operation, it maintains the membrane potential at a relatively stable value. For our purposes, we can assume that the sodium-potassium pump begins once the cell has been depolarized from −75 mv to −70 mv. In other words, the sodium-potassium pump "kicks in" when the potential of the cell reaches −70 mv due to the Na^+ and K^+ leakage. As an analogy, ideally, a ship is watertight. In reality, however, ships do leak. A slight leakage is acceptable if it is maintained at a low level. If the leakage becomes too great, however, it is important to eliminate it. The water pumps (bilge pumps) are activated to do the job. In a very leaky boat the bilge pumps are turned on when the water inside the boat reaches the maximum allowable limit. Once the pumps are active, the water level is maintained at a constant level. In the analogy, the sodium-potassium pump is activated when enough Na^+ and K^+ ions have leaked in to increase the internal potential from −75 mv to −70 mv. The sodium-potassium pump maintains a constant resting state by pumping the leaking Na^+ out and returning the K^+ to the inside. The sodium-potassium pump is nearly always active. The only time the active transport system is not working is during the brief durations when action potentials are being produced. The generation of the action potential is the next discussion.

Conductance and the Action Potential

One of the important aspects of the neural operation has been alluded to but not addressed specifically. It should be apparent that ionic movements across the membrane determine both the resting potential and the action potential. However, what has not been stated is that the membrane of the axon itself is sensitive to the voltage differential across it. The axon membrane is **potential sensitive.** This means that the "pores" or gates that allow the different ions to pass through the membrane are opened or closed as a function of the potential across the membrane.

During the resting state, the potential-sensitive gates of the membrane are open only to the flow of K^+ ions (ignoring leakage). The onset of an action potential begins when a graded potential at the axon hillock reaches the threshold value of –50 mv. At threshold, the potential-sensitive Na^+ gates open wide to allow a rapid influx of Na^+ into the cell. The initial increase in internal potential closes the potential-sensitive K^+ gates. The rapid influx of Na^+ into the cell continues until the depolarization reaches the +55 mv peak spike value. The consequent rapid increase in potential has an almost immediate second effect on the potential-sensitive gates for Na^+ ions. At the peak of the spike (+55 mv), the gates close to the passage of Na^+. An instant later, the gates open for the efflux of K^+ ions from the cell. The efflux of K^+ returns the cell to near resting potential. Said differently, the K^+ gates are open and the Na^+ gates are closed when the cell is at rest (–70 mv). When the neuron is depolarized and reaches threshold, because of the graded potential at the axon hillock, the Na^+ gates open and the K^+ gates almost immediately close. This sequence is then reversed when the internal potential reaches +55 mv. At the peak of the spike, the Na^+ gates close and the K^+ gates reopen. The recovery portion of the action potential that follows the maximum spike potential (+55 mv) is due to the efflux of the K^+.

Figure 1.14 shows a hypothetical view of the potential-sensitive gates during rest (Point 1), during a generator potential (Point 2), during the initiation of an action potential (threshold at Point 3), during the action potential (Point 4), and during the recovery or decline of the action potential (Point 5). Although the gates are shown diagrammatically opening and closing in unison, this simultaneity does not actually occur. It is just difficult to draw gates opening and closing with microsecond offsets. The insert at the bottom of Figure 1.14 indicates the electrical activity at the various points. The result is, of course, an action potential. The hyperpolarization is shown at Point 6. This hyperpolarization occurs where the internal potential becomes more negative than the resting potential. This is due to the "overshoot" of K^+ ion efflux. Point 7 reflects a state of rest identical to that at Point 1.

The conductance of an action potential is a relatively simple concept. It is like the burning of a fuse. Once a fuse has been lit, the heat of the ignited portion raises the temperature of the area adjacent to it. When the powder in the zone next to the flame reaches its flash point, it too bursts in flame. The flame at this new point then raises the temperature of the powder next to it, and this powder now ignites. The flame, therefore, moves steadily down the fuse burn-

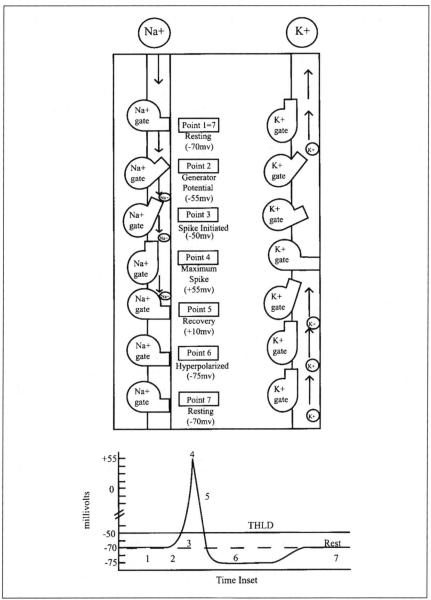

Figure 1.14. Diagrammatic View of Na⁺ and K⁺ Gates and the Movement of Ions During the Generation of an Action Potential

ing the powder as it goes. The activity of the neural impulse is similar. During the occurrence of a spike, the influx of Na^+ causes a voltage change across the cell membrane as it flows into the cell. The voltage change affects the membrane permeability to Na^+ in the neighboring area and Na^+ begins to enter.

When the threshold value of -50 mv is reached the Na^+ gates open wide, and the spike is conducted to the neighboring area of the membrane. In sum, the influx of Na^+ causes the gates for Na^+ to open in the area of the axon next to the spike. The influx of Na^+ is followed by an efflux of K^+. The exchange of ions flows down the membrane in a manner analogous to that of the fuse.

It is interesting to note another analogy of membrane conductance and fuses—namely, conductance time. The speed at which the flame moves down the fuse is dependent, to some degree, on the actual size of the fuse. The larger the fuse, the faster it conducts the flame to the dynamite. In neural conduction, the size of the axon is also a factor in the speed of conduction. The larger the axon diameter, the faster it conducts.

There is, finally, one comment necessary to complete the story. Some neurons have myelination and nodes of Ranvier. The flow of action potentials in myelinated neurons is increased in speed because of the special mechanism of saltatory conduction. The myelin acts as a cover that is resistant to the passage of ions through the membrane. Thus, for the neuron to conduct, the action potential must leap from node to node. The speed of conduction is increased when a neuron has myelin. Finally, the size of the neural impulse (spike) is nondecremental. This simply means that the magnitude of the spike does not decrease as it is conducted down the axon. In the present example, the "height" of the spike is maintained at $+55$ mv from beginning to end.

Dysfunctions

The nervous system is a very delicate and tender structure. As we progress through the book, selected diseases and accidents are discussed relative to a normal functioning system. The common everyday experiences and news reports, unfortunately, cover a large range of neurological problems. It is not the goal of this section to examine the vast array of situations and conditions that can occur. Rather, these sections of the book, found in nearly every chapter, are directed toward a brief introduction and excursion into some commonly known, and some not so commonly known, dysfunctions (Brodal, 1981).

A serious neurogenic problem is the **cerebrovascular accident (CVA)**, commonly known as a stroke. The irretrievable loss of neural tissue because of a stroke is one of the most serious problems an individual can encounter. The brain, which makes up approximately 2% of the total body weight, requires 17% of all the cardiac output and uses 20% of the oxygen consumption. Nearly 2 million U.S. citizens suffer neurological impairment because of cardiovascular disease alone. The brain is quite susceptible to interruptions in the blood and oxygen supply.

A CVA refers to neurological symptoms and signs that occur because of diseases from blood vessels that serve the brain. The CVA can occur because the vessels become closed (occlusive CVA), or because the vessels burst (hemorrhagic CVA). In either case, the effect on brain cells can be life threatening and traumatic. The occlusive CVA is thought generally to be due to atherosclerosis (clogging of the arteries due to fatty deposits) and thrombosis (blood clots). The hemorrhagic CVA is due to genetic aneurysm, weaknesses in the vessel wall, or hypertension (high blood pressure). Often when a hemorrhagic CVA occurs there is a loss in consciousness, possibly due to changes in the intracranial pressures.

The symptoms of a CVA vary according to the region of the brain in which it occurs. The symptoms presented by the patient provide clues for diagnosing the location of the CVA within the brain. For example, if the loss of neural cells occurs in the right parietal lobe, there is often a loss of perceptual abilities with disturbances in the ability to accomplish spatial tasks such as copying maps, pictures, or diagrams. Occasionally there is a severe difficulty in finding your way around in the environment, called topographagnosia. You should keep in mind that the functions affected seldom are controlled by a single region of the brain. The specificity you find for particular functions refers to certain regions of the brain that are more concerned with one set of functions than others. Most functions require integrated actions from several regions of the cortex as well as lower centers within the brain. Broca's and Wernicke's areas (see Figure 1.2) are examples of specificity, yet it is clear that without the input from the auditory sensory system, the areas are restricted in their function. It should be clear at this point that if a CVA were to occur in the area that produces speech, Broca's area, the individual's speech is drastically affected. A similar CVA within Wernicke's area results in the loss of the ability to understand verbal communication.

A loss of neural cells within the precentral gyrus, just in front of the central fissure in the frontal lobe, results in the loss of voluntary movement. A stroke within the motor area of the left hemisphere, for example, results in the loss of movement in the right half of the body. A lesion or a loss of cells due to CVA, or a heavy hit to the head by a boxer, in the posterior parietal cortex usually leave deficits in learning tasks associated with somesthesis. For example, a CVA in the left hemisphere often shows verbal and language deficits, agnosia or the inability to perceive even though the sensory channel is functional.

Loss of neural cells in the right hemisphere can result in striking effects. There sometimes is a complete lack of appreciation for all sensory inputs from the contralateral side of the body and from the opposite portions of the environment. Patients often fail to dress, wash, and undress the side of the body that is contralateral to the neural loss. Such a behavior is called the neglect syndrome.

A final example of a CVA within the temporal lobe is that the loss of neural cells, whether they are few or many, is a serious event. The loss of central neural cells is permanent. The peripheral nervous system, on the other hand, has regenerative capabilities. Peripheral nerves do regenerate.

A CVA within the superior temporal lobe in the right hemisphere usually leads to deficits in auditory pattern recognition. Should the stroke occur within the medial or inferior portion of the right temporal lobe the result is a visual learning deficit for patterns. The general outcome of temporal lobe losses is that loss in the left lobe eliminates the ability to process verbal material and loss in the right hemisphere eliminates the ability to process sensory pattern information.

A short comment or two needs to be inserted here regarding the regeneration or replacement of central nervous system cells. The first statement has to do with the "tenderness" of neural lifetimes. You are born with the maximum number of neurons you will ever have. The only sure thing in your life is that you continue to lose neural cells through the normal attrition of everyday living.

Second, a question is probably hanging around at this point concerning how it is that people can recover after a traumatic insult to the central nervous system. Not many years ago very little was known about how such "repairs" came about. This does not mean that we now fully understand how the brain comes to take up the slack of injured and destroyed neurons. What is recognized, however, is that the brain has a remarkable ability to take over functions of the neural cells that are destroyed. Not all functions, of course, are recoverable. It depends on the extent of the injury or stroke. The brain has shown a high degree of what is called **neural plasticity**—that is, the ability to do some considerable reorganizing or remodeling, both structurally and functionally. Because the brain may not produce new nerve cells after a stroke, lesion, or other disease, it is necessary to examine other mechanisms of recovery. It has long been recognized that the initial improvement, over the first few days or weeks, is likely due to the decrease in the edema (i.e., retention of fluid or swelling of the brain), resorption of the blood, and the recovery of the injured cells. The continual recovery of a patient over an indeterminate period requires another explanation.

Without doubt, many people have viewed the recovery following severe brain damage with amazement. The reasons for partial or total recovery of literally millions of damaged brain cells require some explanation. A complete answer, however, is not yet available, although research on brain functions and structures has suggested three possibilities to account for recovery.

One idea is that the neural elements that have not been affected by the insult or damage caused by the CVA take up the slack by sprouting new collaterals. The new collaterals make both structural and functional connections with neural elements that, before the damage, were in contact with the destroyed cells. That is, there may be a new pathway provided and thus the functions may be reintroduced.

A second alternative for the recovery is that of "unmasking." This idea simply means that the death of brain cells can lead to the revelation of unknown or seldom used pathways that accomplish the same function as the cells that were destroyed by the CVA. Pathways and cells, which were functional before the death of the cells, come to be primary rather than secondary when the initial primary group of cells is destroyed.

The third possibility, one that surely is involved to some extent, is that of learning. If learning occurs in normal individuals, as we certainly know it does, it requires that the brain be capable of modifying its structure and circuitry in some manner. It makes sense to assume that the improvement that comes about is the result of such learning processes even if it is in a defective or damaged nervous system. What the exact rewiring is and how plasticity is accomplished still remains to be determined. There are, certainly, amazing things on the horizon when it comes to the brain.

The problems that can occur with the neuron are mostly degenerative diseases and viral invasions. One of the more unfortunate, and fatal, of such degenerative diseases is that commonly referred to as Lou Gehrig's disease or amyotrophic lateral sclerosis (ALS). This disease progressively attacks the motor neuron and causes muscle atrophy due to the lack of innervations. The cause of the disease is presently unknown. *Amyotrophic* is derived from the neurogenic atrophy of the muscle. *Lateral sclerosis* refers to the hardened spinal cord observed during autopsy. This is due to the proliferation of the glia cells, astrocytes, and the scarring of the lateral columns. The disease does not affect sensory neurons or, somewhat surprisingly, the motor neurons associated with the viscera and glands. The search for the cause and a cure continues. The investigations are presently focused more in the exploratory and understanding stage than in the preventative and or curing position.

Summary

The nervous system is a continuous entity that is partitioned, for the sake of discussion and study, in two parts: the peripheral and central nervous systems. The peripheral nervous system is made up of 12 cranial and 31 pairs of spinal nerves. The spinal nerves each innervate a particular part of the body surface. The body surface served by a single spinal nerve is called a dermatome. The spinal nerves diverge and mix with peripheral nerves so that the severance of a single spinal nerve causes only a partial loss of sensitivity.

The central nervous system is partitioned in two parts: the spinal cord and the brain. These two parts function as a unit and are, in fact, structurally a single continuous system. The spinal cord receives information from the environment via the afferent axons that enter the dorsal horn. Efferent information is sent to muscles and glands via the ventral horn. The division of the spinal nerves in two functional sections is known as the Bell-Magendie law. The spinal cord both conducts as well as integrates information it receives. The conductive aspect of the cord is done by the pathways that ascend and descend via the dorsal column, spinothalamic tract, pyramidal tract, lateral spinothalamic tract, extrapyramidal tract, ventral column, and Lissauer's tract. Both the dorsal column and the lateral spinothalamic tract are sensory in nature and send information to higher nervous centers via the thalamus. The dorsal column first-order afferents enter the spinal cord and ascend ipsilaterally to the medulla within the brain stem. The second-order fibers then cross the midline and ascend via the medial lemniscus. Each hemisphere of the brain, therefore, processes sensory information from the contralateral side of the body; the left hemisphere processes information from the right side of the body and the right hemisphere receives and processes information from the left side of the body. The third-order fibers leave the thalamus and project to their final destination in the postcentral gyrus of the cortex. The integrative aspects of the cord are done by the interneurons within the spinal gray matter (butterfly shaped). Layers 1 through 5 of the interneurons integrate and modulate the information as it passes through the cord on its way toward or away from the higher centers of the brain.

The two hemispheres of the cortex, separated by the **longitudinal fissure** are structurally and functionally connected via a large band of fibers called the **corpus callosum.** Each hemisphere is composed of four lobes: frontal, parietal, occipital, and temporal. Each lobe has been identified with sensory and motor functions. The motor system is found in the frontal lobes (precentral gyrus) and the somesthetic sense is in the parietal lobes (postcentral gyrus). The fissure of Rolando (central fissure) divides the frontal and parietal lobes. The occipital lobes, located posterior to the parietal lobes, process visual information. The temporal lobes, separated from the parietal and frontal lobes by the Sylvian sulcus, processes auditory information.

This chapter has taken a rather large, complex, and continually growing body of literature and presented a very simplified story of the chemical and electrical events that are the basis of neural operation. Because the story is necessarily brief and incomplete, some liberties were occasionally taken to ensure, within the author's capabilities, that the fascinating operation of neurons were clear. As an aid for your understanding, an overview of the cell operation is given next to highlight the main points discussed:

1. The neural membrane is semipermeable. It contains gates or channels through which positive and negative ions may flow.

2. The voltage potential across the membrane, from inside to outside, is approximately −70 mv when the neuron is not "active." The −70 mv within the cell, relative to the outside, is determined by the K^+ ions. The cell, at this point, is at the resting potential.

3. The difference between the −75 mv and the resting potential of −70 mv is due to the leakage of Na^+ and K^+ ions into and out of the cell.

4. When the leakage is sufficient to increase the −75 mv to a value of −70 mv, the cell initiates an active process to maintain the resting state. The active transport of the Na^+ and K^+ ions—Na^+ out and K^+ in—by the sodium-potassium pump ensures that the cell does not become depolarized (go to zero).

5. The positive value of +55 mv occurs at the maximum point of the action potential because of the sodium influx.

6. Chlorine does not enter the activity of the neuron in terms of the resting potential and action potential. Calcium also does very little to affect the state of the neuron. The Ca^{2+} ions are important, however, when it comes to synaptic transmission.

7. The membrane changes permeability in response to voltage changes across it. In other words, changes in potential across the membrane opens the Na^+ channel to allow Na^+ to rush in because

of concentration and electrical gradients (passive transport). The K$^+$ channels are almost immediately closed during the Na$^+$ influx. The brief influx of Na$^+$ is approximately a millisecond in duration. At the peak of the spike (+55 mv), the Na$^+$ gates close immediately followed by the reopening of K$^+$ channels.

8. The reopening of the K$^+$ channels allows the K$^+$ ions to "escape" to the outside due to high electrical and concentration gradients. The efflux of the K$^+$ to the outside of the cell causes the return of the negative internal potential.

9. The efflux of the K$^+$, in fact, results in a hyperpolarization of the cell to a value below the –70 mv resting state.

10. The sodium-potassium pump begins operation following the action potential to prevent the eventual "running down" of the cell. The tremendous number of ions inside and outside the cell almost ensures that there can be thousands of spikes before the cell becomes depleted and all the Na$^+$ and K$^+$ become equal across the cell membrane. The sodium-potassium pump is not in operation at the point when an action potential is being actively generated.

11. The conductance of the action potential down the axon is dependent on the size of the axon and whether or not it is covered with myelin. The large myelinated neurons conduct the action potential, nondecrementally, at a rapid rate. Small diameter unmyelinated neurons conduct at a slower rate.

Suggested Readings

Brodal, A. (1981). *Neurological anatomy in relation to clinical medicine* (3rd ed.). New York: Oxford University Press.

Heimer, L. (1983). *The human brain and spinal cord: Functional neuroanatomy and dissection guide.* New York: Springer.

Hodgkin, A. L. (1964). *The conduction of the nervous impulse.* Springfield, IL: Charles C Thomas.

Hodgkin, A. L. (1992). *Chance and design: Reminiscences of science in peace and war.* Cambridge, UK: Cambridge University Press.

Kandel, E. R., Schwartz, J. H., & Jessell, T. M. (1995). *Essentials of neural science and behavior.* Norwalk, CT: Appleton & Lange.

Kimelberg, H. K., & Norenberg, M. D. (1989, August). Astrocytes. *Scientific American,* pp. 88-95.

Peters, A., Palay, S. L., & Webster, H. de F. (1991). *The fine structure of the nervous system: Neurons and their supporting cells* (3rd ed.). New York: Oxford University Press.

Posner, M. I. (Ed.). (1989). *Foundations of cognitive science.* Cambridge: MIT Press.

CHAPTER 2

Synapses and Receptors

Before we can address sensory processes, we need to consider the function and structure of connections between neurons. That is one of the goals of this chapter. The *synapse,* Greek for "junction," is the point at which a neuron interacts with another element of the body. The element may be, most likely is, another neuron. However, the interaction can also be between the neuron and a muscle, a gland, or an internal organ. We focus on the neuron-to-neuron interaction. The other goal of this chapter is an introduction to the operation and identification of the sensory receptors (Mountcastle, 1980). A statement you saw in the previous chapter is quite true: No receptor = no sensation.

A Brief Review

The synapse is deceptively simple in its function. The details, however, are a little more complex. To understand the function of a synapse and how it provides us with sensations and perceptions, we must consider several factors. First, we need to have the structure of the synapse and its divisions firmly in mind. Second, we must examine how synaptic potentials differ from action potentials. Once these preliminaries are set, we can scrutinize the operations within the synapse. These latter circumstances are especially interesting and lead to serious considerations of how memories and perceptions are formed.

Chapter 1 introduced the connections among neurons. We begin this chapter by briefly reviewing the different structural synapses found in the brain (Eccles, 1964, 1976). The first kind of synapse occurs quite often. It is the **axosomatic** synapse. The other three mentioned previously are **axodendritic,** between an axon and a dendrite; **axoaxonic,** between two axons; and a unique combination, the **axodendritic-axoaxonic.** This latter one is a combination of two different combinations. Nothing is simple in the nervous system.

Figure 2.1 displays the four major features of a typical axodendritic synapse:

1. Presynaptic terminal (**end bouton**) of the axon
2. Vesicles within the end bouton
3. Synaptic cleft
4. **Receptive membrane** (postsynaptic cell)

The **presynaptic** and **postsynaptic** portions of the synapse are separated by a gap or space called the **synaptic cleft.** The presynaptic terminal contains packets of neurotransmitters in vesicles at the active zone of the terminal. The neurotransmitter is released in the synaptic cleft when action potentials arrive and Ca^{2+} enters the cell. Across the synaptic cleft, at the postsynaptic membrane, is another active zone called the postsynaptic density. This region contains the neurotransmitter binding sites. In summary, Figure 2.1 indicates that neurotransmitter synthesis occurs in the soma and is transported to the presynaptic terminal for storage in vesicles. When Ca^{2+} enters the cell, an exocytosis (movement of neurotransmitter out of the vesicle) of a neurotransmitter, for example, acetylcholine (Ach), is initiated. The neurotransmitter is released in the synaptic cleft where it diffuses across the space and binds with a neurotransmitter receptor in the postsynaptic membrane. The result is the opening of ion channels and the generation of a postsynaptic potential. These steps are repeated at each synapse. More details of this process are provided in the following sections.

Potential Sensitivity

One of the primary concepts presented in the previous chapter was that ion channels in the membrane of the axon are potential or **voltage sensitive.** For the neuron to conduct an action potential, there had to be sequential openings and closing of the Na^+ and K^+ channels of the membrane. As the channels opened and closed, the action potential flowed down the axon. The action potential was not generated, however, until the cell, at the axon hillock, was depolarized and reached the neuron's threshold. Once the resting potential of the cell had increased to the threshold level, the Na^+ gates opened, the K^+ gates

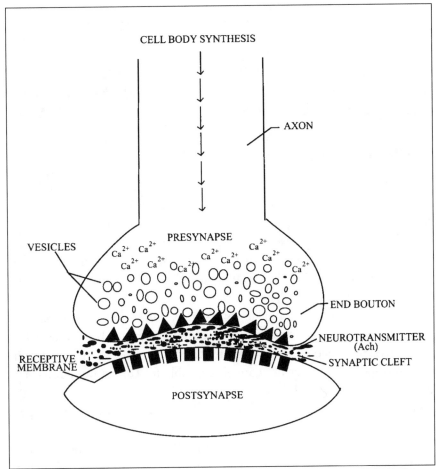

Figure 2.1. Synapse Showing the Presynaptic End Bouton, Synaptic Cleft, Vesicles, Neurotransmitter, and Postsynaptic Membrane

closed, and a spike was generated. The spike occurred because the voltage changed across the axon membrane and opened the gates for Na+ to enter. This activity was followed by the closing of the Na^+ gates and the simultaneous opening of the K^+ gates. This latter action has the effect of repolarizing the cell. The important element of the discussion was that the entire sequence of conducting events was dependent on the cell membrane being voltage sensitive. The gates for Na^+ and K^+ open and close *sequentially* as a function of the membrane's sensitivity to the voltage difference across it. It is the sensitivity of the axon membrane to the voltage across it that permits conduction of the action potentials.

In the subsequent discussion, however, we learn that the voltage sensitivity is primarily, but not entirely, restricted to the axon. Although the majority of axons are potential sensitive, specific classes of ion channels are not responsive to voltage fluctuations. These channels are chemically sensitive and are mainly located at the soma and dendritic extensions. Chemically responsive synapses are also located at the axoaxonic synapses.

Calcium Influx

The membrane of the axon is voltage sensitive and permits the Na^+ and K^+ to influx and efflux, respectively, through their rapidly opening and closing gates. A question arises, however, about other ions. We know that calcium, Ca^{2+}, slowly leaks into the axon because of the strong concentration and electrical gradients. We also know that the Ca^{2+} ions are mechanically removed as Na^+ leaks in. However, Ca^{2+} does nothing to aid in the generation or propagation of action potentials.

One of the reasons for the lack of participation by Ca^{2+} is that there are relatively few Ca^{2+} channels in the axon of most neurons. If the number of channels is few, then the Ca^{2+} ions are limited in their effect. At the axon terminal, however, the number of channels available for Ca^{2+} is numerous. The consequence of this fact is important. The arrival of action potentials at the axon terminal opens the gates wide for the Ca^{2+} ions. When the gates are open, the calcium enters rapidly.

In the action potential, it is not the influx of Na^+ (the "up-shoot" portion of the spike) that unlocks the Ca^{2+} gates—rather, it is the efflux of K^+ during the recovery portion of the spike. The Ca^{2+} channels open and permit the influx of Ca^{2+} during the decline in the spike. This sequence of events makes perfect sense. The Ca^{2+} ions are concentrated outside the cell and have a positive valence. When the Na^+ is rushing in, the inside of the cell becomes depolarized, and the spike becomes positive. The positive valence keeps the Ca^{2+} out. However, when the K^+ ions leave the cell, the inside of the cell becomes negatively polarized and the concentration and electrical gradients for Ca^{2+} lead to the influx of Ca^{2+} into the cell. The result is a large surge of Ca^{2+} at the presynaptic terminal (end bouton).

The influx of Ca^{2+} is a critical event in the release of neurotransmitters by the vesicles. The Ca^{2+} acts as a catalyst to change the presynaptic terminal so that the vesicles move to the synaptic membrane and fuse with it. The vesicles then deposit their contents (the neurotransmitter) in the cleft. The Ca^{2+} acts as the intermediary between the arrival of the action potentials and the release of the neurotransmitter.

Neurotransmitter Release

The movement of the vesicles to the synaptic cleft, at the "request" of the Ca^{2+}, is a critical event in the communication of one neuron with another. The fusion of the vesicle with the presynaptic membrane has been carefully studied. The number of action potentials at the terminal determines the quantity of Ca^{2+} released. The more action potentials that arrive at the terminal, the more Ca^{2+} influx there is. The amount of Ca^{2+} influx is, in turn, directly related to the amount of neurotransmitter jettisoned in the cleft. The vesicle, with the Ca^{2+} acting as a catalyst, moves to the synaptic cleft, fuses with the cell membrane, and releases a packet of neurotransmitter molecules in an all-or-none fashion. Each vesicle stores a single **quantum** of neurotransmitter, and each quantum contains thousands of molecules. *Quantum* is the terminology used to designate the entire package of chemicals stored and released by a single vesicle. The release of a quantum of neurotransmitter, and its effect, is known as the quantal hypothesis. This hypothesis assumes that the arrival of 1 action potential at the axon terminal causes the release of 1 to 5 quanta (1 to 5 vesicles) in the synaptic cleft. If, for example, the average spontaneous activity of a neuron is 5 spikes per second, there is continuous release of transmitter substance in the synapse at a rate between 5 and 25 quanta per second. This translates to 5 to 25 vesicles expelling their contents every second. Because there are about 30,000 to 40,000 vesicles in each end bouton (the number varies with the synapse), it takes about 20 to 25 minutes to deplete all the vesicles of their cargo if no action is taken to replenish them. There is, of course, something done.

Replenishing the Vesicles

The delivery of the transmitter to the synaptic cleft by the vesicle is the beginning of several possible events. The fate of the neurotransmitter molecules as they are released in the cleft depends, to a certain degree, on chance. Some molecules are, for example, immediately deactivated by an enzyme specifically designed to accomplish the task. Other molecules diffuse across the gap, encounter the postsynaptic membrane, and bind with their appropriate receptors. In this latter case, the contact and binding with the receptors causes the postsynaptic membrane to modify its configuration. The change in the membrane configuration is due to the opening and closing of ion channels and an ionic exchange across the postsynaptic membrane. The ionic influx/efflux results in the **postsynaptic potential.** Once the membrane has changed configuration and opened or closed the channels, the neurotransmitter has done its job. The transmitter molecules then break away and diffuse back to the synaptic cleft.

At this point, either the neurotransmitter molecules can be destroyed by the enzyme specifically designed to neutralize them or they can diffuse across the cleft and return to the presynaptic cleft where a process of **re-uptake** occurs. The neurotransmitter molecules are taken back to the presynaptic terminal and "loaded" back in a vesicle for reuse. More interesting, the period of time between the arrival of the action potentials at the presynaptic terminal and the change in the postsynapatic membrane causing an influx or efflux of ions at the postsynaptic membrane takes only 0.2 to 0.5 msec. The majority of this time is due to the "slow" influx of the Ca^{2+} ions into the presynaptic terminal.

Postsynaptic Potentials

The ionic exchange at the postsynaptic membrane occurs because of the neurotransmitter binding with specific molecular receptors in the membrane. The ionic exchange yields either an excitatory (depolarizing) or an inhibitory (hyperpolarizing) potential within the postsynaptic cell. This alteration in voltage is referred to as an **excitatory postsynaptic potential (EPSP)** when the membrane is depolarized or an **inhibitory postsynaptic potential (IPSP)** when the inside of the postsynaptic cell is hyperpolarized. Whether the potential is excitatory or inhibitory depends on the neurotransmitter, its specific receptor, and the ions that are involved in the efflux or influx across the associated ion channels.

Excitatory Postsynaptic Potentials

Recall that Na^+ influx results in the inside of the cell becoming positive relative to the outside. In an axon, this is the up-shoot portion of the action potential. When the Na^+ channels close and the K^+ channels open, the spike declines and the cell returns to its negative resting potential. By following this logic, it can be demonstrated how an EPSP occurs. The EPSP generation happens when the neurotransmitter reacts with the postsynaptic membrane and the postsynaptic receptor protein changes the membrane characteristics and opens **cation** (positive ion) channels. For this discussion, we assume the cation is Na^+. The influx of Na^+ depolarizes the postsynaptic cell in the immediate vicinity of the synapse. The size of the depolarization, of course, depends on the amount of Na^+ influx into the cell. The amount of Na^+ is dependent on the number of Na^+ channels opened by the neurotransmitter and receptor protein interaction. The more neurotransmitter released by the vesicles, the more Na$^+$ channels are opened on the postsynaptic cell. This sequence of events results in a local **graded potential** within the postsynaptic neuron. *Graded* simply means that the size of the potential varies and is dependent on the amount of neurotransmitter released. The adjective *local* is also important because the activity in the postsynaptic cell is restricted to the area where the synapse is located. The local graded potential is also electrotonic in its effect. *Electrotonic* means that the potential instantly moves or spreads from its initiating source at the synapse and declines in size as it is gets farther from the synapse.

Figure 2.2 displays the sequence of events leading to the EPSP and also shows, graphically on the left and diagrammatically on the right, the relationship among the variables associated with the presynaptic and postsynaptic potentials. The relationship shown in Figure 2.2(a) is between the number of action potentials arriving at the axon terminal and the number of quanta released in the synaptic cleft by the vesicles. Although the relationship is not linear, the important aspect to understand is the image shown in the graphical display. The graph shows that as the number of impulses arriving at the presynaptic terminal increases, the amount of neurotransmitter excreted in the synaptic cleft also increases. Diagrammatically, at the end bouton labeled A, two spikes have released six quanta of neurotransmitter. At end bouton B, the nine action potentials have yielded a significant increase for neurotransmitter released by the vesicles. Figure 2.2(b) continues this representation by showing that as the number of quanta increases more Na$^+$ channels get opened.

Figure 2.2(c) takes the sequence to the next stage and shows the association among the number of open Na$^+$ channels and the **amplitude** of the EPSP. This figure reflects a positive change in membrane potential, at the postsynaptic membrane. The increase in the graded local potential, for example, caused at neuron E is 10 mv. The increase caused by neuron F is 20 mv. Because the change is an increase from the resting potential, from –70 mv to –50 mv for example, the potential is an excitatory one—namely, an EPSP. Finally, Figure 2.2(d) graphically displays the relationship between the number of action potentials at the presynaptic terminal and the magnitude of the EPSP generated at the postsynaptic neuron.

Now consider Figure 2.3. This figure displays two axons with their terminals functionally connected to the same dendrite by means of separate dendritic spines. The presynaptic terminals are spatially located close to each other. When both synapses are active, each one produces an EPSP at its

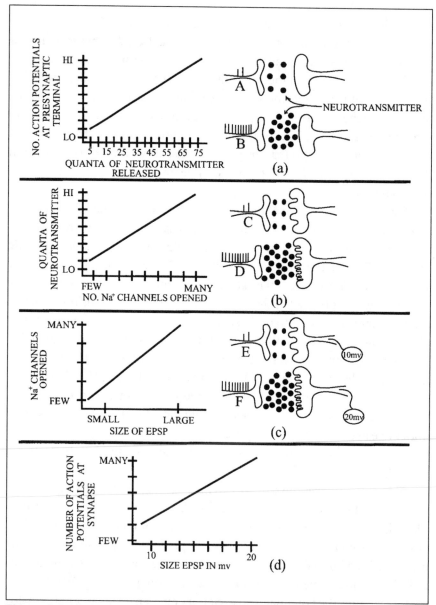

Figure 2.2. Diagrams of Neural Activity at the Synapse

NOTE: (a) relationship between the number of action potentials and amount of neurotransmitter release in quanta, (b) relationship between amount of quanta released and open N+ channels, (c) relationship between number of open N+ channels and the size of the postsynaptic potential, and (d) relationship between frequency of action potentials and size of the postsynaptic potential.

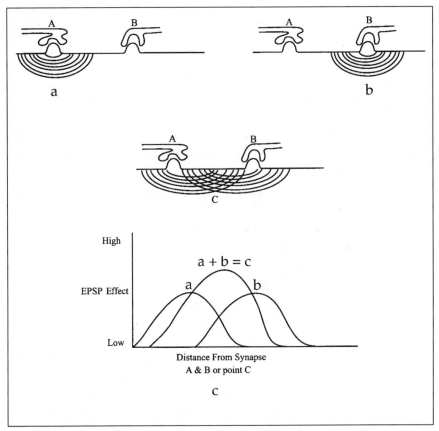

Figure 2.3. Spatial Summation

NOTE: (a) activity at Synapse A alone, (b) activity at Synapse B alone, and (c) spatial summation of the activity from Synapse A and B.

respective dendritic spine. Because the magnitude of any EPSP varies as a function of distance from the initiating source, the EPSP is larger directly beneath the spine at the point of synaptic activity. The EPSP dissipates and declines in magnitude as a function of distance from the initiating source. Figure 2.3(a) shows the magnitude of the EPSP when Axon A is active and B is inactive. Figure 2.3(b) shows the magnitude of the EPSP when the situation is reversed; namely, B is active but A is not. Figure 2.3(c) displays the postsynaptic effect when both Axons A and B are active. The effect of the EPSPs from two synapses is an algebraic summation where they overlap. The algebraic summation of graded potentials near each other spatially is known as **spatial summation.** The spatial summation of activity from several weak EPSPs can result in a relatively large potential on the dendritic process. Thus, what one axon terminal cannot do alone, several can do together. If all the potentials are EPSPs, then there is power in numbers. An alternative method of increasing the magnitude of the postsynaptic potential is by **temporal summation.** We already know that axons can have a greater effect on the postsynaptic membrane by repeated firings of action potentials. As noted earlier, the more action potentials that arrive at the terminal, the more neurotransmitter substance released. The rapid arrival of action potentials at the presynaptic terminal results in an accumulation of neurotransmitter at the postsynaptic membrane. The more neurotransmitter, the larger the postsynaptic potential. The arrival of many spikes in a short interval of time results in a larger postsynaptic potential. This is temporal summation.

A reminder needs to be added at this point regarding the EPSP and the ions related to its generation. For ease of discussion, it was assumed that the EPSP was the result of only Na^+ ions entering the postsynaptic cell. This is, in fact, a true statement of the situation. However, there is more to the story. The binding of the neurotransmitter to the postsynaptic receptors has an additional effect. Some K^+ ions also leave through the postsynaptic membrane at the same time the Na^+ ions are entering.

The efflux of K^+, at first glance, appears to counteract the Na^+ influx and reduce the EPSP. The K^+ does in fact slow the rate at which an EPSP is generated. The Na^+ influx into the postsynaptic neuron is, however, dominant and easily overcomes the K^+ efflux. Although K^+ is leaving the cell, the EPSP is generated because of the greater ionic influx of Na^+.

Inhibitory Postsynaptic Potentials

The inhibitory postsynaptic potential is dependent, just as the EPSP is, on the particular neurotransmitter and the receptor. The sequence of events outlined earlier for the EPSP is repeated for the IPSP with only a single, but important, exception. The IPSP is the result of different ions passing through the postsynaptic membrane. The influx of Cl^- into the cell, because of its valence, decreases the postsynaptic cell's voltage below its usual resting value. The IPSP occurs when the neurotransmitter opens the channels permeable to Cl^- ions, permitting Cl^- influx and the generation of the graded potential at the synapse. A second way in which the IPSP may be generated is to open more channels for K^+ ions, making it possible for more K^+ ions to leave, and thus decreasing the internal potential at the postsynaptic membrane. The postsynaptic cell would then become hyperpolarized at the synapse because of the efflux of the K^+ ions. The efflux of K^+ would lead to an IPSP, just as the influx of Cl^- results in an IPSP.

The IPSP is as important as the EPSP in the function of a neuron. Spatial and temporal summation also occurs for IPSPs. The summation, either spatial or temporal, leads to an increased hyperpolarization of the postsynaptic cell.

A final comment is necessary about the EPSP and IPSP. The two types of potentials are in constant conflict. Usually, the synapses on any one neuron are not all excitatory (EPSP) or all inhibitory (IPSP). In fact, each neuron is steadily and continually being hyperpolarized and depolarized at thousands of synapses. The receiving neuron is, as a result, under siege either to depolarize and send a message (bursts of spikes) to the next cell or to be completely silent, hyperpolarize, and cease communicating with other cells. The situation is resolved when an "algebraic summation" of the entire synaptic input is done. The receiving cell computes a continuous "running average" of the total EPSP and IPSP activity at any one moment. If the depolarizations outweigh the hyperpolarizations and the resultant algebraic summation is sufficiently positive for the cell to reach threshold, the depolarizations outweigh the hyperpolarizations, then a communicative signal is generated at the axon hillock. The communicative signal is, of course, a burst of action potentials sent by the axon terminal. The story is a familiar one. The neuron communicates via the action potentials discussed in Chapter 1.

Chemical Sensitivity

The EPSP and IPSP generated by the movement of ions across the postsynaptic membrane is directly dependent on the quantity of neurotransmitter chemical released by the presynaptic terminal and the receptor sites on the postsynaptic terminal. The opening and closing of ionic channels for the generation of the EPSP or IPSP does not occur because of variation in the voltage at the postsynaptic membrane. Although the influx of Na^+ and K^+ causes a voltage change at the postsynaptic terminal, the voltage change does not affect the channels through which the ions pass. Unlike the axon, which is voltage sensitive, the channels on the dendrite and soma do not open or close as voltage changes. The dendrite and soma membranes are **chemical sensitive.** This means that the only event that opens or closes channels on a dendrite or soma are specific chemicals. The chemicals are the neurotransmitters that bind to the receptors at the postsynaptic membrane. This unique event, chemical sensitivity at the postsynaptic membrane, is critical in the function and communication of neurons. The postsynaptic channels open and close because of the neurotransmitter and receptor binding. This synaptic function allows for memory, perception, and learning. Indeed, the plasticity of the nervous system occurs at the synapse.

Neurotransmitters

About 60 years ago when scientists first discovered neurotransmitters the belief was that the neurotransmitter was the determining factor for communication at the chemical synapse. Since then, however, it has become clear that the predominant variable is not the neurotransmitter. The key to the operation of the synapse now appears to have three critical ingredients:

1. the specific neurotransmitter,
2. the receptor proteins with which the neurotransmitter binds, and
3. the specific **ionic channels** that open or close because of the binding.

The channels open or close as a function of which receptor is available at the postsynaptic membrane and which transmitter is available to bind with it.

The last step, the generation of the EPSP or IPSP, is often more complex because of a second messenger. Briefly, a **second messenger** can be thought of as a sequence of chemical reactions that occur following a neurotransmitter docking with its receptor. The activation of the receptor by the neurotransmitter initiates the second messenger chemical sequence that opens or closes ion channels. The generation of the postsynaptic potential can, with a second messenger, entail a more elaborate reaction than the mere opening of membrane channels by the docking of a neurotransmitter with its postsynaptic receptor. With or without the second messenger, however, the result is the same: a postsynaptic potential.

Keep in mind that the same neurotransmitter can initiate both an EPSP or an IPSP at different synapses. Whether the potential is excitatory or inhibitory depends on how the postsynaptic membrane responds to the neurotransmitter and which ionic channels are opened or closed because of the binding. In the case of vision, for example, the same neurotransmitter initiates an IPSP on one postsynaptic cell while simultaneously initiating a depolarizing EPSP at a different cell (Schnapf & Baylor, 1987).

TABLE 2.1   Neurotransmitters

Transmitter	Comments
Acetylcholine (Ach)	Found in nerve-skeletal muscle junctions, cortex, basal nucleus, involved in Alzheimer's disease.
Dopamine	Involved in motor and reward behavior. Loss of dopamine leads to Parkinson's disease. Too much has been suggested to be a cause of schizophrenia.
Enkephalins	Transmitters that are opiate-like in their function. Bind to receptors that alleviate pain and mimic opiate drugs.
GABA	An extensive inhibitory transmitter, found primarily in the brain.
Glutamate	Major excitatory transmitter in the brain. A principle transmitter in vision.
Glycine	Inhibitory transmitter in the spinal cord and brain stem.
Serotonin	Changes in serotonin are associated with sleep, mood, and whole brain activity.
Substance P	Group of several peptides. A major transmitter in pain perception.

Some scientists have estimated the number of neurotransmitters within the central nervous system to be over 100. The number of transmitters that are well understood, however, are probably fewer than 12. Table 2.1 lists some of the more well known substances with comments on their actions in the central nervous system. Although many of the transmitters are chemically related and thereby structurally similar, their effect on the postsynaptic membrane is often quite different. In addition, the synthesis of each individual transmitter depends on specific biochemical processes within the neuron, the surrounding area of the cell, and even on general protein synthesis and metabolism. The transmitters of specific interest are acetylcholine (Ach), dopamine, serotonin, gamma-aminobutyric acid (GABA), glycine, glutamic acid (glutamate), enkephalins, and substance P (Barondes, 1994; Jacobs, 1994; Snyder, 1986).

Introduction to Receptors

Take a moment here to do an experiment. The experiment is discussed later in the chapter. Close your hand and make a fist. Now get a pencil with a sharp point on it. Slowly drag the point of the pencil very lightly across the back of your fist several times. Do not press too hard. Just let the weight of the pencil apply the pressure. As you drag the pencil point lightly across the back of your hand, you will feel cool sensations at different spots. Each time the pencil point touches the same place on your fist the cool spot appears. How did the stimulus, the pencil moving across your fist, turn neural impulses into a cool sensation? The answer lies in how the receptors in your skin respond to the stimulus in the world—our next topic.

The World About Us

We begin our discussion by presenting a classification of environmental stimuli. As we continue through the chapter, we encounter a variety of different receptors. These, too, are classified. The goal is to answer the question about how receptors respond to an environmental stimulus and change it to nervous impulses. This goal introduces classifications, the **doctrine of specific nerve energies**, and receptor transduction. Throughout the chapter, we consider the manner in which the nervous system encodes the stimulus information.

We already know that our world is full of physical energies. Some we respond to, some we do not. Scientists have organized these physical "energies" in five distinct classes:

1. Electromagnetic radiation (visible light, X-ray, radar, radio, gamma rays, etc.)
2. Pressure stimuli (a touch or pressure on the arm, sound pressure changes, etc.)
3. Thermal stimuli (heat and cold)
4. Chemical stimuli (NaCl, ozone, perfumes)
5. Gravity

You probably recognize some of these classifications from everyday experiences.

More interesting, four of these classifications are capable of eliciting feelings from the skin. More specifically, the application of electricity (electromagnetic) clearly makes an impression, as will a very strong invisible light (sun and tanning booths). A mechanical deformation of the skin or the movement of a hair results in a sensory response (a spider on the arm or a lover's caress). The application of a nondamaging thermal stimulus, either above or below skin temperature, elicits a sensation of warm or cold. Finally, a chemical (for example, an acid) can yield a painful response. Later on, we look at some of these stimuli more closely. However, first, we need to consider a classic idea—one made prominent by Johannes Müller.

The Doctrine of Specific Nerve Energies

We begin with the fact that the ancient philosophers did not overlook external objects and stimuli. They saw the world, heard sounds, tasted grapes, and smelled the roses. One conception of how our perceptions came to be was a simple "like-begets-like" notion. For example, if a tree existed in the world and we perceive a tree, then the tree must be regenerated within our own mind. How else could we see the world? Another example, which took decades to correct, was the implanted air theory of how we hear. It was well known that sound traveled through the air. If you were to hear, so the theory went, you had to have air within your ears. This implanted air theory found support in the fact that the middle ear, located behind the eardrum, was hollow. The middle ear was assumed to have air implanted during fetal development. Thus, the external air could match the internal air and "like begets like." The sound waves in the environment were simply regenerated in the implanted air and you heard sounds. These ideas, as unique and quaint as they are, came under some serious attack as physiological research became more rigorous.

The discovery that nerves were not filled with air and the investigations of the brain as the source of enlightenment brought great strides in knowledge. One of the ideas, believed by many in the early 1800s, and made respectable by Müller, was that the external world is conveyed to the brain by "specific nerve energy." Müller's formulation and exposition of the "doctrine" is broken down to the following two points. First, we do not perceive the external stimulus directly. The external stimuli, whatever they may be, activate nerves. The nerves themselves conduct the activity to centers within the brain. The nerves are intermediaries between the external world and the "mind's eye." We do not see "objects"; rather, we sense the activity of our nerves. Second, there are separate nerves for each sensory modality. In accordance, each of the classic five senses has its own nerve. Regardless of how the nerve is stimulated, it sends information to the brain, and the sensation is interpreted as belonging to that modality each time.

In summary, the doctrine states that there are nerves for each sensory quality. When a sensory nerve is stimulated, regardless of what the external stimulus may be, the sensation is always the same and depends on which nerve is activated. The visual nerve produces visual perception. The auditory nerve, when stimulated, produces hearing. The doctrine of specific nerve energies assumed that each sensory system operated on the same neural principles but yielded different perceptual qualities. The doctrine of specificity is, after more than a 150 years, still correct in many ways. It has also been revised in many ways.

So, where does this leave us at this point? We have five major classifications of stimuli in the world and these stimuli, somehow, activate nerves and nerve fibers. The sensations we experience appear to depend on which nerve is stimulated and where in the brain it is sent. This outline seems elementary until you recall the prior question. How did the stimulus, the pencil moving across your fist, turn neural impulses into cool sensations?

Receptors and Specificity

We can address the "cool spots" phenomenon now. It is clear that the stimulus is the light pressure caused by the pencil as it moved across the skin. The sensation reported was cool feelings. What has gone unstated here is that there are really two sensations available. You felt, but did not report, the "touch" of the pencil being drawn across your fist. So there were two sensations occurring, light touch and cool spots. The important point is that between the stimulus and the sensation, touch and cool spots, there is a missing component. The missing ingredient is one of nature's most intriguing and specialized concoctions: a receptor.

A **receptor** has only one function: **transduce** a stimulus to neural impulses. Once the neural impulses reach the brain, an interpretation may occur. *Transduce* simply means to change. Therefore, the receptor's function is to change one source of energy into another. The receptor is the interface between the environment and the nervous system. Some receptors transduce when struck by photons of light, some respond to chemical molecules, and some respond to pressure on the skin. A receptor transduces or changes physical energy into neural impulses. If an ant crawled on your hand, the receptor would respond to the changing depressions on the skin caused by the movement of the insect. The ant could also cause a mechanical deformation by bending a hair as it crawls toward your wrist. The receptor's job is to change the physical stimulus to information that the nervous system can use. When the stimulus has an effect on the receptor and impulses are sent to the brain, we may become aware of our environment.

Specificity Examined

For decades, the doctrine of specific nerve energies has been a pragmatic, although criticized, concept. It deals fairly well with four of the five classic senses: vision, hearing, smell, and taste. A large problem occurs, however, when you realize that there are more than five senses. The doctrine encounters some considerable difficulty with somesthesis or touch, pain, **proprioception** (body position in space) and kinesthesis (movement of the body and sensations from joints, muscles, and tendons). *Touch,* for example, is really a label that encompasses a variety of different sensations. Scientists realized a century ago that there was more to touch than just the "feel of something on the skin." There was always a need to examine the doctrine more closely. In the 1800s, with the birth of the doctrine, it was still evident that there were things such as pain, pressure, warmth, cool, vibration, and tickle. We also clearly knew, then as now, where our arms and legs are located in space without looking at them. Pain is an unavoidable sensation. The problem was, however, difficult because the doctrine did account for a lot of available data. How do you organize and investigate such a mosaic?

Investigators attempted to expand the doctrine by including several specific sensations within the touch modality. The expansion brought with it an anatomical assumption that there must be specific receptors and pathways for each sensory experience. Given these assumptions, investigators began to eagerly seek the receptors and paths associated with specific sensory experiences. For example, the cool spot, by this logic, had to have a special "cold receptor" at the place in the skin where the cool feeling occurred. To test this notion, investigators began looking through the microscope at tissue excised from the back of their own hands. The search was on. Who could find the cold receptor?

A criticism of the specificity theory was that the same receptor was not always found at every cold spot. Some cold spots had a Krause end bulb and some had something else, or occasionally investigators could not find anything except a few free nerve endings. After several years of literal painstaking research, the investigators compiled the results shown in Table 2.2.

The Krause end bulb apparently did not really signify cold. Furthermore, the search for warm spots was initially exciting because investigators believed they had found these spots when they identified the Ruffini end organ. However, this receptor, too, was not restricted to warm. Table 2.2 lists some of the known receptors and their assumed sensory modalities. The receptors, ac-

TABLE 2.2   Receptors and Sensory Modality

Receptor	Modality
Free nerve endings	Light touch and pain, warmth and cold
Hair cells [TR]	Audition and vestibular
Hair follicle	Pressure and movement
Krause end bulb [MN]	Tactile perception
Meissner's corpuscle [MN]	Light touch, tactile localization, and smooth texture
Merkel's discs [MN]	Light touch (skin deformation & pressure)
Muscle spindles [MN]	Proprioception
Olfactory neurons [MN]	Olfaction
Pacinian corpuscle [MN]	Deep pressure, joint movements, vibration
Rods and cones [TR]	Vision
Ruffini endings [MN]	Kinesthesis and tactile
Taste cells [X]	Gustation

NOTE: TR: true receptor, MN: modified neuron, X: taste receptor (see text, pp. 77-79).

cording to the "modified" specificity theory, were supposedly responsible for the sensations listed in the right column of the table. Notice that the table shows receptors associated with more than one sensory experience. For example, free nerve endings, not even a receptor, are associated with warmth, cold, and pain. In addition, they are related to kinesthesis and proprioception. Herein lies the problem with the specificity theory. The same receptors and pathways can and do lead to different perceptual experiences. This is a clear contradiction to the classic specificity doctrine.

The doctrine does have, nevertheless, utilitarian importance today. As we learn, the diagnosis of disease is often based on the responses and perceptions a patient reports to a physician. These subjective feelings suggest different diseases and physical maladies to a good diagnostician. We pursue these classical lines of thought in the pages that follow. Indeed, even today, medical training continues to use the doctrine as a time-honored approach to sensory processes; particular pathways carry specific sensory information and perceptual experiences. When these pathways are disrupted, particular sensory and motor deficits are then presumed to exist.

If the specificity theory is not perfect, what is the alternative? That is, if each sensation does not have a specific receptor, path, or brain center of its own, how does our brain put together the neural impulses and differentiate a touch from a tickle or a pain? The answer put forth is that sensory organization and perception is the result of the pattern of neural activity from a multitude of sensory inputs. This approach to the interpretation of afferent inputs is referred to as the **pattern theory.** Because the neural impulses generated by any one neuron are identical, however, a question arises concerning the pattern theory. How are bursts of neural impulses interpreted as a neural representation and a sensation of red, cinnamon, pain, tickle, and even sexual pleasure? We start to answer these questions by asking a more basic question. What is a neural code?

Neural Codes: A Perspective

The question of how the brain processes information is a classic one that has no complete answer. We can consider, nevertheless, some of the ingredients that factor into the way in which an environmental stimulus is encoded to create a perceptual experience. This list, keep in mind, is undoubtedly incomplete and a final inventory is not available.

1. First on the list is the well-established frequency-intensity principle. As noted in Chapter 1, under many conditions the number of impulses generated by a neuron increases as a function of the stimulus intensity. Clearly then, part of the encoding must be based on the number of impulses reaching areas within the brain where a perceptual synthesis is produced. The synthesis is by the cortical processor, wherever it may be in the cortex.

2. Another ingredient in the encoding is the size of the action potentials themselves. Although all action potentials from any individual neuron are, in fact, the same size, there are many different neurons within the system. This suggests the possibility that the magnitude of action potentials, even though they are constant in size for any one neuron, may vary in size across different neural elements. This is, in fact the case. It is not readily apparent whether these different-sized spikes enter significantly in the formula for neural encoding. However, the fact that they exist implies that they may be different for a reason other than random variation and different neural resting potentials.

3. A third possibility in the equation is the speed of neural conduction. This factor is no doubt used as a signal by the higher neural centers of the brain. The speed of conduction, you recall, is a direct function of the diameter of

the axon. The large myelinated fibers, such as the A-delta, conduct rapidly while the unmyelinated axons like the C fibers convey the information at a more leisurely rate. Thus, some action potentials arrive sooner than others, even though they may be stimulated at the same moment in time.

4. One important consideration in the coding process is the actual number of neural elements (neurons) activated by the stimulus. Not only does a strong or intense stimulus cause action potentials to generate at a higher rate (frequency-intensity principle), but the stimulus usually activates more neurons as well. Thus, not only does the number of active elements enter the calculus, but the number of action potentials generated by each neuron is also an important contributor to the equation.

5. Another critical consideration is the target destination of the axon. The encoding of the information is no doubt dependent on where the information is sent. This particular part of the coding of afferent information is directly associated with the specificity idea. If the neural path ends in the visual cortex, then it is unlikely that the individual reports feeling a bug on her arm. Although if she sees it, she may imagine she feels it.

6. Another player in the encoding process is the synapse. Synapses differ in their plasticity, processes, size, number of spines, and of course the types of neural transmitters and receptor sites. That the synapse is an integral part of the electrochemical encoding of the sensory experience should come as no surprise. The modulation of the neural inputs by the transmitters and the introduction of drugs (legal and illegal), disease, and mental pathology are obvious indications that sensory encoding is affected by synaptic function.

7. An extremely important concept that enters in the encoding of sensory information is that of a constant neural background of activity. The fact is that neurons are seldom quiet in the absence of obvious stimulation. The ongoing "spontaneous" activity plays a significant role in the encoding process by the brain and the nervous system. You need only to realize that as long as you are alive, the nervous system is in a continuous commotion; it never rests. This means that, during sleep or play, a ceaseless neural activity is present. This activity is the background against which incoming afferent information is judged. Any change in the circumstances of a neuron or group of neurons is a meaningful indication to the brain that a possible change has occurred in the environment. The pivotal aspect of this concept is that the pro-

cessing mechanisms of the central nervous system notes any change in an ongoing activity. An increase or decrease in neural activity is both quantitative and qualitative data for the brain.

8. The final participant in the encoding of afferent stimulation is the receptors themselves. Receptors are the first elements in the chain of events leading to a conscious experience. They have the initial say as to whether anything is encoded and is subsequently experienced. If a receptor fails to respond, then there can be no recognition of the external world. The stimulus must have an effect on a receptor or the organism is unaware that a stimulus exists or a change has occurred.

An important aspect of nearly all receptors is that they adapt. Adaptation is a decrease, and in some cases a complete cessation, of a receptor's response to a constant unchanging stimulus. For example, when you first put on your watch this morning, the receptors responded to the pressure, bending, and deformations on your wrist. You were aware that the watch was on your wrist and that it was secure. However, if you let your arm rest, and not move it, for a couple of minutes or so, you soon discover that you cannot tell whether your watch is on your wrist or not. You have to look to see or move your arm and stimulate the cutaneous receptors (Iggo & Andres, 1982). This is because the receptors under the watch have stopped responding, adapted, to the constant pressure. Once a change occurs, you move your wrist, then you are aware of the watch once again. These particular phenomena, adaptation and response to change, are most important in receptor function. The operation of receptors and their ability to transduce energy from one form to another is the next step in the story.

Receptor Transduction

The transduction of environmental stimuli to neural activity by receptors is our first step in becoming aware of the world. Receptors are classified in three broad divisions. The first is the **true receptor** class. This type of receptor is a separate cell unlike any other in the human body. The true receptor has no axon or dendrite; rather, the cell's response to an **adequate stimulus** is to change that stimulus to neural activity by means of a **receptor potential.** An adequate stimulus is the single best stimulus in the environment that can cause a receptor to generate a receptor potential. Other stimuli can cause the receptor to generate the receptor potential, but they cannot accomplish the task as easily as the "best" or most adequate stimulus. For example, electromagnetic radiation or light is the adequate stimulus for the receptors found within the eye. Shining a light in your ear, however, does not make you hear. Light does not activate the receptors even if the light actually reaches the receptors. Nor does yelling in your eye make your eye respond. You may stimulate your visual system by another means, however. By pressing on your eyeball, you can initiate visual sensations. Pressure is just not the adequate stimulus for vision.

Receptors produce changes called receptor potentials. A receptor potential is functionally the same as the generator potential discussed in Chapter 1 and the postsynaptic potential discussed previously. In most respects, receptor potential, generator potential, and postsynaptic potential are interchangeable. They are not action potentials but are all graded local potentials.

Receptor potential is named because it is produced by a special classification of cells, the receptors. The characteristics of the receptor potential are similar to the generator potential and the postsynaptic potential. The potential varies in magnitude as a function of the stimulus intensity. The greater the intensity of the adequate stimulus, the greater the receptor potential.

As noted earlier, the receptor potential is a local or graded potential and is electrotonic in effect. That is, when the potential is generated by the adequate stimulus, it spreads or expands toward the base of the receptor and, if it is a true receptor, toward synapse with a **primary sensory neuron (PSN)**. The primary sensory neuron is the first neuron in the series leading to higher nervous centers. When the receptor potential initiated by a stimulus reaches the base of the receptor a neurotransmitter is released.

The synapse between the receptor and the primary sensory neuron is the first functional contact between the nervous system and the physical environment that we can experience. *Functional* in this context means that we become aware of the physical universe only when action potentials are initiated by the receptor's transduction of the physical energy. This is, in many ways, the point at which conscious experience may begin. The sensations and experiences depend directly on the action potentials produced in the sensory neuron by the receptors. The number of action potentials propagated is, in turn, a function of the stimulus intensity and the magnitude of the receptor potential. The true receptors are found in vision, hearing, and the vestibular system.

The second class of receptor is the **modified neuron.** This type of receptor is exactly what the label implies. It is a specialized neuron that has modifications or accessory laminae appended to the peripheral or distal end of an axon. The accessory layers on the neural fiber allow the neuron to respond to an adequate stimulus, generate receptor potentials, and produce the necessary action potentials without a synapse. Table 2.2 lists examples of these types of cells.

The final classification of receptors is, in reality, not a receptor at all. It is a neuron that has no accessory layers. It is neither attached to nor associated with any receptor. It is a neuron that has its distal arborizations embedded in tissues of the body (e.g., the skin, muscles, or joints). These neurons, which vary in diameter, are classified as thermoreceptors and nociceptors. The thermoreceptors are, as you suspect, neural fibers that respond selectively to changes in temperature on the skin. The nociceptors, as Table 2.2 indicates, are the **free nerve endings** that respond to noxious stimuli of various sorts. We examine these particular sensory responses when we discuss temperature and pain in more detail.

The taste receptor is special. It fits none of the three categories just discussed. It transduces the multitude of chemical stimuli in the gustatory sense. The true receptor classification does not strictly fit this unique cell, nor does the modified neuron classification. In addition, the taste receptors are not neurons either. The taste receptors are quite interesting because they have no dendrites or axons yet they generate small action potentials. Even more interesting, they are continually degenerating, and then new ones are regenerated. Taste receptor cells are discussed in a later chapter.

A further difficulty with these simple three classifications becomes apparent when you consider the actual point of transduction in the olfactory system. The olfactory receptor cell, usually considered a modified neuron, in reality has the active transduction mechanisms located in "receptors sites" on hairlike cilia that extend in the nasal cavities. This unique situation is discussed in a later chapter on olfaction.

Introduction to Transduction Mechanisms

The methods of transducing physical stimuli to neural impulses differ with the various receptor types. The general transduction method is, however, outlined here as a preliminary for ensuing discussions.

We begin by noting that each receptor or nerve ending, when affected by its adequate stimulus, responds by changing its membrane permeability. The change caused by the environmental stimulus is the initiating event in sensory activity. For example, a depression of the skin such as the light touch of a pencil may deform the accessory layers of a Pacinian corpuscle wrapped about a nerve ending. This can lead to membrane changes in the axon. The mechanical deformation alters the permeability of the membrane to Na^+ and K^+ ions. The influx of these positive ions causes the internal potential of the axon, the primary sensory neuron, to shift toward zero and depolarize to initiate action potentials.

On the other hand, if the receptor is a true receptor, the adequate stimulus initiates a receptor potential that spreads through the entire receptor cell. If the receptor potential is of sufficient magnitude, it initiates action potentials in the primary sensory neuron at the synapses located at the base of the receptor. In this latter case, sometimes a second messenger is involved in the cascade of events leading to the receptor potential. The second messengers are other ions and molecules that act to facilitate the opening of the channels and promote the influx or efflux of ions through the receptor's cell membrane. These messengers are discussed in more detail when we encounter these particular receptors in later chapters.

Dysfunctions

It is important to keep in mind that memory, thoughts, and perceptions are dependent on the activity of many pathways and the interactions of a multitude of neurons. It is neither the single synapse nor the single cell that forms the final product of living, loving, and learning, as a psychologist once said. What is important is the combined effects of millions of neurons and the thousands of synapses formed by each neuron. The brain functions with a complex involvement of pathways and nuclei (groups of neurons) to provide the richness of memory, thought, and perception. When synapses misfire, or a malfunction at the junction occurs, the "normal" quickly becomes the aberrant. Some of these deviations are outlined here. The discussions are not complete, and the list is not extensive. What is intended is that you gain an appreciation for the possible disasters that, unfortunately, do occur.

We begin by asking, what can go wrong at a synapse? Let us consider some of the possibilities:

1. The transmitter is not synthesized.
2. Action potentials are not arriving.
3. Calcium does not enter the terminal.
4. Vesicles are not full.
5. Re-uptake of transmitter substance does not occur.

6. An enzyme or other chemical substance removes the neurotransmitter at the cleft.

7. Another substance mimics the transmitter and fills the receptors so receptors do not respond when the "real" transmitter is released.

8. The transmitter fails to be released because another drug blocks the exocytosis.

9. The receptors are continually active because the transmitter substance is not removed from the cleft and more neurotransmitter is released.

10. Another drug interferes with the second messenger.

11. Other substances weaken the transmitter within the synaptic cleft by chemical alterations.

12. Neurotransmitter leaks out of vesicles.

13. The ions that influx into the postsynaptic cell are removed or reduced in concentration.

14. The presynaptic neuron degenerates due to injury, disease, or the ingestion of an exogenous substance. There is no synapse.

15. The postsynaptic neuron dies and degenerates because of injury, disease, or drug abuse. Once again, there is no synapse.

This list is probably not complete. However, it does present a formidable catalog of undesirable events. An unfortunate list of diseases, behavioral aberrations, emotional deficits, and perceptual difficulties can arise from some of these calamities. Here are just a few.

Alzheimer's Disease

Alzheimer's disease usually strikes the elderly (over 60), although it can occur in younger people. It results from the degeneration of neurons and the depletion of Ach in the brain. Because Ach is a significant transmitter in the brain, the elimination of the transmitter produces a severe memory deficit. The disease begins slowly with the slippage of memory of everyday events and slowly accelerates until, just before death, no memory remains of places, events, friends, or family. The loss of Ach and the subsequent memory degeneration is catastrophic. Once the dissolution of the neurons and the loss of Ach begin, it is continual and nonrelenting in its effects. Although a cure for

Alzheimer's is not presently available, there is hope in the future. Scientists and pharmaceutical companies are testing, on both animals and humans, drugs that give promise for the future. The experimental testing now being done with a small group of Alzheimer patients suggests that a drug can, if not cure, at least slow the relentless progress of the disease.

Schizophrenia

Schizophrenia entails all or some of the following phenomena: loss of contact with reality, emotional disorders, hallucinations, distortion of reality, indifference, paranoid ideas, delusions, incoherence, illogical thoughts, and grossly disorganized personality and behavior.

What is it that has caused at least 1% of the world's population to display such classic signs of mental illness? Is schizophrenia learned? Is it a change in the synapses? Is it genetic and part of the legacy from the family? All the answers are not yet available. Yet there is a strong hypothesis concerning the effects of neurotransmitters on the behavior of schizophrenic individuals. This hypothesis, the dopamine hypothesis, suggests that indeed a direct and close association exists between dopamine and the symptoms of schizophrenia. The data suggest that dopamine may overactivate one type of receptor within particular areas of the brain. As noted previously, a neurotransmitter can have different effects at different receptors. Thus, it appears that dopamine may be affecting one receptor (D1) in a normal manner, yet causing a deviation at a second location (D2). The use of antischizophrenic drugs, **neuroleptics,** alleviates the schizophrenic symptoms by blocking the dopamine D2 receptors. The alleviation of the symptoms, although a significant improvement in the mental health field, does not cure the schizophrenia. The individual must continue to take the neuroleptic drugs or the symptoms return. Although the neuroleptic does remove hallucinations and delusions, there are other symptoms that do not respond as well (shyness, social withdrawal). Furthermore, there are possible severe side effects in an individual who continues to receive neuroleptic therapy. The decrease in dopamine, via the blocking of receptors, can lead to Parkinsonian effects, hormonal imbalance, and **tardive dyskinesia.** The latter condition is an involuntary movement of the mouth, tongue, arms, and legs. If tardive dyskinesia occurs, it is difficult to correct; in most cases, it cannot be reversed. It is an **iatrogenic** disorder that is produced when a physician prescribes a neuroleptic drug over too long a time period.

Parkinson's Disease

Parkinson's disease is a neurological deficit that affects motor movement. It is the third most common neurological disease of humans and affects 500,000 people in the United States. The mean onset of the disease is about 58 to 60 years. The symptoms are motor rigidity, movement difficulty in arms and legs, and limb tremor. The cause is the depletion of dopamine due to the degeneration of neural cells in the brain that produce this neurotransmitter. During the early investigative period of neuroleptic drugs for schizophrenia, the appearance of Parkinsonian symptoms was an indication to the physician that the "correct" dosage level had been achieved. The schizophrenic patient lost the psychotic symptoms about the same time that the Parkinsonian symptoms began to appear. The neuroleptic reduces dopamine. Therefore, when motor rigidity began to appear in the patient, the physician knew that the dosage was sufficient and beginning to have an effect. The treatment for Parkinson's affliction lies in the use of a compound known as L-DOPA. This compound is a precursor to the production of dopamine. Although L-DOPA is not a cure, it does alleviate the symptoms in most patients for a period of time. The drug, after a period of time, loses its effectiveness.

Dysfunction Summary

The number of problems and dysfunctions of the nervous system is very large indeed. Although outcomes of our attempts to improve the deleterious effects of disease, injury, and aging are often short of the mark, there are approaches to brain function that lead to optimistic expectations. It is clear that the basis for living, loving, and learning is the smooth and coordinated activity of the brain. The continuous release of neurotransmitters, the conduction of action potentials, the interaction of our sensory systems with the external and internal world are continuous wonders. Associated with this marvel is the question of how the brain stores the information once the information is received. The answer to this question is still a mystery; however, new clues and intriguing hints are coming from research laboratories every day. Studies investigating environmental experiences and brain activity have shown variations in synaptic formations, new dendritic spines, and changes in ionic conduction across the neural membranes. The modulation of cellular function is a means of information storage (memory). The cache of information is modified by new information arriving each moment. It is an awe-inspiring phenomenon when you realize that a change in the environment can occur and, in about a second, the event can be permanently stored in the brain and available for recall at any moment. It is just as interesting to note that some items of information may appear repeatedly, yet not be recalled longer than a few seconds. The questions are many and the answers are slow in coming. However, research continues to open new avenues and explain amazing facets within the brain.

It is important to recognize that many different types of dysfunctions can and do occur because of receptor malfunction or death. The common ones come to mind: blindness, deafness, vertigo, and loss of smell and taste. These are discussed in more depth in each chapter associated with the particular sensory system.

Summary

This chapter has dealt with several of the components necessary for our daily task of interacting with environmental stimuli. The information provided in this chapter is fundamental to the understanding of how we perceive the world. The idea, however, that our perceptions of color, pitch, music, tickle, ice cream, and fresh mown hay are all "in our head" is often viewed by students as amazing—perhaps even unbelievable. Yet when you consider the fact that we, and all the other creatures of the planet, must have some means of interacting with the physical universe, the concepts presented here are perfectly logical.

As we noted in Chapter 1, the world is full of nothing but stimuli (electromagnetic, thermal, chemical, pressure and gravity), and all living organisms have evolved to exist within their particular ecological niche. To do this, they had to develop the necessary structural and functional apparatus to allow them to sense their environment. Their sensory apparatus consists of specialized receptors, neural pathways, and neural mechanisms for integration, synthesis, and analysis.

The receptors became very specialized because they responded best to their specific adequate stimulus. Yet, not every receptor and sensory fiber evolved to provide just a specific and unitary experience. The specificity idea was broadened in scope and now recognizes that processing information by the brain (and spinal cord) is often accomplished by unique patterns of neural activation and inhibition. The patterns themselves are the source of our different perceptions (the taste of an apple versus the taste of an orange).

These patterns of input, initially transduced to action potentials by the receptors, are interpreted and processed by the more central mechanisms.

The neural code is complex and still not entirely understood; it is clear that the frequency, timing, number, speed, discharge pattern, adaptation, and population activity arriving at various nuclei within the nervous system underlies our perception of the world. The complexity is enough to ensure a continued interest by scientists for years to come.

Suggested Readings

Barondes, S. H. (1994) Thinking about Prozac. *Science, 263,* pp. 102-103.

Iggo, A., & Andres, K. H. (1982). Morphology of cutaneous receptors. *Annual Review Neuroscience, 5,* 1-31.

Jacobs, B. L. (1994). Serotonin, motor activity and depression-related disorders. *American Scientist, 82,* pp. 456-463.

Mountcastle, V. B. (1980). Sensory receptors and neural encoding: Introduction to sensory processes. In V. B. Mountcastle (Ed.), *Medical physiology* (Vol. 1, 14th ed.). St. Louis: Mosby.

Snyder, S. H. (1986). *Drugs and the brain.* New York: Scientific American Library.

CHAPTER 3

Somatosensory System

Overview of the Chapter

In Chapters 1 and 2 the basics of the somatosensory system were introduced. Chapter 1 related the afferent paths leading into the spinal cord and the central nervous system. Chapter 2 outlined the receptor transduction associated with the somatosensory system. We begin this chapter with an overview of the afferent pathways as preparation for a more detailed examination of the processing that occurs along the route to the cortex. Following the overview, we begin our discussion of the cutaneous inputs by examining more closely the important characteristics of the receptors and neural fibers. Chapter 2 alluded to the attributes of the receptors and neurons. Following the present discussions, we briefly examine the thalamus and then turn our attention to the qualities of the somatosensory cortex. As we progress we associate, where possible, particular sensory experiences with the physiology and structure of the nervous system.

Because of the many different experiences you can receive from the skin and bodily tissues, it is difficult to organize and present a coherent picture without dividing the system in smaller parts. You must intellectually dissect the somatosensory system in several different slices to appreciate its complexity and functional beauty. One approach has been to divide the topic of the "body sense" (somatosensory) in three overlapping but distinct views: the cutaneous (responses originating from the skin), proprioception and kinesthesis (sensory inputs from muscles, joints, and internal organs), and pain. This approach makes logical sense and is followed here. We divide the "body sense" in smaller segments as we proceed.

Somatosensory Paths Revisited

Figure 3.1 shows the two major afferent somatosensory pathways from the skin to the cortex. These paths, the dorsal columns and the lateral spinothalamic tracts, conduct neural activity to the cortex by way of the thalamus. These pathways provide the information that could be interpreted as several different kinds of sensations (touch, tickle, pressure, pain, hot, cold, burning, limb movement, body position, wetness, and flutter or vibration). These paths conduct the tactile information that enables us to know that a block of wood is square and not octagonal in shape. It is also the somatosensory system that informs the people with visual impairments that the special grouping of six small bumps on the metal panel (braille) in the elevator mean the fifth floor. The same neural paths, in many cases the same types of receptors, also convey afferent information about illness, diseases, and accidents (e.g., appendicitis, heart attack, lesions and contusions, trauma, kidney stones, nausea, stomachache, etc.). In addition, our ability to know where our arms and legs are in three-dimensional space is the result of many of the same receptors and some of the same neural paths we find assigned to our skin. The ability to know where your body is located in the environmental space is critical. If you are to move about the planet without having to continually monitor leg and arm position every moment, then instantaneous and automatic knowledge is essential. This knowledge is gained through a sophisticated feedback system under the auspices of the somatosensory system.

The input to the central nervous system, via the dorsal column, begins with the receptor and the initiation of action potentials conducted by the first neural element. This neural element is the primary sensory neuron. It is the first neuron in the afferent path of every sensory system that immediately follows (or is part of) the receptor. The primary sensory neuron enters the dorsal column and synapses in the nuclei of the medulla. The second synapse in the dorsal horn pathway occurs in the **ventral basal nucleus** of the thalamus. From the thalamus, the third-order neurons project to the SI and SII areas of the parietal lobe.

In the lateral spinothalamic tract, the initial synapse occurs within the dorsal horn of the spinal cord rather than the medulla. The second-order neuron in the spinothalamic tract crosses the midline within the spinal cord and then ascends to the thalamus. It is here, in the thalamus, that the second synapse occurs for the fibers in the spinothalamic tract. Like the dorsal column pathway, the spinothalamic tract has its last synapse, before the cortex, in the ventral basal nucleus of the thalamus. From the thalamus, the third-

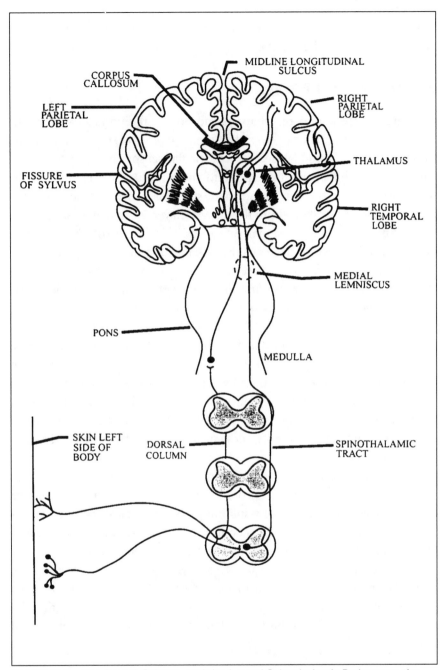

Figure 3.1. The Dorsal Column and the Lateral Spinothalamic Pathway to the Cortex

order neurons travel to somatosensory cortex SI or SII located at and near the postcentral gyrus of the parietal lobe.

Receptors and Fibers

As we have noted in previous chapters, most of the receptors located within the skin can be stimulated by several different qualities of stimuli. The receptors are not specific and labeled for a particular sensory experience. This is true even though they usually respond to one stimulus more readily than to others; for example, they have an adequate stimulus. When it comes to the cutaneous receptors located within the different layers of skin, it is, once again, easier to partition the discussion in categories. This division of labor can then be further refined, where necessary, by classification in subcategories.

The partition begins with three groupings of cutaneous receptors. These classes are the **mechanoreceptors, thermoreceptors,** and the **nociceptors.** The mechanoreceptors are those that respond to pressure, movement of hairs, and depression of the skin. The thermoreceptors, on the other hand, are not really receptors at all. In fact, they differ very little from free nerve endings. There are no modifications on the terminal portions of the neuron. Thus, the terminology concerning what is and what is not a receptor becomes, at this point, rather fuzzy. A fiber is actually referred to as a thermoreceptor, a cold receptor, or a warm receptor when there are no true or modified receptors to be found. As we learn, however, these naked neural fibers are particularly sensitive to temperature variations of the skin. The last classification within the cutaneous sense, the nociceptor, is similar to the thermoreceptors in that they too are neither true receptors or modified neurons. The nociceptors are fibers that have the capability of responding to physiological insults and injuries (Burgess & Perl, 1973). The chemicals released by damaged or diseased organs and tissues act as stimuli and instigate the action potentials necessary for the perception of pain. Chapter 4 addresses in more detail the specific sense of pain. For the moment, we focus on the more peripheral aspects of the system. Figure 3.2 shows a diagrammatic view of several receptors within the three classifications of receptors: mechanoreceptors, thermoreceptors, and nociceptors.

Mechanoreceptors

Authors who have undertaken the discussion of mechanoreceptors have approached the task from different perspectives. Some have partitioned the

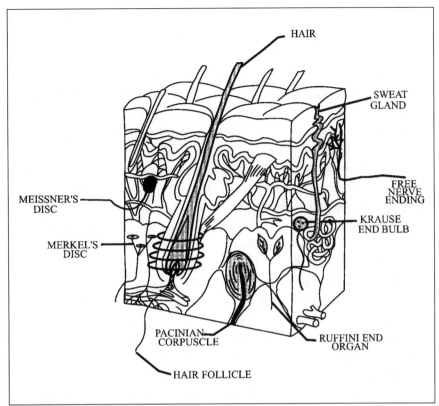

Figure 3.2. Sensory Receptors of the Somatosensory System

NOTE: Meissner's disc, free nerve ending, Krause end bulb, Pacinian corpusle, Ruffini end organ, Merkel's disc. The hair follicles are wrapped in free nerve endings (basket nerve ending).

mechanoreceptors in two different groups. The division is based on a functional feature of the receptor known as **adaptation.** A receptor that continues to respond to a nonchanging stimulus as long as the stimulus is present is a rare receptor. In fact, when an adequate stimulus first encroaches on a mechanoreceptor there is a rapid and brief response. This initial response, if the stimulus is constant and unchanging, is followed by a steady decline in receptor activity. This decline in activity, in both the receptor potential and in the generation of action potentials, is adaptation. The rate or time required for a mechanoreceptor to adapt or stop responding to a nonchanging constant stimulus is the functional feature dividing the mechanoreceptors in different groups. Figure 3.3 shows two classifications of adaptation, **fast adaptation** (FA) and **slow adaptation** (SA).

Fast-Adapting Mechanoreceptors

As implied previously, the FA mechanoreceptors respond to the movement and pressure applied to the skin with a fast transient response. In the FA mechanoreceptor, the quick burst is always followed by a rapid decline in activity even though the stimulus is still present as shown in Figure 3.3(a). The FA cells respond specifically and nearly exclusively to change. If a mechanical pressure is applied with a constant nonchanging force, the cell initially responds and then rapidly adapts and ceases to react. This results in a lack of awareness of the environmental stimulus. An example of such a cell is the myelinated fiber that is circumferentially arranged around the base of a hair. This is a free nerve ending wrapped around a hair follicle as shown in Figure 3.2. These fibers respond only when the hair is moved.

Another FA cell is the Pacinian corpuscle. The Pacinian corpuscle is found throughout the surface of the body on hairy as well as **glabrous,** hairless, skin. This modified neuron is one of the largest sensory cells in the human body. Even though the Pacinian corpuscle is visible without magnification, it is still quite small. It is approximately one half the size of the period at the end of this sentence. The large size of this receptor has enabled scientists to examine it in detail.

The Pacinian corpuscle is oval shaped and composed of layers (laminae) like an onion. The depression of the cell by a stimulus, as shown in Figure 3.3(a), results in a rapid depolarization of the fiber and a quick transient burst of action potentials. If the stimulus is maintained, the Pacinian corpuscle quickly adapts. The removal of the stimulus once again results in a transient burst of action potentials and a similar rapid adaptation to the constant nonpressure, see Figure 3.3(c).

Two other modified neurons in the mechanoreceptor class are the Krause end bulb and the Meissner's corpuscle. These two mechanoreceptors are found only on glabrous skin such as the palms of the hand, within and around the dermal grooves (fingerprints) found on fingers, lips, and on the soles of the feet (Johansson & Vallbo, 1983). These two modified receptors, in addition to free nerve endings, are also found in the most sensitive and pleasurable areas of the body: the erogenous zones and the genital organs.

The popular media claim that there is a "genital corpuscle" located within the sexual organs is most likely a mistake in labeling. There is no special sensory receptor for the sexual organs; in contrast to popular belief, there is no vaginal "G" spot to stimulate a female orgasm. In males, the greatest sensory innervation is found in the glans penis with many fewer receptors found

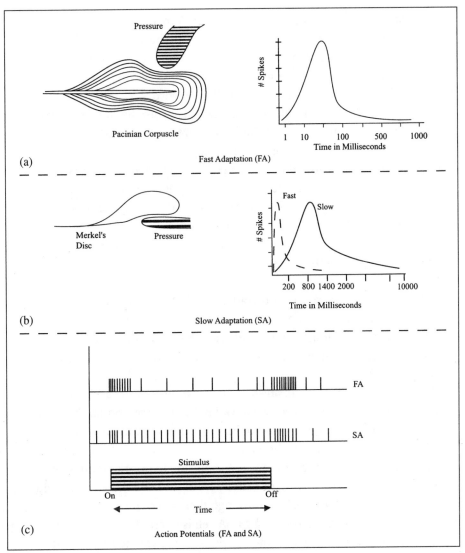

Figure 3.3. Adaptation of Receptors

NOTE: (a) Fast adaptation by Pacinian corpuscle. Other fast-adapting receptors are free nerve endings, A-delta fibers, Krause end bulb, and Meissner's disc; (b) slow adaptation by Merkel's disc. Other slow-adapting receptors are Ruffini end organs, and C-fibers, and (c) action potentials as a function of the fast- and slow-adapting receptors.

on the penile shaft and scrotum. The physiological responses of the sensory cells include both FA and SA mechanoreceptors with high rates of discharge to displacement-elicited stimulation. The female genital organs are innervated with the same morphological receptor types found in the male. These receptors respond, as you may suspect, to stimulation by pressure and displacement. The densest gathering of sensory receptors in the female is in the external structures of the genital organs. The clitoris, homolog of the male penis, has the greatest sensory innervation. There are also receptors, fewer in number, located in areas other than the clitoris. These sensory receptors are found in the labia and vaginal vestibule. The vagina, in contrast, has few sensory receptors and is innervated to about the same degree as the digestive tract and the colon. The afferent supply of sensory receptors at the cervix is substantially more than what is found in the vagina. The vagina, it appears, is clearly not the principal source of female sexual orgasm. The afferent responses from the genital area enter the spinal cord through the dorsal root and ascend to higher centers by way of the dorsal column.

Slow-Adapting Mechanoreceptors

Although there are several slow-adapting (SA) mechanoreceptors, we restrict our discussion to a small set of three. These three are **Merkel's cells, Ruffini end organ (endings),** and an enigmatic unmyelinated nerve fiber often associated with the perception of pain, tickle, and occasionally itch, the **C-fibers.**

These SA mechanoreceptors respond to constant pressure and any maintained deformation of the skin in two ways. First, as in all receptor fibers, there is an initial transient or quick burst of activity when a stimulus first occurs. This is seen in Figure 3.3(b) as the sharp rise in the number of action potentials that occur just after stimulus onset. In addition to this rapid burst of activity, there is also a long period of activity from the cell following stimulus onset. This is seen in Figure 3.3(c). Although there is a slight decrease as time passes, the characteristic response of an SA cell is to remain active as long as the stimulus is present. This sustained response is the second segment of the SA activity to an unchanging stimulus.

An unusual and unique response characteristic of SA cells is that they can be altered by the application of thermal stimuli. The thermal sensitivity, although not the adequate stimulus, increases the firing rate of SA cells to mechanical stimuli. When a cold stimulus is present and a mechanical stimulus (weight or pressure) occurs, the SA cells increase their firing rate. The SA cells are more responsive to pressure stimuli when they are cold than when they are warm. This increase in response accounts for the cold silver dollar illusion. We perceive a cold silver dollar as heavier than a silver dollar at the usual room temperature. The illusion occurs because the SA mechanoreceptors increase their firing rate to mechanical pressure (the weight of the dollar) when the dollar is cooled. This increased firing rate is interpreted by the central nervous system (the brain) as a heavier object on the surface of the skin. In other words, the perception of a heavier weight occurred because of a relatively larger burst of activity from an area of the skin that was cool when the mechanical event happened. This increased activity accounts for Ernest Weber's silver dollar illusion.

Thermoreceptors

Temperature is a unique sense in many ways. For example, the sensation of cold is sometimes surprising. There is, however, more to the sensation of temperature than just the assessment of environmental events. Our very existence is dependent on the continual monitoring and correcting of our internal body temperature. The response to cold weather and warm sunshine are only part of the story.

Although the skin contains the necessary mechanisms to detect and initiate action potentials, the impulses leaving the periphery are just the initial messages from thermal fibers. Fibers and thermoreceptors are also found, for example, in the hypothalamus, spinal cord, and internal organs (the gut) as well as in the external covering of the body (the skin). Those in the skin, referred to as the cutaneous thermoreceptors, are directly involved in the autonomic responses associated with maintaining our internal body temperature within the normal range of 36° to 38° Centigrade.

The use of **Centigrade** to measure temperature usually runs against our everyday expectations. This is probably because the weather forecasts on the radio, on television, and in the newspaper use the **Fahrenheit** scale. The two measures, however, are easily translated from one to the other. The change from degrees Centigrade to degrees Fahrenheit, and vice versa, follows a simple formula. To change Centigrade to Fahrenheit, multiply the degrees Centigrade by 9, divide the product by 5 and then add 32°. To change from Fahrenheit to Centigrade, you simply reverse the mathematical process: subtract 32°, multiple by 5 and divide the product by 9. This simple conversion yields 96.8° and 100.4° Fahrenheit for internal body temperatures of 36° and 38° Centigrade. A simple rule of thumb to help in quick conversions is to remember that 35° Centigrade equals 95° Fahrenheit. Using this reference, you then simply add or subtract 9° Fahrenheit for every 5° change in Centigrade.

There is considerable variation in normal body temperature. Although 98.6° F is the accepted norm, it is just that, a norm. The human temperature varies from individual to individual and depends on where and when you take the measurement. Rectal temperature is approximately 0.5° higher than an oral measurement. Likewise, the temperature varies with time of day and, in the female, the menstrual cycle. Finally, you should keep in mind that our pets do not have the same "normal" body temperature that we do. This is particularly true if your pet is an amphibian (temperature varies with the environment) or a dog (average body temperature near 101° F).

When you measure the temperature of the human skin, for example on the arm, and simultaneously record the neural responses from a thermo-receptor, you discover an interesting relationship. The fiber from which you record shows a rate of activity that varies directly with the temperature of the skin. For example, once the temperature stops rising the response of the fiber levels off and is maintained at a constant firing rate.

The fiber activity follows the temperature of the stimulus. This activity occurs for both the warm and cold temperature fibers—namely, the warm thermoreceptor and the cold thermoreceptor. The two classes of fibers, warm and cold, have been examined for a fairly wide range of stimulus values, from about 15° C to 55°C. The results show that the cold fibers have a primary response range between about 15° C and 40° C with a maximum near 26° C. There is also a range of temperatures that are paradoxical in their effects. The perception of cold can occur when the stimulus is very hot (above 45° C). As-sociated with this cold perception is the finding that cold fibers respond at a high rate when temperatures are between 45° C and 50° C. This unusual expe-rience, a cold feeling with a hot stimulus, is **paradoxical cold** (Long, 1977).

The increase in activity for warm thermoreceptors, above the normal spontaneous rate, begins when the temperature of the skin reaches approxi-mately 30° C. The activity of the fibers follows the temperature of the stimu-lus and continues to increase to a maximum activity near 45° C. The warm fi-ber activity decreases rapidly and ceases responding entirely near 50° C. Figure 3.4 shows the relationship between temperature and warm and cold fi-ber thermoreceptors. An interesting aspect of these two functions is the point at which they cross. At this point, there are relatively low levels of activity from both types of fibers and the temperature of the skin is slightly below normal (32° C). You should also note that there is also a phenomenon called paradox-ical heat (Hamalainen, Vartiamen, Karvanen, & Jarvilehto, 1982). This is sim-ply the feeling of warmth when the skin is moderately cooled. Once again, the general rule of sensory systems becomes evident: The senses are designed to respond primarily to environmental change. Sometimes, however, the change may be unexpected.

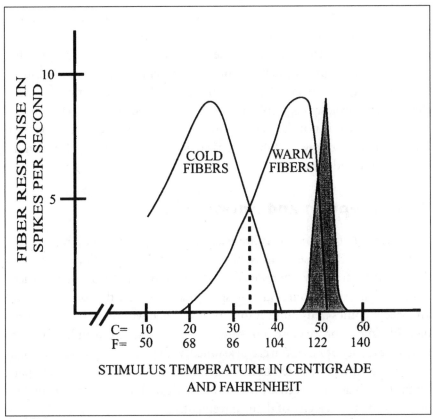

Figure 3.4. The Response of Warm and Cold Fibers as a Function of Temperature

NOTE: Paradoxical cold is shaded.

In the case of skin temperature, if the individual is in a moderate climate and the skin is near 32° C there is little need to send information to the "higher ups" (the central nervous system). On the other hand, should you leave a warm environment in the winter to find firewood outside, you immediately notice the variation in skin temperature. First, your body begins to shiver to generate body heat and "chill bumps" (goose pimples) make their appearance. Goose pimples are the result of the **pilomotor reflex** handed down from our ancestral past. Birds' "fluffing" their feathers during the winter is a direct example of this reflexive action. The fluffed feathers produce thermal insulation with air pockets in the feathers. This insulation between the environment and the bird is life preserving. In our case, when we are cold, we almost immediately are motivated to seek warm clothes and shelter.

On the other hand, should the temperature in the room become too warm you are tempted to remove your clothes, fan yourself, while simultaneously trying to be socially acceptable by not displaying perspiration. One of the primary reasons you perspire is, of course, to remove body heat. I am sure you know that it is not the perspiration that produces the well-recognized body odor. It is the growth of the bacteria that gather in the warmth and moist areas of your body crevices.

Proprioception and Kinesthesis

Proprioception and *kinesthesis* are used interchangeably. They refer to the manner in which we sense muscular motion, weight, position, and movement. Usually, it is only when we take a moment to concentrate on the orientation and location of our bodies in space that we realize that proprioceptive knowledge comes to us quite automatically. When we are in the dark (complete blackness) or we close our eyes, we still can move our index finger to touch the tip of our nose. You can also touch, with your eyes closed, your right wrist or elbow with your left index finger. How this is done depends, in part, on the brain's ability to sense the limbs in space and instantly calculate their position and the velocity of their movement.

The receptors responsible for sensing where we are in space and whether our body is actively or passively being moved are found in the skin, joints, muscles, tendons, and ligaments. It was not long ago, however, that it was thought that the required information was derived just from the ligaments and joints. Close examination of the joints had revealed several different types of receptors. These receptors were classified in various ways according to their shape and fiber size. It was generally agreed that Pacinian corpuscles, Ruffini endings, Golgi corpuscles, and free nerve endings provided significant information regarding the position and movement of limbs. The idea that muscles, tendons, and skin assisted in the task was not taken seriously until the 1970s (Grigg, Cineman, & Riley, 1973). The evidence supporting the idea that the joint receptors were almost completely responsible for sensing our limb locations and how fast they move (velocity of movement) came from very convincing experiments.

When we normally extend our arm or bend it, we can perceive the direction and speed of the movement. The receptors within the joints and tendons, if we recorded them during the movement, display firing rates proportional to the angular velocity of the joint rotation. What this means is that a fast movement results in rapid firing of the receptors and slow firing occurs with slow movement. Moreover, when the limb comes to rest, there continues to be a response from the receptors and, even more interestingly, the number of responses issued from the cells depend on the angle of the resting joint. There is a fixed, steady firing rate for each possible joint position; the firing rate is dependent on the joint angle throughout the normal range of movement. Some cells fire at one angle, whereas others fire at a different one. The different fibers appeared to be the code for the angle of the limb. It appears, then, that there is less adaptation for the sensation of limb position. Regardless of what angle the limb assumes, there are receptors that continue to respond at a rate appropriate for the angle.

Given this set of facts, it appeared to be unnecessary to be concerned about possible sensory inputs from the skin, muscles, and ligaments. The muscles, skin, and ligaments may contribute, so the scientists said, but their donation is minimal. This seemed to be the situation until joint replacement therapy came into vogue.

It is interesting to note a conundrum in medicine at this point. *Therapy* is an often-used euphemism for serious invasive medical intervention (e.g., elective surgery, electro-convulsive shock, radiation, or chemical "therapy"). Nevertheless, one of the most interesting effects of the successful surgical joint replacement therapy, aside from the wonders of a workable steel joint, was that even with no physiological joint the patient could respond precisely when asked about the velocity and location of a limb. This occurred when there was a missing joint and no receptors. Clearly, other factors were involved in knowing where the leg was in space. The missing ingredients had to be the intramuscular stretch receptors, the muscle spindles, and tendon organs. The muscle spindles are, in fact, oriented within the muscle tissue such that their discharge rate depends on the tension and length of the muscle. The muscle spindles are, therefore, capable of responding to the movement (velocity) of the limb and to signal a static position (location) based on the uniform tension within the muscle fibers.

In summary, the kinesthetic (proprioceptive) sense of bodily position and motion is generated from the interaction of a number of receptors. The joints clearly provide information about the angle and movement of the limbs in space while the stretch receptors provide a substantial input to the movement and activity of the body.

The overall judgment of body position is the result of peripheral skin activation, the stretch receptors, and tension and movement within the muscles themselves. The total afferent activity creates the heaviness and the illusion of the cold and warm silver dollars. The objects we encounter every day are also the result of this total afferent activity.

Receptive Fields

We have skirted around the topic of receptive fields. It is time to meet the challenge of learning about this ubiquitous issue. Consider for a moment the following far-fetched situation. Every neuron from every somatosensory receptor is activated by a touch anywhere on the body surface. In this unlikely example it makes no difference where on your body you are touched, all the receptors and the primary sensory neurons are activated. Given this situation, would you be able to tell which part of your body was touched? The answer is no. It would make no difference where you were touched, your brain would be bombarded by all the neurons from all over your body. You could not discriminate a touch on the arm from one on your nose.

This extreme example can be contrasted with another illustration that is just as outlandish. Assume that every somatosensory receptor and fiber is connected to its own minuscule area of skin. Each receptor and primary sensory neuron is activated only if you happen to touch its private domain of skin. Furthermore, the area of skin that is assigned to each receptor and primary sensory neuron is not assigned to any other receptor. If the area assigned to each receptor did not overlap with another receptor and were the size of a period then you have very fine (perfect) discrimination. You could tell these two dots (:) apart because they do not overlap and each one has a different path to the brain. You could tell exactly where you had been touched. All the brain needs to do is focus on which neuron was activated to know where the touch originated. These two examples are the extremes of reality. No one receptor has a private field for its response and not all of the receptors and fibers are activated when you are touched. In between these two extremes lies the truth and the definition of a receptive field. The cutaneous system **receptive field** is that area of skin that, when stimulated, causes a receptor or primary sensory neuron to respond.

It follows from this discussion that the smaller the receptive field, the better the discrimination. Likewise, the larger the receptive field, like the whole body, the worse the discrimination. In sum, a receptor or neuron that has a small receptive field is better able to discriminate. The more receptive fields overlap with other receptive fields and the larger they are, the less discriminating is the sensory system.

If, at this point, **acuity** comes to mind, you are on the right track. Acuity is directly related to the receptive field. Consider individuals with visual impairments. They use braille to read the floor numbers in the elevator. Do you think they could read the "bumps" if they were asked to use their elbows or the backs of their hands? Could they do it if they were, in some way, able to rub their backs against the bumps? The answer is no. The reason they could not read the braille is that the receptive fields are too large almost everywhere except the fingertips. The fingertips are blessed with small receptive fields. You can discriminate between bumps organized very closely together only with your fingers. However, because their receptive fields are large and overlap, the elbow, back of the hand, and backs cannot finely discriminate.

As a party game, you may try spelling "I love you," one letter at a time with your finger, on a friend's back. How large do you have to make the letters before your friend can differentiate the letters and decode your message? If you wrote the same message on the arm, do the letters have to be as large?

How do you go about determining the size and location of a receptive field? The answer is easy. Scientists find a receptor or a neuron and record from it. The first thing they find is a "live" cell with a spontaneous activity. Then, while recording from this cell, they search for the receptive field by stimulating the peripheral portion of the sensory system. In the cutaneous sense, they move a pressure device across the skin until they find the location where the cell activity changes. This change in activity, from spontaneous to an increase or decrease in activity, signifies that the area of the skin being stimulated is innervated by the neuron from which they are recording. The task then is simple. Move the stimulus around and draw or sketch out the area of skin that activates the neuron. This area of skin is the neuron's receptive field. By looking at the size of the receptive field, you can make an educated guess about the acuity or discrimination ability at that point. Finally, you should keep in mind that many of the sensory systems have receptive fields.

The Thalamus

The pathway from the skin to the spinal cord has been detailed previously in Chapter 1. The focus of the remainder of this chapter is on the somatosensory portions of the thalamus and cortex.

The thalamus is often referred to as the great relay station of the brain. What this means is that early investigations of the thalamus showed that nearly every sensory system had synaptic terminals within the thalamic nuclei. Figure 3.5 shows the general overview of the thalamic organization.

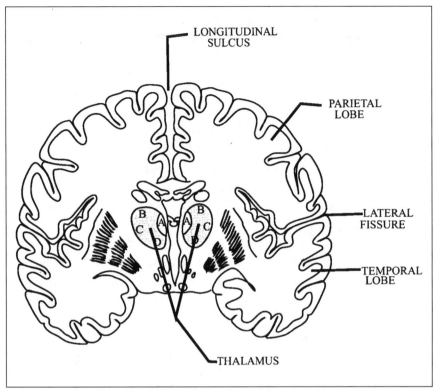

Figure 3.5. Transverse Section of the Brain Showing the General Orientation of Thalamic Nuclei

NOTE: A is medial, B is dorsal, C is lateral, and D is ventral basal.

The thalamus consists of two nuclei, one in each hemisphere, with areas specialized by sensory modality. The area of concern for the somatosensory system is, as noted earlier, the ventral basal nucleus. When the cells within the ventral basal nucleus are examined with microelectrodes, they respond to the pressure and stimulation initiated at the peripheral parts of the body on one side. The thalamus in the left hemisphere receives inputs from the right side of the body and vice versa.

An interesting thing about the microelectrode investigations is that the body image can be mapped onto the ventral basal nucleus. This mapping is precise in that particular parts of the arm, when stimulated, activate the same cells within the thalamus. Likewise, when the leg is stimulated, or the hand or finger, there are separate or different cells that respond according to the location of the stimulation on the body. Thus, a body map is within the brain itself.

Furthermore, the neurons within the ventral basal nucleus have receptive fields associated with the area of the body they represent. The receptive fields, like the ones found for the primary sensory neurons, vary in size and location. Each thalamus contains a distorted neural representation or map of one half of the body. This neural area is called a somatosensory **homunculus.** *Homunculus* is Latin for "little man." The homunculus has, unfortunately, a personality problem. He has, psychologically speaking, a dissociative reaction: Half of him is in the left thalamus, the other half is in the right thalamus. The homunculus, as we learn, is projected to the SI area of the cortex. The cortex is our next stop.

The Somatosensory Cortex

The cortex contains the neural elements that allow us to know ourselves as human. Here is where the "real you" is found. Understanding the cortex is the final frontier of psychology, biology, and neuroscience. As you may suspect from previous chapters, the neocortex, which is required to accomplish this wonderful task, is only as thick as two dimes. Yet nearly every part of the cortex, so it seems, has been studied, drilled, recorded, labeled, scanned, cut, listened to, ablated, stimulated, and dreamed about. In spite of these tremendous efforts, we are still relatively ignorant of the cortex and its true structure and function.

The relatively small portion of the nervous system known as the somatosensory cortex is no different. We know some about its features, but there is much more to learn. However, that is an endeavor that awaits you and the generations to come. For now, it is our task to learn something about the somatosensory cortex based on our current knowledge.

One of the most interesting approaches to understanding the brain, and the cortex specifically, was the pioneering studies by **Wilder Penfield** and his colleague (Penfield & Rasmussen, 1950). They operated on humans using local anesthetics in an attempt to correct epileptic seizures. They shaved the head and removed portions of the skull to expose the patient's brain. Once the brain was exposed, the patient was stimulated while laying on the operating table wide awake and alert. The patient felt no pain because the cortex has no pain receptors. The stimulus to the cortex was done with microelectrodes and brief electrical shocks. While they were stimulating the patient's cortex, they asked the patient to talk to them about any experiences as the brain was stimulated. Although these experiments may appear to be brutal or inhumane, they were not. Although the surgery was devoted to the cure of epileptic seizures, while the operation was being performed the surgeons gained research knowledge by asking the patient about what was felt when they stimulated different areas of the cortex. As noted previously, brain stimulation produces no pain for the patient. Figure 3.6 shows some of the results from their research and displays the cortical somatosensory homunculus and the important concept of cortical magnification in sensory systems. The magnification accounts for the distorted features of the homunculus shown in the Figure 3.6. **Cortical magnification** means that the most important features of a sensory system require, and receive, the largest portion of the cortex. The homunculus reflects the importance of such items as the opposable thumb, the fingers, lips, and tongue. An analog of the sensory homunculus is found in the motor cortex of the precentral gyrus of the frontal lobe. The cortical magnification also occurs in the motor cortex. There are significantly larger portions of motor cortex associated with the control and manipulation of fingers and the organs of speech. In fact, the hand and face are each about the size of the projection area of the entire trunk and leg together. Clearly, the projections from the small receptive fields on the fingers and face have enlarged as they progress toward the thalamus and the cortex. The cortical magnification reflects the importance of the innervated area. An interesting difference between the SI and SII cortical areas is that the SII area receives inputs from both sides of the body. The homunculus is complete and not divided as shown in Figure 3.6.

The cortex, as thin as it is, has been examined in minute detail (see Kaas, Merzenich, & Killackey, 1983; Kaas, Nelson, Sur, & Merzenich, 1981; Pons, Garraghty, Friedman, & Mishkin, 1987). The results of these investigations show that regardless of where you look, the cortex can be partitioned in a structural and functional organization. The cortical tissue has columns and layers that have functional significance. There are still some controversies and unknowns regarding the somatosensory system. There are, however, some fairly firm data that support the following conclusions.

First, the cortex is arranged as functional units of neuronal columns. The columns are oriented perpendicular to the surface of the cortex. The columns, approximately 0.3 mm wide, contain cells that respond in the same manner and have similar receptive field sizes. Research suggests, but not entirely supports, that each column is excited by receptors of a single type (e.g., mechanoreceptors). There are, however, few data to support the possibility that there are columns of cells that respond only to thermoreceptors or nociceptors. The data, sparse as they are, have nevertheless led to serious contemplation and interesting theories by scientists. Research suggests, for example,

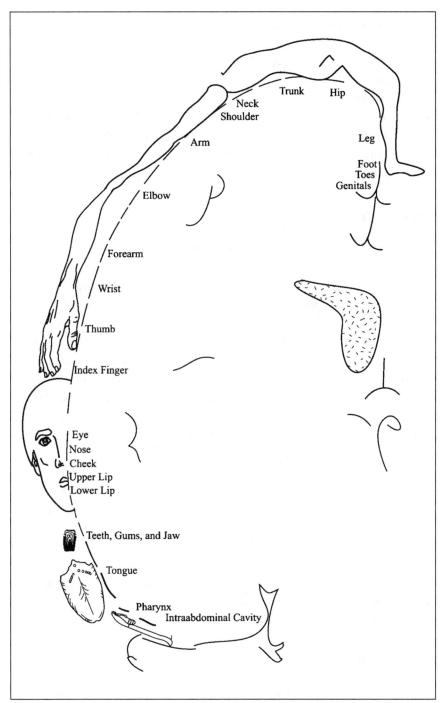

Figure 3.6. Somatosensory Cortex Reflecting the Cortical Magnification in the Brain

that some of the cortical columns function as cellular aggregates to extract features from incoming information. That is, the perceptual features of the environment (pressure, tickle, warmth, cold, etc.) have been theorized as being extracted by the individual columns found in the cortex. Whether the theory will be supported by research is currently in doubt. Other points of view suggest that the six laminar layers of cortex rather than the columns may function to produce the perceptual reality. It is probable that both the columns and the vertical spread of cortical information across several layers will be the outcome.

Dysfunctions

The spinal cord is, as we know, well protected within a bony structure typically called the "backbone." Protection of the neural and vascular system is one of the primary functions of the spinal column and the skull. Unfortunately, the integrity of the spinal column is occasionally breached as a result of trauma such as automobile and motorcycle accidents, knife and bullet wounds, acute fractures, dislocation of vertebrae, and spinal cord diseases, tumors, inflammatory conditions, or degenerative discs. The consequences of these events range from minor pain and irritation to complete disability and, in some cases, death of the individual. We briefly examine some of these concerns.

The immediate result of a complete transection of the spinal cord, at any level, is the loss of all sensations and voluntary movement below the cut. In addition, depending on the location of the cut, there is often a loss of voluntary control over the bowels and bladder. The initial trauma usually results in a loss of all automatic responses, reflexes, due to "spinal shock." After a period of a few weeks, the reflexes often return in an exaggerated form. The limbs become spastic and often assume a fixed rigid posture. Bladder and bowel control becomes automatic in response to moderate filling.

The sensations of pain, touch, vibration, position of the limbs, temperature, and all feeling below the cut are permanently gone because of the severed pathways leading from the body to the brain. The transection of the efferent pathways from the brain to the muscles prevents any voluntary movement. The muscles eventually atrophy.

The complete transection of the spinal cord represents an extreme condition. It has, unfortunately, happened to some individuals. The extent of the injury, usually from an accident rather than disease, and the location of the transection determine the ultimate outcome. If the transection should occur above the shoulders near Cervical 4 or 5 of the spinal cord, see Figure 1.2, the individual is quadriplegic, with the loss of movement and sensation in all four limbs. If the accident has severed the paths at a lower level, the individual becomes paraplegic, with the loss of the use of two limbs.

In the case of complete transection of the spinal cord, the effects are permanent. There is no recovery of sensations or voluntary movement. Neurons within the central nervous system do not regenerate or regrow. Once they have died, they are gone forever. There is, however, hope. Research continues and amazing results are predicted for the future.

A hemisection (where one half the cord is severed) or a less severe accident leads to less traumatic effects on behavior and the individual's life. If, for example, a knife wound were to occur on the right half of the spinal cord, a hemisection, the results are less catastrophic, but nonetheless quite debilitating. A hemisection on the right side of the spinal cord, a cut entering the right lateral side and severing pathways until the median of the cord is reached, results in the following functional deficits:

1. loss of ipsilateral, the same or right side, voluntary movement because of the severed efferent fibers coming from the brain,

2. loss of sensory input regarding body and limb position on the right side, a severed dorsal column pathway, and

3. loss of some sensory information from the left half of the body due to a severed spinothalamic tract.

Summary

The body senses are diffuse and sophisticated. We learn to judge where our bodies are in space by focusing on, perhaps unconsciously, unique sensory systems. The slow-adapting and fast-adapting receptors and fibers are typical of sensory systems in general because they adapt and they respond primarily to stimulus change. The input is processed beyond the periphery by the central mechanisms within the thalamus and somatosensory cortex. The flow of information is continuous through the dorsal columns and the spinothalamic tract. This flow is modified, amplified, rejected, and interpreted as it courses through the nervous system. The receptive fields of each cell aid in the interpretation by providing sharp acuity (small receptive fields) and bursts of activity dependent on stimulus intensity (or velocity in the case of movement). Finally, the overall somatosensory system is intimately related to another powerful attention-getting system—pain. This is the topic of the next chapter.

Suggested Readings

Burgess, P. R., & Perl, E. R. (1973). Cutaneous mechanoreceptors and nociceptors. In A. Iggo (Ed.), *Handbook of sensory physiology, vol. 2. Somatosensory systems.* Heidelberg: Springer-Verlag.

Kaas, J. H., Nelson, R. J., Sur, M., & Merzenich, M. M. (1981). Organization of somatosensory cortex in primates. In F. O. Schmitt, F. G. Worden, G. Adelman, & S. G. Dennis (Eds.), *The organization of the cerebral cortex: Proceedings of a neurosciences research program colloquium.* Cambridge: MIT Press.

Penfield, W., & Rasmussen, T. (1950). *The cerebral cortex of man: A clinical study of localization of function.* New York: Macmillan.

CHAPTER 4

Pain

Pain is an enigma. It can occur from apparently nothing. It may be absent when it should be present, and it may only appear when you think about it. There are no direct pathways to a cortical pain center. The brain itself has no pain receptors, and the placement of electrified needles in your arm (acupuncture) may make pain go away. Drugs can help to remove the pain, sometimes. Cutting afferent pathways, such as the spinothalamic tract, may relieve pain. However, deafferentization, loss of afferent sensory input, may cause pain. Pain, in fact, may really be in your head, other than a headache. Pain that occurs in a limb that is no longer attached is called phantom limb pain (Melzack, 1992). The approach here to the discussion of pain begins with a few "truths" and looks at a theoretical model to account for the known facts. However, as we go along keep in mind that not all of the facts are yet available and much is yet to be figured out.

Pain: One Definition

As the previous paragraph suggests, the definition of pain is not necessarily a sensation that is evoked by tissue damage. The classic approach to sensory processes works with some senses, but is clearly out of context when it comes to pain. The International Association for the Study of Pain (Merskey & Bogduk, 1994) sculpted the following definition:

> Pain is an unpleasant sensory and emotional experience associated with actual or potential tissue damage, or described in terms of such damage.

Pain is always subjective. Each individual learns the application of the word through experience related to injury in early life. It is unquestionably a sensation in a part of the body but it is also always unpleasant and therefore also an emotional experience. Many people report pain in the absence of tissue damage or any likely pathophysiological cause, usually this happens for psychological reasons. There is no way to distinguish their experience from that due to tissue damage, if we take the subjective report. If they regard their experience as pain and if they report it in the same ways as pain caused by tissue damage, it should be accepted as pain. This definition avoids tying pain to the stimulus. Activity induced in the nociceptor and nociceptive pathways by noxious stimulus is not pain, which is always a psychological state, even though we may well appreciate that pain most often has a proximal physical cause. (p. 209)

The definition indicates that there is much more to pain than the destruction of physical tissue. In the face of such a definition, it may appear strange that there is still a "classical" approach to the sensation of pain in modern medicine. That is, the medical profession still depends on classical pathways and the idea that pain is principally derived from disease. The concept of specificity implies paths and receptors that elicit pain. Pain is clearly one of the most important symptoms relied on by physicians as they search for an appropriate diagnosis and treatment. Clinically, often physicians still consider pain as a sequence of receptors, fibers, and spinal pathways to the brain. Medical schools use this view as a means of introducing students to the procedures necessary to diagnose pathology.

Given the reliance by physicians on subjective judgments provided by innocent patients, it is no wonder that the accurate diagnosis of disease is a difficult task. Sometimes there is no disease. The pure psychological and subjective nature of pain can lead to error in diagnosis and treatment. The once common idea that tissue damage activates pain receptors and these, in turn, transmit impulses to the pain center is no longer an uncontested fact. The evidence is abundant that central processes such as learning and psychological expectation play significant roles in the perception of pain. There is no doubt, of course, that there are fibers that respond to noxious stimuli and these fibers, large myelinated A-delta and smaller unmyelinated C-fibers, conduct inputs to the central nervous system. It is this classic pathway, shown in Figure 4.1, that we turn to now.

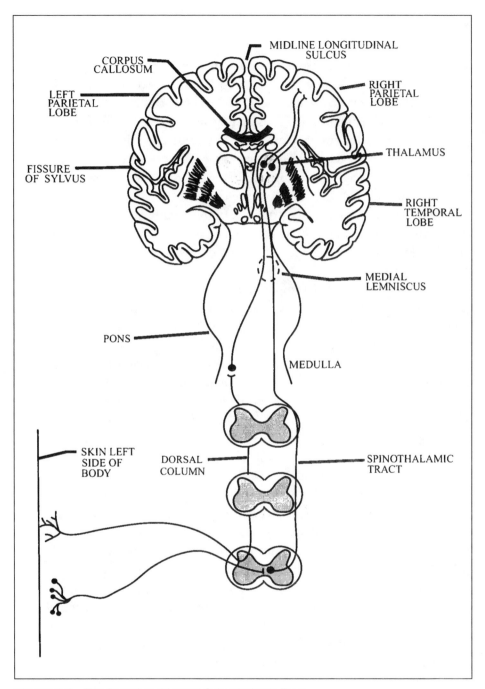

Figure 4.1. The Dorsal and Lateral Spinothalamic Tract

Classic Paths

The A-delta and C-fibers respond to pressure, temperature, and chemical stimuli. The chemical stimuli can result from external forces (e.g., acids) or the chemicals extruded by injured cells. There are several groups of agents that **produce** nociceptor activity. These **endogenous** substances are the **peptides (bradykinin)**, the **amines (serotonin, histamine)**, and the archindonic acid derivative (**prostaglandin**) These agents are often generated by injury to cells. Some of these agents are normally released because of hormonal actions. Menstrual cramps, for example, are caused by the prostaglandin released just before or during menstruation. In this regard, aspirin and other similar over-the-counter pills block an enzyme used to synthesize prostaglandin. The blockage of this enzyme is the method by which aspirin reduces the pain of menstrual cramping.

The fibers, because they respond to such a diverse stimulus input, are known as polymodal nociceptors. The response of these fibers to several sources of "adequate" stimuli indicates that the interpretation and modulation of the input is required by the central mechanisms. That is, the barrage of inputs are interpreted by the individual in view of the individual's learning, the situation, and expectations. An example of this often occurs when, for example, an individual notices blood on the floor and wonders who is hurt. Then he notices his own hand and realizes that he is the injured person. Only after conscious awareness of the injury does the pain begin. If the finger is bleeding, the expectation is that it probably hurts, so it does. It is the central processes, inhibitory and excitatory, which aid in the determination of pain. Once the fusillade of impulses arrives at the dorsal horn of the spinal cord, there are many opportunities for the central neural mechanisms to have a significant effect on the processing.

Figure 4.2 shows, in cross section, the lamina within the dorsal horn. The classical specificity approach to pain requires cells within the nervous system to respond and relay the information received from the nociceptor inputs. Some of the cells are in Laminae 1, 2, and 5 in the dorsal horn in the spinal cord. Layers 1 and 2 have a special name, the **substantia gelatinosa (SG)**. These cells, and those in Layer 5 are responsive to the A-delta and C-fibers coming into the central nervous system from the periphery, viscera, joints, muscles, and tendons.

The spinal neurons, Laminae 1, 2, and 5, are also responsive to descending pathways from the brain stem and cortex. The descending paths are both inhibitory and excitatory in their effects. Spinal neurons are modulated by af-

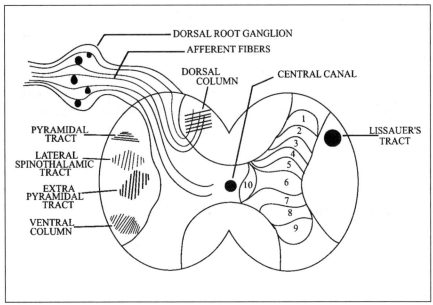

Figure 4.2. Cross Section of the Spinal Cord

ferent inputs from the skin, viscera, joints, and tendons. Modulation means that the spinal and central cells can be either enhanced or inhibited by descending activity. These A-delta fibers can excite as well as inhibit spinal cell groups. The C-fibers can also activate and inhibit these central spinal neurons.

The C-fibers, in addition to their inhibitory effects on cell groups, release a neurotransmitter called **substance P.** Although A-delta fibers have not had their neurotransmitter substance identified, whenever C-fibers are found, you find substance P. This neuropeptide is classified as a classic pain-eliciting neurotransmitter. The release of substance P leads to pain, pain-modulated behavior, and strong affect. Descending fibers in the spinal cord modulate the synapses that occur in the dorsal horn. These synapses are made between the incoming A-delta and C-fibers and the substantia gelatinosa cells in Lamina 5. If impulses from these spinal cord laminae are conducted further into the central nervous system, so conscious perception of pain can occur, then the pathway is usually thought to be through the classic spinothalamic tract. The spinothalamic tract projects to the medial lemniscus and the thalamus. The thalamus is the location where, in the past, the final "pain center" was once thought to exist. The third-order synaptic connections exiting the thalamus extend to the somatosensory cortex (SI) in the parietal lobe.

It is evident from the existing physiology that pain appears to have a typical sensory path with polymodal nociceptors. It is also evident, as noted previously, that learning and social and personal expectations can alter the abundant interactions that occur. Furthermore, of all the sensory systems, pain is the one modality that nearly everyone has at one time or another wished did not work. If such a wish were permanently granted, however, it would be very maladaptive. The search for pain relief has a long history. We examine this search after we examine a theoretical model. The model provides a coherent approach to our understanding of pain.

The Gate Control Theory of Pain

In 1965, Ronald Melzack and Patrick Wall published the gate control theory of pain. The theory is based on research as well as intellectual thought concerning the research literature and was unique to the field of pain. The theory postulated mechanisms in which widely diverse experimental results could be explained, and most important, suggested new avenues of investigation and pain relief (Wall & Melzack, 1994). The theory, it is fair to say, has been the most influential theoretical contribution to the understanding of pain to appear in the last 50 years. Figure 4.3 shows the theory and sequentially displays it, from 4.3(a) to 4.3(d), as it is discussed in the text. The final configuration is shown in Figure 4.3(d). The points where excitatory and inhibitory synapses occur are noted by the positive (+) and negative (−) signs, respectively.

The gate control theory postulates that **analgesia,** relief from pain without a loss of consciousness, can occur by the modulation of sensory and central mechanisms. You should keep in mind as we discuss the theory that the discussion is centered on the spinal cord. However, it is evident from recent studies that the theory can also be applied to the higher centers of the central nervous system—the thalamus and brain stem.

We begin the discussion with the afferent inputs from the **A-delta** and **C-fibers** (Figure 4.3[a]). These fibers are located in nearly every part of the body and come from the viscera, muscles, tendons, joints, and skin. They enter the spinal cord and make synaptic connections with interneurons in the laminae. These two types of fibers differ in several key ways. First, their thresholds are different. The A-delta fibers have low thresholds relative to C-fibers. This means that a mild or weak stimulus can activate the A-delta fibers but leave the C-fibers inactive. Second, the fibers differ in diameter and myelination. The A-delta fibers are large and myelinated. The C-fibers are small and unmyelinated. This difference ensures that the A-delta fibers conduct

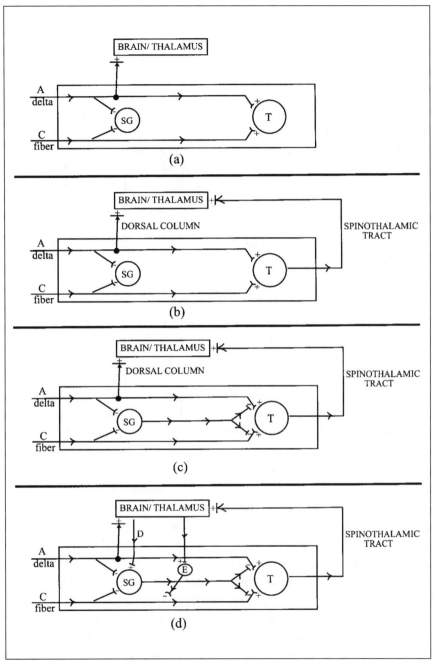

Figure 4.3. The Gate Control Theory of Pain

NOTE: (a) A-delta and C-fibers entering the spinal cord and synapsing on the SG and T-cells, (b) A-delta ascending to the higher centers by way of the dorsal column, T-cells activity ascending via the lateral spinothalamic tract, (c) the SG shuts the gate by axoaxonic inhibitory sysnapses, and (d) efferent paths from higher centers.

action potentials rapidly and the C-fibers more slowly. Third, they differ in the duration of their response. The A-deltas are more transient in their response to a stimulus than are the C-fibers. The C-fibers have a sustained response to a stimulus. As long as the stimulus is present, the C-fiber continues to generate action potentials. The C-fibers are slow-adapting nociceptors, whereas the A-delta fibers are fast-adapting nociceptors. Finally, the destinations of the two fiber systems differ. The A-delta have two branches: one ascends to the thalamus immediately on entering the spinal cord, the other branch almost simultaneously makes synaptic connections with cells in Laminae Layers 1, 2, and 5 of the dorsal horn (labeled SG and T in Figure 4.3[a]). In contrast, the C-fibers are assumed to make contact with the same three laminae in the dorsal horn, without an ascending branch. The C-fibers synapse on the SG and T-cells but do not branch to the thalamus. These different response characteristics and anatomical connections are intimately involved in the variety of pain perceptions.

Figure 4.3(a) shows the A-delta axons making synaptic connections with the substantia gelatinosa (SG) and the **T-cells.** These cells, SG and T, are both excited by the A-delta. The C-fibers also connect to the SG and T-cells. The SG is inhibited by the C-fibers and the T-cells are excited.

Figure 4.3(b) shows an expanded model of the theory. The output of the T-cells ascends to the thalamus by way of the spinothalamic tract. In addition, the A-delta fibers branch and ascend to the thalamus ipsilaterally by way of the dorsal column pathway. Thus, what occurs when the A-delta fibers are activated is a barrage of impulses ascend rapidly toward the thalamus and eventually to the cortex (in milliseconds). Almost simultaneously, the other branch of the A-delta fibers synapse with the SG and the T-cells. Figure 4.3(b) also shows the C-fibers. The functional continuity of the C-fiber pathway, however, is terminated at synapses on the SG and T-cells. The activity, initiated by the C-fibers, ascends to the thalamus only by way of the T-cell axons in the spinothalamic tract and medial lemniscus.

An important and critical aspect of the theory is the "gate" that modulates the perception of pain. The gate is assumed to be the cells of the substantia gelatinosa (SG). According to the gate control theory, the activity of the SG determines in great measure the perception of pain. The axons of the SG cells are added to the model in Figure 4.3(c). The SG axons make inhibitory presynaptic connections on the afferent C- and A-delta fibers. These synapses are the axoaxonic types we learned about previously. The authors, Melzack and Wall, did not ignore the possibility of postsynaptic connections with the

T-cell somas and afferent axons. For purposes of discussion, however, only the presynaptic terminals are shown in Figure 4.3.

These presynaptic connections from the SG are inhibitory in nature (note the – signs). Thus, by theoretical design, the SG cells, when activated by the A-delta fibers (note the + at the A-delta-SG synapse), inhibit the activity of the transmission cells. The inhibition occurs, of course, because the neurotransmitter (not yet positively identified, but possibly serotonin) inhibits the activity of the A-delta and C-fibers just before their synapse on the T-cells. In short, the A-delta fibers activate the SG and the SG, in turn, inhibits the activation of the T-cells and the transmission of spikes up the spinothalamic tract. The decrease in T-cell activity results in a decrease in perceived pain. The C-fibers, on the other hand, inhibit the SG (note the – where the C-fiber synapses with the SG). Thus, the activation of the C-fibers functionally opens the gate by preventing the presynaptic inhibition produced by the SG (Figure 4.3[c]).

Finally, as Figure 4.3(d) shows, there is the central nervous system component to the theory. Ample evidence in the research literature suggests that the central nervous system can modulate the spinal neurons. This means that there must be a pathway from central nervous system to the spinal cells; specifically there must be a descending path with synapses on the cells located in Laminae 1, 2, and 5. These descending fibers, labeled "D" in the model, are assumed to connect to the SG cells and activate them in an excitatory manner (note the + at the synapse). Excitatory synaptic activity on the SG, arriving from the descending fibers, closes the gate and reduces pain by activating the SG. In addition, the descending fibers make contact with a group of cells labeled "E." This cell group is also excited by the descending fibers. The output of the E cell inhibits the C-fibers with axoaxonic synapses. This inhibition decreases the C-fiber's effect on the T-cell and reduces the T-cell activity.

Gate Control Theory in Action

Recall in Chapter 1 there was a short discussion concerning a painful bump to the head. That injury can be examined in light of the gate control theory. There were four aspects of the injury to consider. First, is it possible that a bump may go unnoticed? Why is an injury ignored? Second, once the injury is noticed, a sharp pain is perceived for the first time. Third, why did the initial penetrating pain get replaced by a dull throb? Fourth, why did the pain seem to decrease when it was rubbed? Rubbing an injury and stimulating the area from which the pain is coming logically seem to cause more rather than less pain. The answers to these questions can be explained by the gate control theory.

First, not noticing an injury suggests that there are central mechanisms at work. These mechanisms, attention for example, prevented T-cell activity by activating the descending paths to the SG and E cell groups. The descending fibers, by activating the SG, shut the gate and inhibit the T-cells. In addition, the descending fibers most likely inhibited the C-fibers with the axoaxonic activity of the E cells. This inhibition prevents the release of substance P and produces a subsequent decline in the barrage of impulses sent to the conscious cortex by the T-cells. In sum, the activation of the descending paths by central mechanisms inhibits the sensation of pain by closing the gate and preventing the release of substance P by the C-fibers. The initial activity of the A-delta was brief and ignored by the higher mechanisms.

Second, the initial shock of seeing the injury can bring an almost instantaneous release from the central inhibitory mechanisms. That is, the realization that an injury has occurred removes the inhibition at the SG and E cells. The initial rush of action potentials causes a sharp, **epicritic** pain. The slow throbbing pain that follows is the result of the C-fiber activity. The A-delta fibers adapt while the C-fibers continue to send messages. The continual barrage by the C-fibers opens the gates to pain by inhibiting the SG. This allows a continual barrage of activity to arrive at the T-cells; hence, a ceaseless and perpetual dull **protopathic** pain is felt.

Finally, why does the pain decrease by rubbing it? The answer to this lies in the differential effects of the two afferent fibers, A-delta and C. By lightly rubbing the wound, the A-delta fibers are activated but the C-fibers are not. This occurs because the threshold for the A-delta fibers is lower than the threshold for the C-fibers. The excited A-deltas stimulate the SG cells. When the SG cells are activated, they close the gate by inhibiting the inputs to the T-cells. Thus, even though there may be an increase in activity from the A-delta fibers, the closing of the gate results in an overall decrease in the barrage of activity submitted to the higher centers. In short, by activating the A-delta fibers, the C-fibers are effectively blocked (inhibited) and the transmission-cell activity decreases accordingly. The decrease in T-cell activity is significantly larger than the slight increase in A-delta activity. The effective activation of the A-delta fibers is like removing the C-fibers from the system.

To test your understanding of the theory, consider your pet dog. When she injures her foot chasing the ball, she very likely lies down and licks her injury. How does the gate control theory account for this behavior? The dog licked her wound and relieved the pain because the light touch of her tongue activated the A-delta fibers. The A-delta fibers activated the SG cells in the substantia gelatinosa. The SG became active and sent bursts of action potentials to the axoaxonic synapses just before the T-cells. The T-cells' activity was reduced because of the inhibition, so fewer impulses were sent to the central processor. Licking reduced her pain.

Pain and Drugs

The search for pain relief is centuries old (Davis, 1982). In fact, it is thousands of years old. Since the beginning of human misery, the shaman (a tribal doctor) has searched for herbs, roots, berries, juices, and incantations to remove disease and pain. The search really has no known beginning and probably has no end. However, here are just a few highlights of the journey. One drug that has a long history, aside from alcohol, is the extract from the poppy. The use of the poppy extract dates back over 6,000 years. Ancient Greeks used opium, the Romans indulged in its use, and the Chinese used it while building the continental railroad in the United States in the mid-1800s. At the turn of the century, the Europeans had "opium dens" for the exclusive purpose of becoming intoxicated with the drug. The recognition that opium was a potent addictive substance, however, caused difficulties in its medicinal use.

A scientific analysis of the chemical actions of the poppy extract was finally achieved near the beginning of the 19th century. A chemical substance, **morphine,** was derived from the poppy. Morphine, named after Morpheus the Greek god of dreams, was initially thought to be a wonder drug that alleviated pain while not being an addictive substance. Morphine was used for several years before it was fully realized that it was just as addictive as opium. Soldiers returning from the Civil War were addicted to the morphine that had been injected to relieve the pain of battle wounds. The chemical isolation of morphine, however, was just the beginning of the explosion of chemicals derived and extracted from plants for the relief of pain and recreational euphoria. In the next few decades, the pharmacology profession, the branch of science that attempts to discover the chemical composition of compounds and their effects on the body, synthesized digitalis from the foxglove plant, cocaine from the coca plant, and quinine from the bark of the cinchona tree.

About 1875, another chemical derivative of the poppy came in existence. This new drug was **heroin.** It was initially believed to be nonaddictive. In 1886, the Bayer Company introduced aspirin to the public and two years later, they became the first company to offer a cough medicine with the "nonaddicting" mixture heroin. It was widely advertised as nonaddicting and better than other cough medicines containing codeine. For example, the label from a cough medicine called Glyco=Heroin (Smith) said, "Scientifically Compounded. Scientifically Conceived. GLYCO=HEROIN (SMITH) simply stands on its merits before the profession, ready to prove its efficacy to all who are interested in the advances in the art of medication." It took over 25 years for the medical profession to recognize the plight of many patients who became addicted. One of the reasons for the long delay was that the heroin was administered orally as a cough medicine. Its effects are much less potent when administered orally than when injected intravenously. In addition, the psychological expectation of euphoric feelings were not socially prevalent. One of the important aspects of the drug, however, was that it relieved the pain that patients felt to be among the worst. The deep, dull, diffuse, burning, long duration pains associated with such interminable diseases as cancer were lessened. How these drugs operate on the pain system was the next important question to be examined.

Opiate Receptors

Certainly, we do not have opium "receptors" because of our evolution. (Please keep in mind, at this point, that *receptor,* when used in reference to opium derivatives, refers to the chemical binding of the substance to a cell membrane or neural tissue rather than a receptor cell.) If derivatives of opium affect us, as they clearly do, then the derivatives of opium must be binding to the membranes of cells that normally exist. We were not born with receptors designed specifically for opiates. The exogenous derivatives must use the normally available receptors employed by our own endogenous neurotransmitters. The search for these specific opium receptors was successful. The search was extended over several countries by numerous scientists. The investigations yielded agonist and antagonist compounds that led to significant discoveries of receptor function (Snyder, 1986). An **agonist** is a compound that elicits a distinct and measurable change in the biological organism. In the case of opiates, morphine is an agonist that acts to remove pain and induces euphoria and a relaxed state. An **antagonist,** as the "ant" prefix suggests, is a chemical compound that prevents or reverses the effects of a specific agonist. An antagonist for morphine and heroin is a substance called **naloxone.** The common treatment for a heroin overdose is the immediate injection of naloxone. Experiments using morphine as an agonist and naloxone as an antagonist revealed several receptor sites. The sites where morphine and heroin act to relieve pain are Laminae 1 and 2 of the spinal cord and similar cells within the brain stem and thalamus. The cells within the spinal cord and brain stem include the substantia gelatinosa. The area of the thalamus that responds to the opiates is the ventral basal nucleus. Many other areas within the brain have receptors for opium derivatives. Some receptors were found in brain areas associated with euphoria, respiration, blood pressure, emotions, hormonal states, nausea, and vomiting. The side effects are obvious here. The pain may be relieved but there can be serious and deadly effects with an incorrect dosage.

The discovery of opiate receptor sites urged investigators to continue searching for the endogenous chemical compounds associated with the opiate receptors. It simply was not logical that nature had intended the opiate receptor sites to be just for our pleasure and drug addiction using morphine and heroin. The search was accomplished by taking advantage of the agonist and antagonist information already available. For example, one of the clues to the puzzle was the fact that morphine inhibits intestinal muscle contractions. Because this is so, brain extracts that contain opiate-like substances should prevent intestinal muscle contractions. For example the common drug, paregoric, is often used to treat diarrhea because it is an alcohol extract of opium. The logic is that paregoric constricts the intestinal muscles and reduces the diarrhea. Moreover, if a brain extract is found that prevents muscle contractions because it has opiate characteristics, the effects of the brain extract should be reversed when the antagonist naloxone is applied to the muscle. That is, the opiate brain extract should first inhibit the muscle contractions and then, after naloxone is applied, the effect of the brain extract should be blocked and the muscles should contract once again. This logic worked. Brain extracts that responded as expected were discovered (see Kandel, Schwartz and Jessell, 1995). An example of their procedure is diagrammed in Figure 4.4. Once they had found the brain extracts (chemicals), they isolated two substances and named them **enkephalins** after the Greek derivative, meaning "from the head." About the same time, other investigators, using different methods, isolated brain extracts which also had morphinelike characteristics. These other isolated substances were called **endorphins** (from *endo*genous m*orphine*). *Enkephalin* and *endorphin,* are now used interchangeably. Enkephalin and endorphin refer to any molecules or substances produced by the body that yield opiate-like responses.

Drugs and the Gate Control Theory

According to the gate control theory, for a drug to have a positive analgesic effect, it must be administered in such a way that the gate is closed and the T-cell barrage of activity is reduced. There are two common ways to adminis-

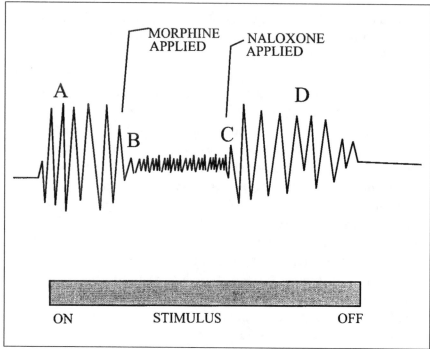

Figure 4.4. Opiate Antagonism by Naloxone

NOTE: (A) muscle contractions elicited by stimulation, (B) muscle inhibition caused by morphine, (C) naloxone releasing muscle from inhibition, and (D) resumption of normal muscle contractions.

ter these drugs, orally or by injection. When the drug is ingested, it must make its way past the digestive system and into the bloodstream to be delivered throughout the body. In the case of the spinal cord and brain, the chemical has to cross the protective blood-brain barrier. Assuming the drug passes these tests, it must then, by some means, close the "correct" gates and relieve the pain. By "correct" gates I mean, for example, closing the gates located in the spinal cord does not relieve the pain that originates in the brain stem. Moreover, the correct dosage must be administered. The dose must be large enough to relieve the pain yet not cause respiratory failure.

A most efficient means of pain reduction by drug action appears to be by way of the relatively recent developments in drug implantation systems. The permanent implantation of a slow-release drug system permits a localized long-duration application of pain-relieving substances. For example, a spinal segmental implant of morphine, implanted at a specific level in the spinal cord, is reversible by naloxone and does not affect the motor or other sensory functions. The assumption is that the implanted morphine has a direct effect on opiate receptors located on the C-fibers themselves. The reduction of the pain is caused by the decrease in C-fiber activity and the decrease in substance P, the pain-eliciting neurotransmitter. In addition, pain has been reduced by an intracerebral injection of morphine. As noted previously, the thalamus and other brain-stem mechanisms have opiate receptors. The injection of morphine into the cerebral ventricular system (cerebral spinal fluids) appears to be a promising approach for intractable pain in the head and upper body—cancer of the mouth, throat, shoulders, neck, and upper thoracic areas.

Electrical Stimulation and Pain Relief

When your puppy licked her leg and you rubbed your head, the light stimulation resulted in a reduction in the throbbing pain. Rubbing was a mechanical stimulation. What would happen if an electric impulse generator were attached near the place where the pain fibers entered the spinal cord? Could you then self-stimulate and reduce the pain by pressing a button? The answer is yes. Indeed, the use of **transcutaneous electrical nerve stimulation, TENS,** was introduced by Patrick Wall and was based on predictions made by the gate control theory (Hansson & Ekblom, 1983; Warfield, Stein, & Frank, 1985). The reduction of constant pain from cancer, for example, by the use of electrical stimulation was an immediate goal. The electric stimulation was assumed to activate the A-delta fibers and consequently reduce the pain. In addition to the TENS, there is a procedure in which electrical stimulation is directly applied to the dorsal column of the spinal cord. Although the mechanism by which analgesia occurs via dorsal column stimulation is somewhat unclear, it appears that the stimulation of the large A-delta fibers is involved. One possible mechanism is the closing of spinal column gates by descending fibers activated by the A-delta fibers that ascend through the dorsal columns. TENS and dorsal column stimulation are now widely used therapies in pain clinics. They are effective in the reduction of pain for some individuals who have incurred physical trauma such as car accidents or gunshot wounds.

The implanting of electrodes within the brain itself has also been attempted as a means of pain relief. The medical profession does not uniformly support intracerebral stimulation as a treatment. In the minds of some scientists, the procedure is in the gray area of exploratory surgery (no pun intended). The technique, based on current knowledge of the pain system, has been successful in some individuals and unsuccessful in others. The electrical stimulation by the implanted electrodes has been in use since the 1970s. Only a few pain clinics perform it and usually only when other means have failed. The logic for intracerebral stimulation is, as you may suspect, based on the closing of pain pathways by way of the theoretical gate. The stimulation, in the thalamus or other neural centers, is assumed to activate the E cells in the descending path (or similar cells in the cerebrum). The descending path, it is assumed, activates the E cells with an excitatory neurotransmitter, serotonin, and the E cells then release an endorphin to inhibit the C-fibers. Indeed, it is this type of stimulation, intracranial, that seems to be effective for **neurogenic** pain relief. Neurogenic pain is a sensation that is perceived as painful because of an injury to the nervous system itself. Deafferentation of neural pathways is such an injury. The TENS approach and the dorsal column stimulation are insufficient in removing the pain involved with the deafferentation. The thalamic stimulation, on the other hand, sometimes provides a measure of relief.

Acupuncture also falls under the umbrella of electrical stimulation because the needles, which are inserted into specific parts of the body, are often electrically stimulated. The explanation for the pain relief with acupuncture is that the neurotransmitters activated by the needles are related to inhibitory systems that include GABA, serotonin, and the endorphins. The acceptance of acupuncture as a means of pain relief has grown in the last 20 years. The evidence that supports its use, when it works, has been scant, but it does appear to have some significant support in the public eye. The data, while still inconclusive, are still being gathered. Ancient Eastern medicine may become more respectable than some scientists originally believed possible. Time and research are going to determine the place of acupuncture in the Western world.

Surgical Management of Pain

Statements that you hear regarding surgery as a method of pain relief often refers to a patient who has pain that cannot be controlled under any other circumstance. The relief of pain by surgery is considered as the very last resort. Why? Because it often does not cure the pain. This is particularly true if there are psychogenic aspects such as psychological tensions. Surgery must be fully justified because no surgical treatment is 100% guaranteed to be effective. This is particularly important because no surgery, ever, is without personal risk for the patient. Cutting and removing viable tissue and organs is the last step. What is cut and removed cannot be replaced.

These comments, I believe, tells it all when it comes to surgery to relieve pain. The rule is one that every neurosurgeon should learn: "Touch a brain, never the same." This rule, of course, applies to the entire central nervous system, whether it is the cortex or the spinal cord. When a surgeon makes an incision in an attempt to remove pain, and it does not work, there is no way to repair the intrusion done by the scalpel.

The most common surgery has been on the pathways carrying the sensory information, the spinothalamic tract and the dorsal column. The dangers are high, and the cure is often near only 50%. The problems that result from surgery are also serious considerations. Box 4.1 shows some common surgical procedures that have been attempted to relieve pain.

Behavioral Techniques and the Placebo

There is no doubt that expectation plays a role in the relief of pain. When an individual arrives at a "pain clinic," the expectations are clearly high. The hope is there. These expectations are by themselves strong motivators for central mechanisms and the reduction of pain. The behavioral techniques when applied, such as relaxation therapy, biofeedback, and hypnosis, are unaffected by the concurrent use of naloxone. This means that the relief of pain is not involved with the opiate system but very likely is under some cognitive control and is often attributed to a placebo effect (Turk, 1994). Whether the relief is a placebo or is due to cognitive elements is, really, irrelevant when it comes to the patient. The pain is gone. That is what counts.

Summary

The experience of pain is a personal and very subjective sensation. Pain is physiological and psychological because learning, society, situations, and expectations can all alter the perception. The gate control theory is a tremendous intellectual tool in the search for understanding pain. Opiate receptors, endorphins, and a complex of neural interactions have all been explored in an effort to find a cure. There is, of course, no single cure for pain. The elusiveness of a cure suggests that many different approaches have to be attempted if you are to live pain free. Aspirin is useful, rubbing the sore is helpful, and sometimes, though rarely, surgery may be of some aid. Acupuncture and placebo both have a place in the arsenal against pain. The wise use of drugs is clearly a strong candidate for pain relief. The pharmaceutical companies have been pursuing addiction-free drugs very seriously. There are, after all, mil-

---

BOX 4.1

Surgical Intervention
for the Prevention of Pain

1. Nerve Section. The severing of a peripheral nerve for the purpose of relieving distal pain.
2. Sympathectomy. Severing of sympathetic ganglions along the spinal cord for the purpose of reducing pain from the viscera.
3. Myelotomy. A sectioning of the spinothalamic fibers in anterior white commissure. This is a partial section of the classic spinothalamic pathway.
4. Posterior Rhizotomy. A severing of a dorsal horn spinal nerve.
5. Cordotomy. A severing of the spinal cord, either partial or complete. Usually a spinothalamic cordotomy.
6. Medullary Tractotomy. Cutting of nerve tracts in the medulla.
7. Mesencephalic Tractotomy. Surgical division of the nerve tracts that pass through the mesencephalon.
8. Thalamotomy. Cutting the subcortical areas of the thalamic nucleus for purposes of blocking pathways through the thalamus.
9. Gyrectomy. The excision or resection (ablation) of a cerebral gyrus, or of a portion of the cerebral cortex.
10. Prefrontal Lobotomy. An operation in which the white matter of the frontal lobe is incised with a leukotome (wire) passed through a cannula (tube). This operation severs the frontal lobes from the emotional centers of the brain (limbic system).
11. Hypophysectomy: Surgical removal of the pituitary gland.

---

lions of dollars at stake. They may indeed find a chemical derivative that functions as an opiate, yet has no unfortunate side effects. However, as of now, that drug is not on the market.

Suggested Readings

Davis, A. B. (1982, Sept./Oct.). The development of anesthesia. *American Scientist, 70,* pp. 522-528.

Kandel, E. R., Schwartz, J. H., & Jessell, T. M. (1995). *Essentials of neural science and behavior.* Norwalk, CT: Appleton & Lange.

Melzack, R. (1992, April). Phantom limbs. *Scientific American,* pp. 120-126.

Melzack, R., & Wall, P. D. (1965). Pain mechanisms: A new theory. *Science, 150,* pp. 971-979.

Turk, D. (1994). Perspectives on chronic pain: The role of psychological factors. *Current Directions in Psychological Science, 3*(2), 45-48.

Wall, P. D., & Melzack, R. (Eds.). (1994). *Textbook of pain* (3rd ed.). Edinburgh, Scotland: Churchill Livingstone.

CHAPTER 5

Olfaction

Olfaction is practically as ancient as life itself. The chemical senses were in full operation when evolution decided to fling the vertebrates onto the beach. There were, then as now, chemicals swirling, flowing, floating, and sprouting in water, vapor, and air. These chemical molecules existed in the environment of organisms that have since become extinct. The chemicals, however, still abound in the seas and atmosphere that surrounds us today (Le Guerer, 1994).

The sensory systems of organisms, humans included, have evolved over the aeons to respond to the chemical messengers that surround us in the air we inhale and the solutions we consume (Schwenk, 1994). The olfactory system is also quite important for prey animals. It is interesting to note in passing, however, that whales and dolphins do not have the sense of smell. The chemical senses are, moreover, the primary mechanism used to initiate sexual behavior and the consequent reproduction of the species in the majority of animals. Before any animal can sexually reproduce it must find, in space and time, the opposite sex. This search is most often accomplished by the use of an excretion called a **pheromone.** A pheromone is a chemical produced by males or females for the purpose of sexual attraction (Halpern, 1987; Holden, 1996; O'Connell & Meredith, 1984). The enticing odor usually arrives in the vapors and the evening breeze. Research has suggested, but data are scarce, that pheromones may occur for humans in much the same way as they do for other animals. The probability of human pheromones is, however, not firmly documented.

Humans have, for better or for worse, culturally removed, covered, and changed their own scent (Stoddart, 1990). They have also altered the smell of the environment. Some of the odors have been derived from secret concoctions—for example, perfumes. Others are available from more natural-occurring events such as the aroma of the fresh baked bread. Some odors result from pollution. As we will learn, odor and memory are also intimately linked.

For centuries, odors and incense have had an appeal in Hindu, Christian, Jewish, and Muslim religious ceremonies. In fact, speaking of secret formulae, during the Dark and Middle Ages odors were purposely concocted from mixtures of burning incense and aromatic plants in attempts to protect physicians, cure the ill, and to ward off the plague. The physicians arrive at the bedside of their sick and dying patients dressed in a costume, replete with a headdress bearing a large beak. It has occurred to some that this could be where *quack* came to refer to the honorable profession of physician and healer. However, true or false, one of the primary skills acquired and used by physicians was the classification of disease based on the smell of a patient's breath, excrement, and wounds. In fact, breath testing has bloomed into a serious diagnostic procedure today. It is not uncommon for intoxicated motorists to be required to "blow 10" in a handheld instrument. Breath collecting and analyzing devices have become important approaches to the diagnosis of diseases by astute physicians and researchers. The systems are rather simple. The patient inhales through activated carbon, with a nose clip to insure breathing is only through the mouth, and exhales into a mouthpiece. The exhaled air passes through a drying apparatus and is trapped for later analysis. The test can reveal malabsorption syndromes such as severe and chronic diarrhea due to disorder in the small intestine, pancreas disorders, peptic ulcers, chronic gastritis, liver disease, and exposure to potential hazardous solvents or petrochemicals (Phillips, 1992).

Yes, olfaction is important. The billion-dollar business of aromatic sprays that ward off the evil lurking within the bathroom has an effect on our behavior. The physiological apparatus that responds to these chemical elements is the focus of this and the next chapter.

The Peripheral Olfactory System

The nose, that fixture of skin and cartilage, is right there in the middle of your face. That is where olfaction begins. Two nostrils, the **nares,** are separated by the median **nasal septum,** the dividing cartilage. Beyond the nares is the nasal cavity. In the human, the cavity rises upward through a complex maze of cartilage called the inferior, medial, and superior turbinate that are sometimes

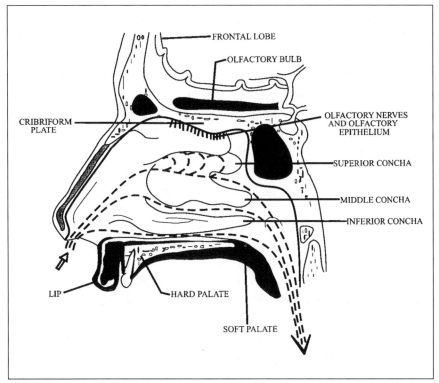

Figure 5.1. The Human Olfactory System Showing the Superior, Medial, and Inferior Concha, Cribriform Plate, Hard and Soft Palate, Olfactory Bulb, and Air Flow to the Lungs

labeled as inferior, medial, and superior concha. Figure 5.1 shows a diagrammatic representation of the human peripheral olfactory system.

When you investigate the nasal cavity, you discover two types of linings: the respiratory and olfactory epithelium. It is the role of the respiratory epithelium to clean the dust from the air, warm it as it passes through the cavity, and provide moisture prior to reaching the lungs. To accomplish the task, the respiratory epithelium is blessed with a rich supply of blood vessels and mucus secreting glands. The glands that produce this mucus are Bowman's glands. The respiratory epithelium can respond, for example, with an automatic and almost immediate copious flow of mucus and with a possibly motor-controlled sensory reflex, whenever one inhales a potent irritant such as pepper, onion, or smoke.

As you breath in, the flow of the inspired air enters the nasal cavity and is divided in three streams on its way to the lungs. The lower, flat ribbonlike flow passes between the hard palate and the inferior turbinates. A second flow passes between the inferior and medial turbinates. The third passes over the medial and around the superior turbinate. This latter path, the one with the least cubic measure of air, comprises approximately 5 to 10% of the total inhaled air. It is this eddy of air that has an opportunity to stimulate the olfactory receptor apparatus embedded within the olfactory epithelium. Estimates indicate that in the normal human breath, only 2% of the total inspired air passes near the olfactory epithelium.

The passage of air through the maze of turbinates has an important purpose. It promotes the interaction of the respiratory epithelium with the inspired air. This close contact of the air with the epithelium, particularly in the posterior portion of the nasal cavity, is important. Located in this area are the **ciliated cells** that continually beat and move in a rhythmic motion. As you read this sentence, these ciliated cells are active. What they do is move the mucus toward the throat where it is swallowed. The continual waving motion of the cilia moves the mucus toward the nasopharynx at a rate estimated to be between 10 and 60 mm a minute. This movement helps maintain the air-mucus interaction and simultaneously maintains a clean passageway for the continually inspired air. It should come as no surprise, then, that an infection or cold will often increase the mucus flow and result in the dripping and runny nose. It is the normal continual cleansing, consequently, that improves the probability that some of the molecules inspired with the vapors of the air will stimulate the olfactory receptors and result in the perception of an odor.

The olfactory epithelium is, by comparison, restricted in size. The olfactory epithelium is confined to an area that has been estimated to be between 1 and 4 cm^2 in size. This portion of the nasal cavity is referred to as the olfactory cleft and is located, in humans, dorsally and posterior to the superior turbinate cartilage. The reason for the *cleft* is that the passageway at the top of the nasal cavity, which contains the receptor apparatus, is actually so narrow that the majority of the olfactory epithelium lies on the lateral and medial wall of each nasal passageway. You may visualize the olfactory epithelium as being about the size of your fingernail, perhaps smaller, and occupying the small inverted "V" at the top of each nasal cavity. Although the epithelium is found medially, dorsally, and laterally at the roof of the cavity, anatomical studies reveal the majority of the olfactory receptors are located on the lateral wall.

The small patches of tissue, the olfactory epithelium, is sometimes called neuroepithelium because the olfactory neurons cover an area about one half the size of a postage stamp and contain a set of three intriguing cells. There is, first, an unmyelinated bipolar neuron associated with the transduction of odors, called the **olfactory receptor.** The other two cells are supporting cells, and **basal cells.** The intriguing thing about the olfactory receptor is that it is not in the classification system used previously. It is more like a modified neuron. Yet it is something more. It is a bipolar neuron that has a life span, in humans, of about 1 to 3 months. A new olfactory receptor is regenerated every 30 to 90 days from its precursor, the basal cell. The basal cell, in other words, divides by mitosis and one of the two halves then becomes an olfactory receptor. This regeneration phenomenon is all the more fascinating because it requires the axon terminal of each newly formed olfactory cell, as it is generated from the basal cell, to migrate to the next neuron in the system and form a new synaptic connection. How the migration occurs and how the existing neurons change to accept a new synapse is presently unknown.

The instigating signal that sends the basal cell to mitosis to become an olfactory receptor is also a mystery. In addition to this regeneration, the actual transduction of chemical molecules to neural action potentials occurs at the cilia located on the **olfactory knob** of the receptor. We discuss this phenomenon more fully in a later section of the chapter.

The olfactory epithelium contains, in humans, approximately 5 to 6 million olfactory receptors. These cells are, of course, at different stages in their short 30- to 90-day life cycle. This number of receptors is significantly fewer than that found in most other animals on the planet. For example, a cat has an olfactory epithelium of approximately 20 cm^2 in size. There are approximately 30 to 50 million receptors per nasal cavity. The rabbit has approximately 10 million olfactory receptors entering each olfactory bulb from the nasal cavity. The cat and rabbit are overshadowed by the dog. The German Shepherd has been estimated to have as many as 2 billion olfactory receptors in a single nasal cavity. The number in the Bloodhound must be at least as many, probably more.

The number of olfactory receptors in these large dogs clearly indicates the importance of smell to these animals. In addition, the location of the olfactory patch has been strategically placed for maximum sensitivity. The main airstream that is inhaled and sniffed by these animals passes directly over an extensive olfactory patch. In humans, recall, the olfactory receptors are located up and out of the way. It requires a healthy sniff by a human to double the number of molecular contacts with the neural transducers. The average sniff lasts, odorwise, only 400 msec, just long enough to about double the receptive contacts. In humans, larger, bigger, and more vigorous sniffs are, remarkably, no better than dainty small ones. It appears that what counts, for us anyway, is that we must sniff to double the olfactory stimulation.

The typical olfactory receptor comprises five primary parts:

1. an elongated cell body;
2. a long peripheral process, the axon;
3. a short process, the dendrite;
4. the olfactory knob or olfactory vesicle; and
5. the 10 to 12 **olfactory cilia** that protrude in the nasal mucus.

Surrounding the olfactory receptors are the supporting and basal cells. Figure 5.2 shows the three cells constituting the olfactory neuroepithelium and **Bowman's gland.** This latter gland secretes the mucus. As mentioned in more detail shortly, the mucus plays a role in the transduction process.

The olfactory knob located at the distal end of the short dendritic process of the receptors accommodates 10 to 12 cilia. The cilia are, moreover, embedded within the mucus. Thus, the inhaled odorant molecules must flow past the olfactory epithelium and be absorbed in the mucus to stimulate the cilia (Cometto-Muniz & Cain, 1990; Cometto-Muniz, Cain, & Abraham, 1998). As noted previously, the cilia themselves are believed to be where transduction occurs. The last part of the olfactory cell, the longer peripheral axon, is unmyelinated and conducts the impulses to the olfactory bulb.

Each unmyelinated axon enters the olfactory bulb by joining approximately 1,000 other axons to form a bundle of axons called the **fila olfactoria.** The fila olfactoria itself is myelinated by a Schwann cell. The fila pass through the perforations in the **ethmoid bone** (also referred to as the **cribriform plate**) and enter the ipsilateral olfactory bulb. The fila or bundles, when they reach the olfactory bulb, then branch and make synaptic contact onto the dendrites of mitral cells. The dendrites of the mitral cells are located in glomeruli (singular = glomerulus).

It is of some interest that the olfactory axons are extremely fragile. As they pass through the cribriform plate heading toward their next destination, the olfactory bulb, a head trauma can virtually wipe out the sense of smell. Remarkably, however, if the trauma is not extensive or too severe, the severed olfactory receptor axons, and smell, can recover by basal cell regeneration. The repair of the sense of smell, depending on damage, usually occurs within 4 to 6 months. The amazing reorganization of the central nervous system in the

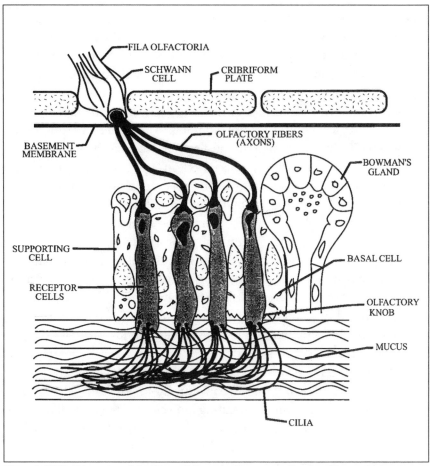

Figure 5.2. Diagram of the Four Olfactory Receptors Passing Through the Cribriform Plate

NOTE: The Schwann Cell wraps the axons and forms the fila olfactoria. Additional supporting cells, mucus, and Bowman's gland are displayed.

face of such traumas continues to be investigated. This reorganization and regeneration is one of the significant exceptions to the rule that damage to central nervous system tissue is permanent. The regeneration of olfactory receptors and the recovery after trauma in adult mammals continues to be studied.

Olfactory Transduction

Olfactory stimuli comprise a multitude of molecules in inspired air. The basic ideas of the transduction process have been discussed theoretically for several hundred years. Only in the past few decades, however, have any substantial data been forthcoming to aid understanding. The transduction of olfactory stimuli to a perceptual odor is just now beginning to be thoroughly examined (Brand, Teeter, Cagan, & Kare, 1989; Finger, Silver, & Restrepo, 2000; Paysan & Breer, 2001; Reed, 1990).

One of the many difficulties in studying olfaction is the investigator's ability to deliver and control a "pure" stimulus to a "clean and ready" olfactory system. The investigation itself must also be accomplished in an "olfactory clean" environment. What is "olfactory clean" to one animal—the human experimenter—may certainly not be "olfactory clean" for an experimental animal about to sniff an experimental vapor. In addition to stimulus control, olfactory clean, and olfactory ready, there is the difficulty of getting to the olfactory receptive system itself if you wish to have neurological recordings. It is at the top of the nasal cavity, covered with mucus, and the olfactory bulb lies on top of the ethmoid bone directly beneath the frontal lobe. Thus, neural recording is not simple. Nevertheless, investigators have persisted and have learned a great deal about the transduction process. The data are in some respects clear and solid. In other instances, there are just shadows merged with a clever hypothesis.

The cilia from the olfactory knob have been examined closely. Several conclusions can be drawn from these investigations. First, the cilia contain the receptor sites for the odor-generating molecules. The many cilia on the olfactory knob play a significant role in the ability of an olfactory receptor to respond to any one molecule. By using the surface areas of the many cilia, the olfactory receptor interaction with the chemical molecules increases severalfold. The cilia and the membranes of the cilia are composed of several different proteins. These proteins are receptor sites that bind the molecules to the cell to start the transduction process. In short, the initial step in odor perception appears to be when the olfactory molecule wends its way through the mucus and binds to a protein site on an olfactory cilium.

The application of odorant to the olfactory epithelium and the resulting binding of the stimulus molecule to cilia receptors initiate the chain of events leading to the generation of action potentials. To initiate these impulses, the olfactory receptors produce a graded receptor potential. At this time it is not clear whether the receptor potential is depolarizing or whether hyperpolarization also plays a role. Nevertheless, the receptor potential does occur when Na^+ and K^+ ions enter the cell through relatively nonspecific channels (Lancet, 1986). The Ca^{2+} ions have also been considered to be a necessary factor in the transduction process; however, their role is not completely understood. The manner in which the Na^+ and K^+ ions gain entrance is, however, usually not the direct result of an odorant molecule fitting in a receptor site in the cilium. In most cases, the stimulus molecule is considered the **first messenger** in a sequence of events leading to the receptor potential. Once the molecule has merged with the cilium receptor, a series of chemical reactions occur within the olfactory receptor itself. This reaction includes a second messenger. It is through the second messenger that the Na^+ and K^+ channels are opened and a receptor potential produced. You may recall that a second messenger refers to a chemical sequence within a cell. The second messenger carries the information necessary to open channels for the Na^+ and K^+. The second messenger reactions are not unique to the olfactory receptor; they also play a prominent role in the transduction process in vision and are involved in hormonal effects and the initiation of action potentials at synapses by some neurotransmitters.

The players in the game of olfactory transduction are the following:

1. the odor generating molecule (first messenger),
2. an enzyme in the cilium membrane named **adenylyl cyclase**,
3. an energy packet, **adenosine triphosphate (ATP)**,
4. the second messenger, **cyclic adenosine monophosphate (cAMP)** and **cyclic guanosine monophosphate (cGMP)**,
5. another protein in the membrane, **protein kinase**,
6. the nonselective ion channels for Na^+ and K^+,
7. another enzyme called **phosphodiesterase (PDE)**, and
8. an end product of the process called **adenosine monophosphate** (noncyclic).

The game is played this way. An odorant is inspired, the mucus assimilates the molecule, and contact is made with a cilium receptor. There may be an **olfactory binding protein** secreted in the mucus of the nasal cavity. Investigators have further hypothesized that the binding protein delivers the molecules to the receptors after binding with them. The olfactory binding protein can be viewed as a "packhorse" that retrieves, from the mucus, the molecules for binding at the cilia. The binding of the molecule with the receptor portion of the cilium's membrane results in the activation of the adenylyl cyclase enzyme within the cell membrane. When activated, the adenylyl cyclase converts the ATP energy packets to the second messenger, cAMP. The cAMP is chemically related to ATP and is called cyclic because the phosphate group that forms a cyclic ring with the carbon atoms. The important consequence of this chemical activity is the amount of cAMP synthesized. The enzyme adenylyl cyclase, once the single odorant molecule activates it, rapidly and continually initiates the synthesis of cAMP from ATP. The production of cAMP continues until the odorant molecule is no longer bound to the receptor. The ratio of cAMP to odorant molecules is estimated to be in the neighborhood of 1,000:1. Thus, the use of the second messenger insures amplification of the effect of the odorant molecule. This amplification allows animals, including humans, to receive an olfactory perception from very few odorant molecules. The cAMP, when manufactured at the urging of adenylyl cyclase, is "free floating" within the receptor cell until it binds with the protein kinase located on the inner portion of the cell membrane. The protein kinase functions as a Na^+/K^+ channel inhibitor when not bound with the cAMP molecule. When cAMP binds with the protein kinase, however, the protein kinase becomes active and changes the shape of the cell membrane. This change in membrane shape opens the channels for Na^+ and K^+ ions. Influx of these positively charged ions results in a receptor depolarization and the generation of action potentials at the axon hillock. The odorant molecule, when it breaks away from the receptor, stops further synthesis of cAMP. The enzyme phosphodiesterase rapidly inactivates the cAMP within the cell by changing the cAMP configuration to the noncyclic adenosine monophosphate. It is not entirely understood how the receptor returns to resting potential. However, that protein kinase returns to its inhibitory state when cAMP has been deactivated. This inhibitory state closes the channels used by Na^+ and K^+ and an active Na^+/K^+ pump returns the cell to its normal resting configuration. Figure 5.3 shows, diagrammatically, the sequence of events leading to the receptor potential. The electrotonic spread of the receptor potential reaches the soma of the olfactory receptor and the impulse generation occurs at the axon hillock of the axon if the receptor potential is strong enough.

cAMP is not the only possible second messenger. Other second messengers and binding proteins may be within the olfactory system. There are probably different second messengers in different animals, and these different second messengers, and their binding proteins, may respond to different odorants in different animals. In addition, it is also possible that one kind of odorant molecule can initiate activity in many different receptors and initiate different "odors" in different animals. This kind of complex interaction clearly suggests that the recognition and identification of odors is the result of a converging system of many on to few. Figure 5.4 illustrates this convergence and complexity. Note how a single olfactory cell can communicate with many cells in the olfactory bulb.

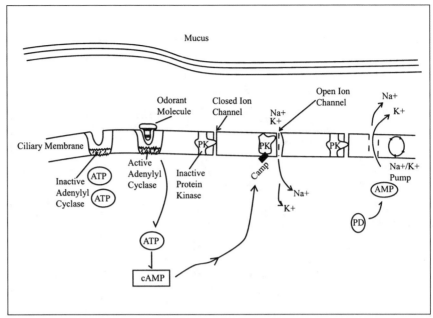

Figure 5.3. Olfactory Transduction

NOTE: The odorant molecule docks in the receptor site, adenylyl cyclase is activated, cAMP is formed from ATP, protein kinase is activated by the cAMP, and Na⁺ and K⁺ ions enter. When the odorant molecule breaks away from the receptor, PD changes cAMP into AMP and the ion channels close.

The Olfactory Bulb

We begin by noting that the olfactory bulb is partitioned in synaptic and nuclear regions. The synaptic region is the outer **plexiform layer.** The nuclear region is called nuclear because it contains the nuclei and cell bodies of neurons within the olfactory bulb. Although the olfactory bulb is not completely understood, the available data indicate that each bulb has at least four major types of cells. These cells are the **mitral, tufted, periglomerular,** and **granule.** In addition, there are a small number of fibers that come from the contralateral bulb. The interaction of these primary cells within the synaptic regions and the location of their cell bodies in the nuclear layer is our primary interest here. Figure 5.4 outlines this discussion.

The outer plexiform layer is our first stop. The axons of the olfactory receptors enter the olfactory bulb and infiltrate complexes called **glomeruli.** A glial sheath is formed around each glomerulus that acts to separate the contents of each glomerulus from neural elements within the bulb. Keep in mind that there are no cell bodies within the glomerulus. The olfactory axons enter

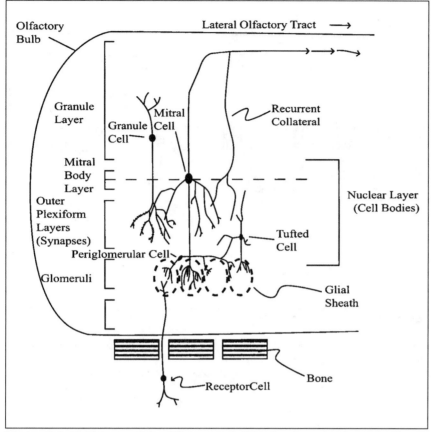

Figure 5.4. A Diagram of the Olfactory Bulb With the Granule, Outer Plexiform, and Nuclear Layers

NOTE: The tufted, mitral, periglomerular cells are also displayed.

the glomeruli, branch profusely, and synapse on the multitude of dendrites in the glomeruli that come from mitral and tufted cells. Investigators suggest that each glomerulus receives different odors (Benson et al., 1985; Shepherd, 1985). The mitral cells, incidentally, were named by a famous anatomist Santiago Ramon y Cajal in the late 1800s. He thought they looked like a Bishop's mitre headdress—hence their name. In addition to the axodendritic connections of the olfactory receptors to mitral and tufted cells, the latter cells also receive dendrodendritic synapses from the periglomerular (PG) and granule cells. At this point, you may note that, if dendrites only receive information from other cells, how can two dendrites communicate? This statement about the dendrodendritic synapse means that some dendrites, in contrast with the usual situation, must be structurally specialized to store and release transmitters. These profuse synaptic complexes form the many glomeruli and, as noted previously, form the outer plexiform layer of the olfactory bulb. The cell bodies of the periglomerular cells, like those of the mitral and tufted cells, lie in the nuclear layer. Each periglomerular cell sends its axon laterally from one glomerulus to another. The periglomerular cells appear to have neural modulatory effects on the inputs to the central olfactory bulb. The mitral and tufted cells, after receiving synaptic connections in the outer plexiform layer, send their myelinated axons laterally out of the olfactory bulb toward the next neural structure in the system. Finally, the granule cells make their contacts with the mitral cells and send their axons laterally in a manner similar to that of the periglomerular cells. The difference is that the granule cells make their connections and receive their inputs a little later in the flow of information. The effects of the granule cell lateral connections are similar to those of the periglomerular cells because they can modulate the incoming flow of activity.

The flow of neural activity within the olfactory bulb is extensive and entails both excitatory as well as inhibitory interactions. Activity is constantly arriving from multiple sources. There are fibers descending from higher central mechanisms as well as projections being received from the contralateral olfactory bulb. In this latter case, the projective path has been systematically studied and mapped. Perhaps one of the most well known projections is that which extends from one bulb to the other by way of the **anterior commissure.** The anterior commissure is, like all commissures, made up of a band of fibers. In this particular case, the anterior commissure has axons from the mitral and tufted cells that extend to areas in the contralateral olfactory bulb homotopic to the sending ipsilateral bulb. Projections go in both directions, and each fiber ends in a region that is homotopic to its origin. That is, the final destination of a fiber is in the same location as its origin, except the synapse is in the opposite bulb. The functional result is that one bulb can influence, directly, the processing of information from the other bulb. In addition, each bulb receives feedback from the contralateral bulb regarding the processing of olfactory inputs. This interaction within the olfactory bulbs, before conscious perception, probably yields blending or synthesis of neural activity from the two bulbs.

In summary, the olfactory bulb has an outer plexiform layer, the glomeruli. The glomeruli consist of synaptic connections among receptor axons and the dendrites of mitral, tufted, periglomerular, and granule cells. The periglomerulus and granule cells form synapses on the mitral and tufted cells. The mitral and tufted cells send their axons centrally to form the lateral olfactory tract leaving the bulb. There is a projection path through the anterior commissure that permits neural interactions between the olfactory bulbs.

Central Olfactory Structures

Figure 5.5 shows the central olfactory projections. The lateral olfactory tract leaves the olfactory bulb and converges on the **olfactory tubercle** and the **pyriform cortex.** In this latter case, the pyriform cortex is not to be confused with the neocortex covering the cerebral hemispheres. The pyriform cortex is a relatively small area of tissue lying at the end of the **hippocampus.** Once the information is received by the pyriform cortex and the olfactory tubercle, it is processed, synthesized, analyzed, and sent to other central mechanisms. The output of the olfactory tubercle extends to the medial dorsal portion of the thalamus. The final path is from the thalamus to the **orbitofrontal neocortex** located in the ventral portion of the frontal lobe.

The pyriform cortex has direct contact with portions of the **limbic system**—namely the **amygdala, entorhinal cortex, hypothalamus,** and the **hippocampus.** There is a parallel path from the lateral hypothalamus to the orbitofrontal neocortex.

It may be, but it is not certain, that conscious awareness of an odor molecule, for example, awareness of a skunk, first occurs in the pyriform cortex. Most likely, however, the perception of an odor requires processing beyond this stage to provide distinct behavioral effects and discrimination of one odor from another. Most of the data seem to indicate that the loss of the orbitofrontal neocortex eliminates the conscious perception of olfaction. Thus, neocortical activity appears to be required before we can identify and consciously recognize a smell. The direct involvement of the limbic system, however, also plays an important role in odor perception. It should be expected that when you consider the emotional, appetitive, and reproductive aspects of smell the limbic system is involved. Indeed, the limbic system makes up the emotional portions of the brain. So do not be surprised when your own memories of a romantic evening are triggered by the scent of a particular perfume or special cologne.

Although you may not believe it, the complexity of the connections within the olfactory bulb and the more central neural centers has been simplified in this presentation. The modulation of the olfactory code by multiple neural structures having enigmatic functions and mysterious interactions have just been touched on. Nevertheless, we have enough information at this point to examine the perceptions of odors. This is the topic of the rest of the chapter.

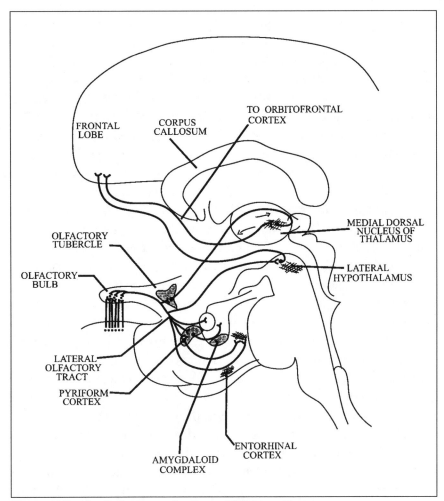

Figure 5.5. The Pathways to the Central Olfactory Centers

Olfactory Perception

Olfaction, from nares to neocortex, is a remarkable and complex system, and there are missing ingredients and many uncertainties in our knowledge of it. Before you started reading this chapter, however, you were not completely ignorant of the world of odor. If your olfactory system were functioning normally, you probably knew the smell of mint and the aroma of coffee. As you pass through life, you will find odors that will remind you of significant events from your past. Interestingly, those events are usually forgotten until a certain odor floats by and stimulates your limbic system and your long-term memory.

The conscious perception of an odor is not determined at the receptor level; rather, it is intimately entwined with cognition, emotion, and the higher-order processes of experience and memory. The perception of an odor, therefore, is rather unusual in the family of sensory systems. One of the more interesting phenomena about odor perception is that an odor can almost instantly key your memory to recall personal events and situations. The reverse, however, does not occur. That is, try as you may, you cannot voluntarily retrieve an odor from your memory. You could attempt right now, for example, to smell the aroma of an orange. You cannot image an odor. You no doubt have little trouble recognizing the odor of an orange if it were physically presented to you. However, unlike vision and hearing, it is not possible to produce, in your mind, the image of an odor. You can quite easily close your eyes and visualize a cool bubbling brook flowing through the canyon in the mountains or visualize the warm sandy beach and the white surf of the ocean. These visual images can be seen in your mind, even when they are not present; you extract and synthesize from visual memories to produce a visual image in your mind's eye. The perception of an odor can occur when there is a chemical stimulus present; however, when we attempt to image an odor that is not present, we have great difficulty. We just do not have a "mind's nose." This one-way path, in which a familiar odor summons a memory but a memory does not generate an odor, is a unique ingredient in the chemical senses in general. This one-way path also occurs in the sense of taste.

It is quite clear that the function of odor perception is to continually monitor the environment and categorize odors in one of two large categories—namely, approach or avoidance. If an odor is new and unfamiliar and is not immediately generalized as pleasant (flower or fruity), it is nearly always considered as unpleasant and placed in the avoidance classification. On the other hand, familiarity does not necessarily mean that there will be an approach to the source. If the odor has been associated with a stressful or unpleasant condition, the assignment of the odor, and the behavior of the organism, will no doubt be toward the negative or avoidance category. These two classes are clearly biologically relevant because we learn to either avoid or approach the source of an odor. Once an odor is detected, the environmental event becomes associated with the odor and is stored in memory. The association of an odor with an environmental event can occur almost instantly.

The reoccurrence of an odor, once it has been encoded, can reproduce, in some cases, the associated memory within milliseconds. This is true even when the memory has not been recalled for decades. The detection of an odor, however, does not always mean we can identify it. This is true even if we have experienced the odor previously and are familiar with it. Being familiar with an odor does not guarantee that we will be able to identify it and put the correct name or label to it.

Common everyday experience suggests that humans can recognize and identify thousands of odors. This folklore, however, is simply that—folklore. In contrast, the data suggest that our identification of odors, under controlled conditions, is quite limited. Estimates of the number of identifiable odors are in the range of 16 to 20. The identifiable odors vary with the individual. One of the large problems investigators have is that we have all had different experiences and associations. Thus, the assignment of an odor label to any particular odor is, to a great degree, very personal. In addition, the complex molecular structure of an odor very often defies a simple label. In addition, the same stimulus can elicit different odors and different labels, by different people. For example, some individuals, perhaps most, could consider the smell of a skunk to be rather aversive. There are, however individuals who find this odor more in the mild to pleasant category. The association of a skunk odor may retrieve fond memories of mountain retreats and autumn vacations. There is no guarantee, just as in the somatosensory system, that a given stimulus will produce a particular perception. The perception of an odor, any odor, is very complex. Odor memory is influenced by similarity, familiarity, memory cues, compatibility of stimuli when mixtures are blended, and a host of psychological factors.

If you pause for a moment, you will realize that the story concerning the perception of odors is not complete. There are many questions to be answered. For example, how many different odors are there? Is there a set of primary odors (Amoore, 1964, 1982)? Can you really cover up one odor with another odor? Is there an odor that can act as an aphrodisiac? Does the human body excrete an odor that another person finds sexually attractive? Does odor sensitivity vary as a function of the menstrual cycle? Do we smell pepper? Do we really need olfactory receptors to smell? Do we lose our sense of smell as we age? Why do some people claim, apparently honestly, not to smell an odor that others find to be overwhelmingly pungent? These last two questions bring up the question of dysfunctions and odor perception. There are difficulties, as you may surmise, in getting answers to these questions. However, we examine the status of each inquiry in the following sections.

How Many Odors Are There?

The answer to this question, although not completely satisfying, is relatively easy. No one knows, so the answer is almost anybody's guess, although an educated guess is that there are more than 400,000 odors that humans can

differentiate. Keep in mind that being able to differentiate one odor from another does not mean you can label or identify each odor. You can probably identify only 16 to 20 odors, but you can tell the difference between thousands.

There are a tremendous number of volatile chemicals that trigger an olfactory experience. Some of the substances are artificial and some occur naturally. Plastic has an odor and so does vinegar, dye used in new clothes, new
books, soap, musty rooms, different kinds of smoke (pipe, cigar, backyard
cookouts), and the "new car" smell. Coffee aroma itself is so complex that it
has over 500 volatile compounds. A list of molecular odors that humans detect is enormous. A compilation of all odors detected by animals and humans
is no doubt unattainable. The list gets larger each day as we mix, mold, pour,
and invent. In addition, there is the situation in which a chemical composition does not have an odor. Carbon monoxide, a poison gas discharged from
automobile exhausts and found in cigarettes, has no odor. The natural gas
used for heating and cooking is also odorless. Utility companies add an odor,
ethylmercaptan, to their product to provide an olfactory stimulus in the event
of gas leaks. This way the leak can be detected by the customer's ever so vigi-
lant nose. An unfortunate exception is the elderly nose. It sometimes has difficulties detecting even offensive aromas.

Are There Primary Odors?

Is there a set of primary odors? That is, can we find a finite number of
classifications in which odors may be placed? We usually assume, for example, that there are three primary colors: red, green, and blue (yellow is not a
primary). The question about odors, then, is similar. Is there a unique number of primary odors, and is there a way of getting some order out of the chaos
of literally thousands of smells? Perhaps.

As noted previously, the function of olfaction is to inform us about our
chemical environment. The simplest way to accomplish this task is to put
odors in one of two categories. These categories are avoidance and approach,
and they lie on a continuum. At one end is avoidance and at the other is approach. Assuming this is correct, investigations of odor have used a metric
scale that individual odors are rated on a scale of pleasantness ranging from
1 to 7. The scale is very subjective and depends significantly on the individual's history and interactions with odors. The scale, however, has been used
for decades. The 1 to 7 scale, known as a Likert scale, has been a familiar device
of psychology. The general result of such investigations has been disappoint-

ing. It appears that we and other animals have an ability to judge a multitude of odors on this scale. Other than pleasantness, however, the evidence does not support the conclusion that there is a set of primary odors. This situation does not prevent us from continuing our search for a reasonable group of primary odors; it has just made the puzzle more interesting.

Masking Odors

If you fail to take a bath after an afternoon jog, could you cover up your sweaty odor by adding cologne? The answer is not a simple one. An artificial odor, such as cologne, added to a strong malodor may increase the malodor rather than decrease it. There is no positive assurance, regardless of what the commercials tell you, that a perfume, cologne, or "lemon fresh" spray will make you or your home free from the odors of mildew, onions, cabbage, dirty diapers, or sweaty bodies. What is perfume and pleasant to one individual, one must remember, may be odoriferous to another. This is particularly true if the combined odor is one that is unfamiliar. As we have noted previously, unfamiliar odors tend to be classified in the avoidance and negative categories. It is possible, of course, to cover or mask one odor with another. If, however, the malodor one wishes to extinguish is strong, the solution to the problem sometimes becomes worse than the problem. This is because to remove the problem odor one must use an overpowering amount of the "fragrance" to clear the air. This self-defeating behavior often occurs when one odor combines with another to produce a formidable aroma.

Aphrodisiacs and Body Odors

There is strong and convincing evidence that animals have keen and sometimes permanent kinship recognition because of their ability to use unique odors. Recent data have suggested that human odors can have a significant effect on our behavior. A mother can recognize her own baby by smelling the child. Likewise, a baby can identify Mom by using his or her nose. We do use our olfactory system in unique ways. This does not mean, however, that humans use odor in their courtship behaviors. The billion-dollar industry in cologne and perfume clearly rejects the hypothesis that we are inert when it comes to examining the scent of individuals in our environment. What is meant here is that our normal body odors, excretions if you will, most likely do not act as aphrodisiacs or human pheromones. This does not imply that we have not searched for aphrodisiacs. The mass media often has stories about new and amazing chemical concoctions that lead to romantic evenings with a desirable mate. In view of all this, you must keep in mind that odor is directly affected by bacteria, diet, and even household surroundings. We carry our chemical environment with us—in and on our clothes, in our hair, and on our body. It is not just the individual's body odor that a Bloodhound uses to find a lost person. Rather, it is the most recent complexity of scents and odors combined. The clothing contains a multitude of odors that make up our "odor print." The emotional and soothing aspects of odors in our clothes can be found in everyday experiences. When a loved one has gone for a long period of time, the smell of that loved one's clothes can often bring a smile and a warm feeling. Indeed, it is common to find solace by sleeping with an article of clothing belonging to that absent person. The odor on the shirt can bring beautiful memories.

Another interesting phenomenon relates to data that associate a female's menstrual cycle with her ability to detect odors. Some of these studies have shown two interesting phenomena. First, odor sensitivity may be the highest (lowest threshold) during ovulation. Some investigations have also shown an increase in sensitivity during menses. The reason for this variation, it has been suggested, is that the olfactory epithelium changes during these two times in the woman's cycle. Another hypothesis for the increase in sensitivity is the normal variations in estrogen levels. Estrogen is highest just before ovulation. This does not, unfortunately, explain the higher sensitivity during menses.

There are two dilemmas with the experiments that study the relationship between odor sensitivity and the menstrual cycle. First, the studies, by necessity, use a small selected sample of odors for their independent variables. The investigators then assume that these few samples represent the vast population of odors we perceive. This assumption is not warranted. You have to be careful in generalizing from samples to populations of odors. Because you find a high sensitivity to one odor during the middle of the menstrual cycle does not imply that odor sensitivity is higher for the thousands of other odors the women perceive. Second, knowing at what point in the woman's cycle odor sensitivity changes is dependent on specific knowledge about the cycle itself. As many women will tell you, counting days or using basal body temperature to estimate exactly when ovulation occurs is not reliable. Thus, knowing the exact point in the cycle where changes in sensitivity occur, if they do, can be quite variable. Some studies have used blood samples to estimate the temporal location of sensitivity changes. This is an improvement in methodology. The first criticism regarding sample size, however, still limits our conclusions about the menstrual cycle and odor sensitivity in general. In summary, the data are interesting but not entirely decisive.

A second interesting finding is known as the **McClintock effect** (McClintock, 1971). This effect is the synchronization of menstrual cycles in women who live together. When women are placed within the same environment over a period of months, for example, roommates in college dormitories, their menstrual cycles begin at nearly the same time each month. When roommates first begin living together, their cycles are independent. After 3 or 4 months, however, menstrual cycles become synchronized. The reason for this synchronization is because the women are sensitive to and respond to each other's body odors. You should keep in mind, however, that these data do not necessarily apply to all roommates and women who live together. There are instances where menstrual cycles are not synchronized even when the women have lived together for years.

Do We Smell Pepper?

The idea that we can smell pepper or that it has an odor may at first appear to be rather ridiculous. It is the popular opinion, of course, that pepper has a taste rather than an odor. The situation regarding this spice, however, is more complex. A question about our ability to smell pepper does have a gram or so of reality to it.

Within the nose, mouth, and eyes there are sensory innervations, free nerve endings that respond to irritating chemicals. This sensory system has been labeled the common chemical sense and is innervated by the V cranial nerve, the trigeminal. The trigeminal has fibers that extend intranasally and intraorally. The sensations attributed to the V cranial nerve are those of somatosensory, pain, and temperature. In addition, these unmyelinated C and myelinated A-delta free nerve endings are also responsive to chemicals that arrive within the cavities of the nose, mouth, and eye. The general response of these free nerve endings, embedded within the epithelium of the oral and nasal cavities, is to initiate reflexive physiological behaviors. Nearly all chemical compounds will stimulate the trigeminal chemoreceptors (free nerve endings) if the concentration is strong enough. Based on the irritant qualities of the chemicals, five different stimulus groupings have been suggested: **pungent spices** (oral), **lacriminatories** (tearing of the eye), **sternutatories** (sneezing and nasal irritants), **suffocants,** and **skin irritants.**

Restricting our discussion now to the interaction of olfaction and the common chemical sense, the sternutatories, we find that there is a wide and diverse reaction to noxious chemicals. The response to an inhaled noxious stimulus is dependent on the stimulus strength. The response is reflexive, and evolution appears to have designed it to minimize the damaging effects of the event. The result may be a small sneeze or a sequence of events that may encompass the individual's entire behavior. A partial list of reflexes include bronchodilation and constriction, bradycardia, secretion of epinephrine, nasal secretions, tearing of the eyes, closure of the glottis and nares (in animals), peripheral vasoconstriction, and a decrease in respiration rate. Clearly, we respond to chemical irritants such as pepper. But are they smelled? This is the next question.

The odor of pepper is often overshadowed by a strong reflex. The usual report regarding odor is that a strong dose of pepper is more of a burning sensation than it is a smell. A very light whiff, however, does produce the herbal pepper odor. This response corresponds with taste perception. Pepper placed within the oral cavity results in a hot burning sensation. This pepper taste blends with the other flavors of our food.

Finally, we come to the question concerning interactions of the trigeminal nerve and the olfactory perceptions. This also incorporates the second question: Can we perceive an odor without olfactory receptors? The popular assumption is that no odor can be perceived if there is a lack of olfactory receptors. The reality of the situation, however, is that the trigeminal nerve endings embedded in the nasal epithelium, act as "odor receptors" and will respond to a large number of odorants. These odors, moreover, need not be intense to elicit a response from the trigeminal nerve. So to answer the question, we will sometimes perceive an odor when the trigeminal nerve is stimulated with an odorant. There is some question, however, as to whether the perception mediated by the trigeminal nerve yields the same odor as that produced by a functioning olfactory system.

When both the trigeminal and the olfactory systems are intact, as they are in most individuals, it is their interaction that appears to be important. The interaction is centrally mediated beyond the olfactory bulb. The interaction is reciprocal because they mutually inhibit each other. In other words, the nasal portion of the trigeminal nerve can inhibit olfactory activity and vice versa. In any event, there is an interaction of the two systems when they are both functional. The modulation of odors by the trigeminal nerve appears to be well established.

Dysfunctions

The loss of odor perception is often not even noticed. The sense of smell in humans is, according to popular opinion, both automatic and unremarkable. Thus, the value of odor perception is often downplayed. This is true even though each year over 400,000 Americans seek help for the loss of smell. The loss of odor perception, anosmia or "smell blindness," is often a difficult disorder to treat and diagnose (Getchell, Doty, Bartoshuk, & Snow, 1991). This is because the loss, unless clearly caused by a head trauma, is directly associated with the loss of taste and flavor appreciation as well as the possible olfactory dysfunctions. In addition, there is the problem of age-related loss of odor perception. The "normal" loss of smell as a function of age has been called **presbyosmia.**

How does one go about noticing that an individual has olfactory difficulties? Infants and children, for example, may be anosmic yet be unable to describe it or let us know of their deficit. This is because they very likely do not know that it is missing, and adults cannot detect their children's loss either. This contrasts vividly with visual or hearing deficits easily determined in young infants and children. The loss of odor perception is sometimes not detected by an individual until high school or beyond.

Some of the most common reasons for anosmia are infections, allergies, sinus problems, viruses, accidental trauma, and even iatrogenic insults by well-meaning physicians. The infections, allergies, sinus problems, and viruses all contribute to possible loss of odor perception by reducing airflow through the nasal passages, destruction of receptors, and in some rare cases the loss of neural paths and centers as a result of disease. The list of possible causes, not all verified by experimental evidence, have been classified in several categories and subclasses. Box 5.1 lists some of the possible causes for olfactory dysfunctions.

Some of the serious diseases that affect olfactory sensations are Korsakoff's syndrome, Alzheimer's disease, Parkinson's disease, Kallmann's syndrome, and Down's syndrome. There may, of course, be many others that are just as serious. Other examples are schizophrenia with olfactory hallucinations, amyotrophic lateral sclerosis, syphilis, cystic fibrosis, and lung cancer.

Korsakoff's syndrome is a loss that occurs because of alcoholism and malnutrition. Not only does the alcoholic have memory problems and the associated liver aliments, there is an associated loss of odor perception. The loss is the result of degenerations within the limbic system. The patient with Alz-

---

BOX 5.1

Some Causes of Olfactory Dysfunctions

Benign tumors intranasally
Benign tumors within the head
Cancers
Chemical pollutants in the air
Congenital and hereditary malformations
Drugs
Endocrine malfunctions
Head trauma
Infections
Lesions of the nose and airway
Medical intervention and surgery
Neurological diseases
Nutritional and metabolic disorders
Psychiatric
Viruses

---

heimer's disease is afflicted with the loss of smell presumably because of the degeneration of areas within the hippocampus and the amygdala. The individual with Parkinson's disease, in addition to the loss of motor control because of dopamine depletion, often suffers from olfactory dysfunctions. The cause of the odor perception loss is unknown. Down's syndrome, or Trisomy 21, is a genetic defect that causes a multitude of severe neural, intellectual, physical, and behavioral dysfunctions. One such dysfunction is often an olfactory deficit. Kallmann's syndrome results from a hormonal deficiency that retards genital development and produces anosmia.

The loss of odor perception because of trauma can occur when the olfactory receptors are injured and degenerate. This usually occurs when a blow to the head causes a shearing of the axons as they pass through the cribriform plate. The basal cells, if they survive, can replenish the system with olfactory receptors, and a partial recovery of odor perception can occur. However, if both the basal and olfactory receptor cells are damaged and degenerate, then a permanent loss in odor perception is quite probable.

Another cause for the loss of smell is medical insult or injury due to surgery on or through the nose. For example, plastic surgery to improve your physical appearance can, if the surgeon is not careful, result in the destruction of the delicate olfactory epithelium. The result is, of course, a good-looking nose that does not work. In addition, an operation on the pituitary gland can cause a loss of smell because the surgical procedure is through the nasal cavities.

Finally, we should remember that the olfactory system is unique and serves us well.

Suggested Readings

Brand, J., Teeter, J., Cagan, R., & Kare, M. (Eds.). (1989). *Chemical senses, vol. 1: Receptor events and transduction in taste and olfaction.* New York: Marcel Dekker.

Finger, T. F., Silver, W. L., & Restrepo, D. (2000). *The neurobiology of taste and smell* (2nd ed.). New York: Wiley-Liss.

Getchell, T. V., Doty, R. L., Bartoshuk, L. M., & Snow, J. B., Jr. (Eds.). (1991). *Smell and taste in health and disease.* New York: Raven Press.

Holden, C. (1996). Sex and olfaction. *Science, 273,* pp. 313.

Le Guerer, A. (1994). *Scent: The essential and mysterious powers of smell.* New York: Kodansha America.

Phillips, M. (1992, July). Breath tests in medicine. *Scientific American,* pp. 74-79.

Reed, R. R. (1990). How does the nose know? *Cell, 60,* 1-2.

Stoddart, D. M. (1990). *The scented ape: The biology and culture of human odor.* New York: Cambridge University Press.

CHAPTER 6

Gustation

A s you eat your breakfast, you may have wondered about the taste of a new cereal or the sweetness of strawberry jam. The gustatory delights in which we all partake are the result of the chemical molecules and their interactions with olfactory and gustatory receptors. We have discussed the olfactory system in the previous chapter. Now we direct our attention to another chemical sense. This one, gustation, is considered to be a lesser sensation to humans. It is not, however, any less important to us than olfaction (McLauglin & Margolskee, 1994). It happens that when we have **ageusia**, which means to have no sense of taste, we quickly discover the importance of gustation. We can also discover the usefulness of taste by studying it.

This chapter begins with an overview of the peripheral portion of the taste system. The periphery includes the oral cavity and the nerves that innervate the taste receptors. After we have examined these structures and functions, we expand our discussion to the more central portions of the nervous system and our cortex. The perception of taste and some of the dysfunctions of taste completes the chapter.

Peripheral Processes

We begin the discussion at the place you most expect, the oral cavity. Not only does the mouth provide us with a most useful orifice for communication, it also acts as the aperture through which our life's sustenance must pass. This latter function is of maximum importance in maintaining our everyday existence. There are, as we know, many substances we should not ingest. We must be careful of what we eat.

An important function of the gustatory sense is to act as a sentry to screen and clear the way for our nourishment. Taste provides a very unambiguous warning. Those substances that have a bad taste should not be eaten. Just as with the olfactory sense, if a piece of meat has bad taste, it probably is bad. Likewise, if we place an item in our mouth that has a bitter or unfamiliar flavor, we usually remove it immediately. Much like the olfactory sense, we approach and avoid foods based on how they taste.

The important structural components of the oral cavity, as far as gustation is concerned, consists of the following components:

1. the **tongue,**
2. the **soft palate** that separates the mouth from the nasal cavity,
3. a thin piece of cartilage behind the tongue, the **epiglottis,**
4. the **larynx** that forms the upper part of the trachea and contains the vocal cords, and
5. the pharynx that makes up the throat between the mouth and the esophagus (Figure 6.1).

Taste Buds and Papillae

The chemoreceptors for taste are organized within **taste buds** located on the dorsal surface of the tongue. Taste buds are, in turn, embedded within small bumps on the tongue called **papillae.** The number of chemoreceptors, or **taste receptors** within each taste bud is estimated to be between 1 and 40. Although the majority of the taste buds are found on the tongue, there are a significant number on other surfaces within the oral cavity. The taste buds that are not on the tongue are located on the surfaces of the epithelium.

Although three types of papillae have been identified and associated with taste, there is a fourth type of papillae, the filiform, which has no taste buds. This fourth type is located primarily in the center of the tongue. Figure 6.2 shows the distribution of the papillae on the human tongue. The papillae that have taste buds are the **fungiform, circumvallate** (also called **vallate**), and **foliate.** The fungiform papillae are found on the anterior two thirds of the tongue. The majority of the fungiform papillae are on the tip and one half of them have no taste buds at all. The foliate papillae are found along the lateral edges of the tongue and have significantly more taste buds than do the fungiform papillae. This means that the foliate papillae have the most taste buds and the most taste receptors. The circumvallate papillae are the fewest in

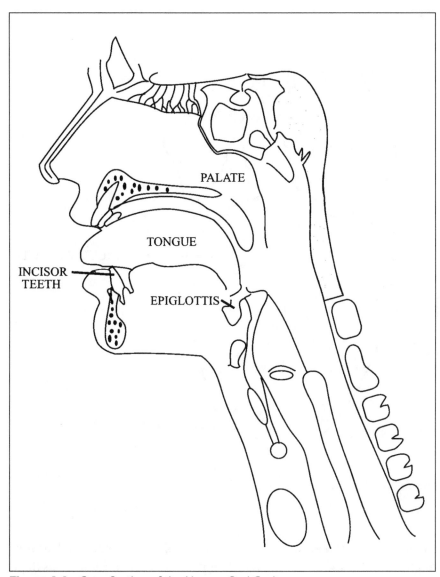

Figure 6.1. Cross Section of the Human Oral Cavity

number, about 8 to 12 in humans and, when viewed from above, form an inverted "V" on the back of the tongue. Although there are relatively few circumvallate papillae, they are larger than the other two forms. They have a characteristic mushroom shape and are seen easily in a mirror. Each circumvallate papilla is surrounded by a trench or circular sulcus. There are, in addition to the taste buds on the mushroom-shaped circumvallate

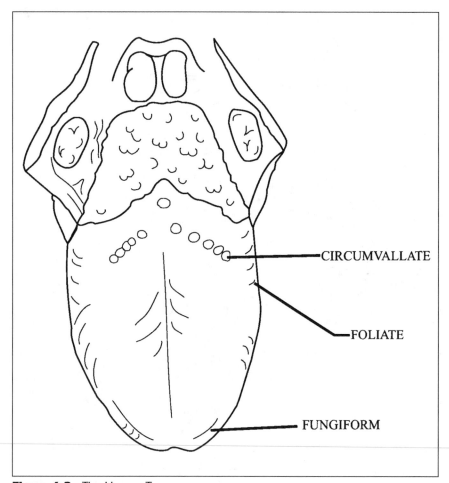

Figure 6.2. The Human Tongue

papillae, a significant number of taste buds within the circular sulcus surrounding each papilla. Although we do not know how many taste buds there are on the human circumvallate papillae, the rhesus monkey has twice as many taste buds on the circumvallate papillae as it does on the fungiform. More than likely, the human distribution of taste buds is similar. Figure 6.3 shows a schematic showing the general anatomy of a taste bud.

Innervation of Taste Buds

The wide distribution of taste buds suggests, as you may suspect, a rather extensive innervation pattern and more than one nerve. The innervation is, in fact, somewhat extended. The fungiform papillae, located on the anterior two

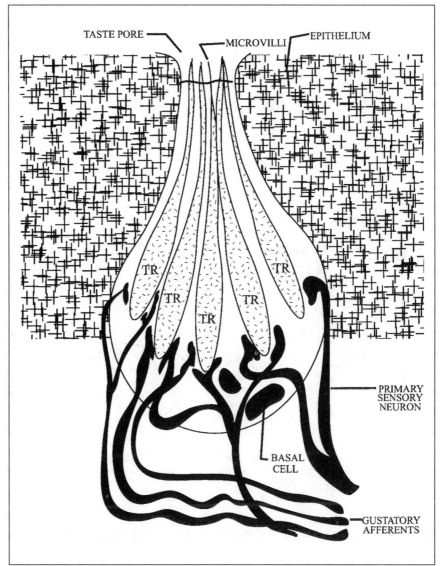

Figure 6.3. General Structure of the Taste Bud Showing the Taste Receptor and Basal Cell

thirds of the tongue, are innervated by the **chorda tympani,** a branch of the facial nerve. The anterior foliate papillae are also served by the chorda tympani. The posterior foliate papillae and the circumvallate papillae are, however, innervated by the **glossopharyngeal nerve,** the IX cranial nerve. A mix of the chorda tympani and the glossopharyngeal cranial nerves serves the soft palate, pharynx, larynx, and epiglottis. A branch of the X cranial nerve, the

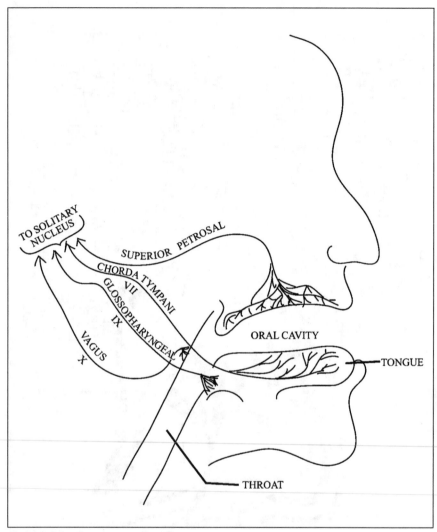

Figure 6.4. The Four Nerves That Innervate the Gustatory Sense in the Oral Cavity

vagus, also is involved. To help confuse the issue, a specific branch of the VII cranial nerve, the **superior petrosal,** serves the nonlingual structures (not the tongue). Figure 6.4 is a visualization of these innervations.

Saliva

Another important variable in gustation is the moisture within the oral cavity itself—saliva. The taste stimuli, most often food substances, that stimulate taste receptors are mixed with saliva during mastication. It is important that this blending occur because it is difficult to taste anything that is not in liquid form. The saliva acts as a solvent for the gustatory chemicals and provides a means of conveying the chemical taste stimuli to the receptors. The chewing and moving of the food substance is, therefore, an important part of the sequence of events leading to taste perception. Even at rest, when there are no externally provided chemical molecules, a covering of saliva bathes the receptor surface and the microvilli located on the taste receptor.

The saliva contains a mixture of electrolytes, glucose, and proteins. The electrolytes, Na^+, K^+, Ca^{2+}, Cl^-, and Mg^{2+}, act as conveyers or conductors of the electrical charge for taste receptor transduction and depolarization. The transduction occurs at the apical membrane of the taste receptor, most likely the microvilli. Microvilli are small extensions of the cell that, when viewed microscopically, appear as delicate "hairs" at the distal end of the taste receptor.

More is said about the transduction process later. The taste receptors are continually bathed in a solution of saliva and electrolytes. This means that if a taste experience is to occur, the stimulus strength must exceed the normal concentration of electrolytes found in the saliva. The saliva provides not only a conductor for the stimulus but a relatively constant baseline that all taste stimuli must exceed for a perception to occur.

Taste Receptors: Unique Cells

The diffusion of taste stimuli to the receptor cells, located within a taste bud, is the initial step in the transduction process. Because most of the taste stimuli are **hydrophilic,** or water soluble, the chemical is carried to the microvilli of the taste receptor. The typical taste receptor is broadly tuned so it responds to many different chemicals. The unique aspect about the taste receptor is that it not only generates a receptor potential but also produces an action potential. The reason why a sensory receptor should have to generate an action potential is not completely understood. One possible reason is that the Ca^{2+} channels, which initiate the release of the neurotransmitter, have a high threshold. The action potential may be required for the influx or movement of the Ca^{2+} to ensure a neurotransmitter release. The rapid voltage change, caused by an action potential but not a receptor potential, may be a key ingredient to the initiation of neurotransmitter release and the activation of the afferent fibers.

In any event, the receptors for taste differ from all other known sensory receptors. Taste receptors generate action potentials. The discovery in 1983 that taste receptors generate action potentials was made initially in frogs but has now been confirmed in other species, including mammals. The action potentials flow the length of the taste receptor, short though it may be, to initiate the release of the neurotransmitter packets into the synapse. The taste receptors are, in this sense, not just passive electrotonic conductors of receptor potentials.

The taste receptor cells, just like the olfactory receptors, show a well-established cycle of birth and death. The uniqueness of the regeneration of the olfactory receptor, which is really a neuron, was noted previously. The taste cells and taste buds are also novel. We have known for many years that taste buds degenerate when the nerve supply is interrupted. The degeneration of the taste buds, with their taste receptors, occurs when the chorda tympani or the glossopharyngeal nerves are severed. This result is not too surprising. The interesting aspect of the degeneration process is that it is reversible. The reinnervation is the result of the regrowth of the sensory nerves. It is one of the astounding features of the gustatory system.

Added to this interesting phenomenon is the continual replacement of the taste receptors within the taste buds during the lifetime of the organism. The half-life of a receptor is approximately 10 days in a rat and assumed to be roughly the same in humans (Bartoshuk, 1978; Pfaffmann, 1978b). The replenishment of the taste receptors differs from the process used in olfaction. In taste, epithelial cells migrate inward from the environment surrounding the taste buds and undergo mitotic division. The division produces basal cells. Then, as taste receptors die, the basal cells differentiate to become the taste receptors. The neural synapses at the base of each taste receptor are, consequently, in a continuous state of flux. As you read this, your old and dying receptors are being replaced with newly formed cells with vigorous new synapses. The continuous change makes you wonder how we taste anything at all.

Taste receptors possess several voltage dependent channels. The flow of the Na^+ and K^+ ions, through membrane channels, is the active ingredient in taste-cell action potentials. The action potentials, in turn, ensure the movement of the Ca^+ ions and the subsequent release of the neurotransmitter at the synapse. The manner in which the depolarization leading to the action potentials in taste receptors is generated is not completely understood. Some taste stimuli act directly on the receptor microvilli to initiate the depolarization of the cell, whereas others are indirect in their operation and use a second messenger.

You should keep in mind as we discuss the transduction mechanisms and the depolarization of the taste receptor that the final answers to the transduction question have yet to be found. Each taste receptor responds to a variety of different stimuli (Sato, 1980). That is, it appears that different stimuli can elicit different taste perceptions from the same receptor cell. This means that each taste receptor has more than one method of transducing stimuli. The sequence of events depends on both the particular stimulus and the taste receptor.

Transduction Mechanisms

The transduction of a chemical stimulus into an action potential begins at the apex of the taste receptor—the microvilli. The events initiated by a chemical stimulus immersed in saliva are classified, for the sake of simplicity, into three steps. There are small and important variations in the way that the steps are produced, but the three-step sequence is generally the same for all taste stimuli (Gilbertson, Damak, & Margolskee, 2000; Herness & Gilbertson, 1999; Kinnamon, 1988; Kinnamon & Cummings, 1992; Pfaffmann, 1978a). First, the receptor cell depolarizes because of the chemical stimulus. Second, the depolarization results in the generation of action potentials. An action potential you recall is due to an influx of Na^+ followed by an efflux of K^+. The flow of the action potential, over a very short distance, leads to the third step, the release of the neurotransmitter substance at the synapse. The neurotransmitter release is caused by Ca^{2+}. The Ca^{2+} initiates the movement of the vesicles containing the neurotransmitter to the receptor-cell membrane. The vesicles, once they blend and merge with the membrane, release their contents into the synaptic cleft. The afferent neuron then initiates impulses that travel to the brain stem. Figure 6.5 shows, diagrammatically, the general principles just described. The more specific transduction process, for different types of stimuli, is diagrammed in Figure 6.6 and discussed more fully in the following paragraphs.

Direct Entry

The most straightforward transduction process that you may envision is when a stimulus enters the receptor directly to initiate action potentials. This occurs when a chemical stimulus mixes with the saliva and enters the apical end of the taste receptor through an ion channel in the membrane of the microvilli. The entrance of the ions through the channel initiates the first step in transduction—the cell depolarization. The **direct entry** approach to trans-

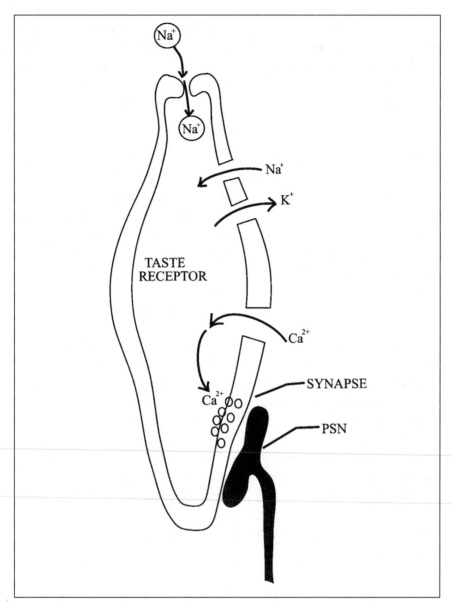

Figure 6.5. *General Principles of Taste Receptor Transduction*

duction occurs, for example, when the chemical stimulus is common table salt, NaCl. Once the stimulus is mixed with saliva, the Na^+ ion enters the cell and depolarization occurs. The action potential is generated and is almost instantly conducted to the basal end of the receptor. At this point, the action

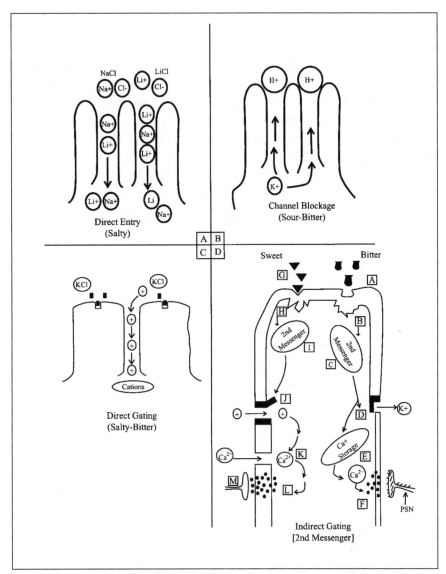

Figure 6.6. Four Modes of Transduction by the Receptor

NOTE: (A) direct entry, (B) channel blockage, (C) direct gating, and (D) indirect gating.

potential initiates the influx of Ca^{2+} and the subsequent release of the neurotransmitter. There is strong evidence that Li^+ uses the same Na^+ channels on the apical microvilli. These channels are involved, of course, in the transduction of salts. Figure 6.6(A) shows the sequence of events.

Channel Blockage

A second mechanism that induces depolarization, and the subsequent action potential within the receptor, is **channel blockage** of the K^+ channel at the apex of the receptor. It is hypothesized, and the evidence is quite strong in its favor, that sour-tasting weak acids initiate the transduction by blocking the K^+ channels with protons found in the stimuli. The K^+ channel is normally open and the K^+ within the cell continually diffuse outward. If the channel is blocked, however, the K^+ quickly accumulates within the cell and depolarizes it. Hydrogen ions (a proton) block the channel. The blocked current results in a membrane depolarization and an action potential. The hydrogen ions are directly related to weak acids. One such acid is the sour juice squeezed from the lemon.

The transduction process in which the K^+ channels are blocked is not restricted to the weak acids. Several investigations support the hypothesis that other substances can block the K^+ channel at the apex of the receptor and can lead to the initiation of the depolarizing event. Some of the substances are quinine, nicotine, and caffeine. These substances produce a bitter taste perception. It is clear that the chemical blockage of a K^+ channel does not automatically dictate the perception. A K^+ blockage can lead to sour or bitter as shown in Figure 6.6(B).

Direct Gating

A third method of initiating the transduction process is by way of a **direct-gating** process. For example, a molecule or ion associated with a stimulus may "dock" or become attached to the microvilli membrane near a Na^+ channel. This docking of the stimulus in close vicinity to the Na^+ channel is assumed to change the configuration of the microvilli membrane and open the gate for the Na^+ or other positively charged ions, cations. This process leads directly to the depolarization of the cell. This is a direct-gated initiation. The Na^+ channel, for example, is opened by the docking of a stimulus molecule onto the membrane of the microvilli. This sequence can be viewed as a "lock-and-key" kind of merging of a stimulus molecule with the membrane of the cell. The docking is assumed to directly change the membrane configuration so Na^+ ions can enter and initiate the depolarization and the transduction process as shown in Figure 6.6(C). The assumed tastes associated with this transduction mechanism are salty and bitter.

Indirect Gating

The fourth and final mechanism leading to transduction uses an indirect-gating process and implicates a second messenger. The initiating event in the chain leading to depolarization begins with the docking of a stimulus molecule and the subsequent change in the microvilli membrane. The docking indirectly opens other channels for ionic exchange by using the second messenger. The docking of different stimuli leads to different chemical reactions within the cell. A second messenger, for example, is called into action by the bitterest compound experienced by humans, denatonium chloride. The docking of the bitter substance (Point A in Figure 6.6[D]) is the initial step in the initiation of the second messenger. The docking of the molecule starts the process by transforming the membrane (Point B). The second messenger (Point C) blocks the K^+ channel (Point D) and depolarizes the taste cell. The depolarization yields an action potential and the release of intracellular Ca^{2+} (Point E). As is the case at presynaptic membranes, the Ca^{2+} is the trigger to release the neurotransmitter (Point F). In summary, experiments reveal that bitter substances initiate, indirectly, an increase in the intracellular Ca^{2+} by means of the second messenger. The eventual release of Ca^{2+}, stored within the receptor itself, initiates the activity in the primary sensory neuron. The specific second messengers involved with bitter are hypothesized to be cAMP (cyclic adenosine monophosphate) and IP^3 (inositol triphosphate). This sequence of events, for the indirect gating by a bitter compound, can be traced in Figure 6.6(d) by following the capitalized letters from A to F.

The transduction process for sweet compounds also suggests indirect transduction mechanisms and the involvement of the same second messengers active in the perception of bitter. The cAMP is the second messenger involved when the stimulus is a natural sweetener (for example, sugar). In contrast, IP^3 has been associated with artificial sweeteners. Understanding of the two processes is not yet complete. The transduction process involved for these two second messengers is, however, different for the sweet stimuli. Figure 6.6(d) shows the two primary differences in the sweet transduction. The indirect gating by the sweet compounds (Point G) changes the membrane (Point H) and affects a second messenger (Point I). The first difference from the bitter sequence occurs with the second messenger. In the sweet case, the second messenger opens channels to cations (Point J) rather than closing the K^+ channels. The influx of cations depolarizes the receptor cell for sweet substances. The cell depolarization leads, as usual, to action potentials and an increased amount of Ca^{2+} within the receptor. The second difference occurs at this point. The increase in Ca^{2+} is due to the action potentials opening Ca^{2+} channels (Point K) in the membrane of the receptor cell. There is an influx of Ca^{2+} and the subsequent release of neurotransmitter by the vesicles (Point L).

In summary, the second messengers, in the case of the sweet substances, are initiated by the docking of the stimulus with the microvilli membrane in a manner analogous to that with the bitter substance. This transduction sequence begun with the sweet molecular docking can be followed in Figure 6.6 (d) using the sequence G, H, I, J, K, and L.

The taste receptor activated by a sweet substance is also the same receptor that is activated by the bitterest substance known to the human tongue. In addition, there is no reason why each taste receptor cannot also respond to sour and salty. Each receptor has the ability to respond to these substances. The perception of taste, clearly, is complex. You cannot make good predictions about a taste perception based on knowing the transduction mechanisms or by knowing the molecular structure of the stimulus.

In summary, as Figure 6.6 shows, there are at least four different approaches to the transduction of chemical stimuli into neural activity. These four approaches are the following:

1. Direct entry—ions from the chemical stimulus enter the receptor directly through channels in the membrane of the microvilli. The result is a depolarization and the initiation of action potentials.

2. Channel blockage—the stimulus substance blocks K^+ channels at the apical membrane of the receptor and results in the depolarization of the cell and subsequent action potential generation.

3. Direct gating—a "lock-and-key" blending of the stimulus and membrane occurs on the microvilli to open cation channels for cell depolarization.

4. Indirect gating—a stimulus binds with proteins within the membrane of the microvilli. The binding then energizes second messengers that, indirectly, depolarize the cell and initiate the action potentials.

Central Processes

The pathways from the peripheral taste receptors to central mechanisms have had a history of difficulties for over a century. The determination of the "correct" pathway has been elusive. The pathways that have the least controversy, based on experimental data and clinical observations of human frailties, are the first-order nerves. They all make their final synaptic termination in the **nucleus** of the solitary tract within the brain stem. The next most recognized path, supported by data, extends from the nucleus of the solitary tract to the ventral basal medial nucleus in the thalamus. There is considerable controversy and uncertainty regarding the remaining pathways. That is, the clinical and experimental data are not conclusive when it comes to determining whether fibers from the oral cavity project ipsilaterally or contralaterally.

The situation becomes more complex because neurons within the ventral basal medial portion of the thalamus respond to a variety of sensory inputs. There are oral somatosensory axons as well as thermal fibers that terminate within the ventral basal nucleus center. Several investigators have discounted the idea that the ventral basal medial portion of the thalamus is restricted to gustation. This complexity continues when you attempt to track the flow of gustatory information to the cortex.

The cortical projections from the ventral basal medial area of the thalamus are presumed, at this time, to reach the cortex and terminate in more than a single area. Just as in the thalamus, there does not appear to be a single cortical area that is restricted to the gustatory sense. The projections shown in Figure 6.7 are, therefore, somewhat uncertain. Some of the clinical data from humans make the uncertainty even more indefinite by suggesting that cortical dysfunctions rarely produce gustatory impairment. These data are in direct contrast to the electrical stimulation data reported by Penfield and Rasmussen (1950) Their data suggest that some epileptic patients have strong gustatory bitter auras just before a severe seizure and the auras can be electrically elicited.

Nevertheless, the fibers from the thalamic regions appear to be ipsilateral in their projections and, based on data from the Old World monkeys, appear to terminate primarily within the **anterior insula-operculum.** Figure 6.7 shows this area of the cortex. The insula-operculum forms the floor of the lateral sulcus. The insula is within the fissure, and the cerebrum overlaying the insula is the operculum. Finally, you should keep in mind that these cortical areas also contain neurons that are responsive to other sensory modalities and, as noted previously, there are other cortical areas that respond to gustatory stimulation.

Taste Perception

The search for an understanding of human gustatory delights has been a difficult and onerous endeavor. It continues to be an arduous and enthralling

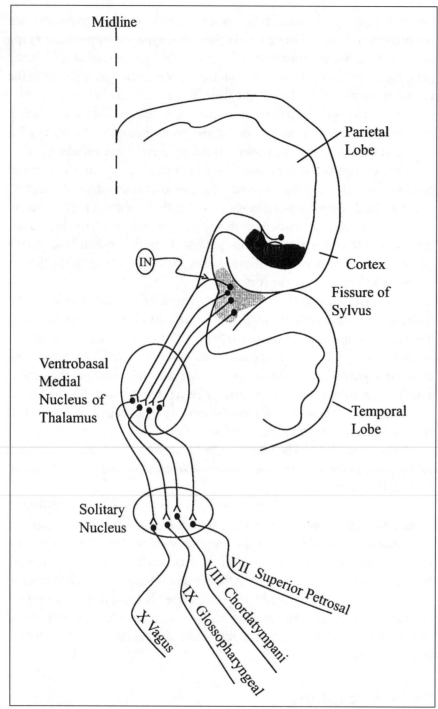

Figure 6.7. Gustation Central Projections

mystery. The reasons for the elusiveness of factual and reliable data have been alluded to in the previous pages. We begin this portion of the chapter by mentioning a few of the difficulties that surround the gustatory sense and then examining some plausible answers to some of the vexing problems.

The idea of using *taste* to mean a separate entity or sensory quality sounds quite practical. There is, however, some concern when taste is closely examined. How does taste, for example, differ from flavor? Is *taste* different from, the same as, or just similar to *savory*? These semantic difficulties are avoided here by assuming that when we speak of taste perception, we are referring specifically to the sensation that results from the sensory apparatus in the mouth and throat. Flavors and savory perceptions of food are much more complex and are discussed later.

Another problem is whether there is a lawful and reliable relationship between **sapid** stimuli, stimuli that lead to sensory activity, and the perceptions they produce. The answer to this problem appears simple and may be found in the domain of psychophysics.

You might think that the generation of input-output functions shows the relationship between the stimulus and response. The input in these functions is the stimulus, and the output is a behavioral response. The question is not simple, however, because of the difficulty in controlling and specifying the stimulus. This is, to a degree, the same kind of problem we encountered with olfaction, somesthesis, and pain. In the laboratory, a large number of different, yet relatively simple, molecular structures yield similar taste responses. In addition, the sapid substances in the real world are rarely found to be as simple as those used in the laboratory. The universe is not as controlled and uncomplicated as the scientist's laboratory environment. A serious difficulty, then, has been the specification of the stimulus. You simply cannot specify a turkey or yam stimulus and know its molecular structure. More easily controlled compounds, such as NaCl, common table salt, are often used. Generalizations about the gustatory process are then hypothesized. This approach is more molecular than that found in nature, but it has yielded significant and interesting data.

Previous discussions concerning receptor transduction provided a clue to the difficulty involved in delineating taste specificity. The classical approach to perception, the specificity (doctrine of specific nerve energies) approach, has not proven to be realistic with gustation. As was noted, each taste receptor can be depolarized by a variety of different stimuli. As a result, it is possible that a multitude of different stimuli may elicit different taste perceptions from the same receptor. The uncomplicated approach to gustatory perception, based on a labeled line theory in which each particular taste has a specific receptor or fiber to the brain, appears to be unfeasible. The situation is not completely bleak, however. There are data available that suggest that some classes of gustatory stimuli, if not all, do indeed follow an invariable pattern and yield reliably consistent taste perceptions. The data suggest, further, that there may be primary taste qualities. These data, and the pattern theory approach, are examined in the following paragraphs.

Primary Tastes

The general definition of a primary taste is a taste that, when it is perceived, is unlike any other. It is unique when appraised and cannot be perceptually analyzed into other taste qualities. In this regard, the physiological data from the experimental animal literature and the subjective testimony of humans have supported the idea of four primary taste qualities. The idea that there may be four primary taste qualities has been around, it appears, since Aristotle. The number of primaries has changed and varied over time, but we keep returning to the four basics. The most likely primary tastes are salty, sour, sweet, and bitter. A relatively recent addition to this list, one that is gathering some support, was originally suggested in the early part of the 20th century. This new taste is **umami.** These four classic qualities, plus umami, are discussed next.

Some investigators have insisted that primary tastes, should they exist, must meet some rather stringent criteria. The idea was that primary tastes should differ from each other on at least one of the following criteria. Each quality or primary taste must have (a) an unique chemical structure, (b) a specific receptor or neural pathway, (c) an unique neural center, or (d) a separate cortical area. This physiological approach to the search for primary tastes is severely limiting. It eliminates the salient point that taste perception is, by definition, a personal and subjective evaluation of the chemical world. Perception is, as always, the result of a neural system that transduces, analyzes, synthesizes, conducts, inhibits, excites, and personalizes the environment. If, however, a particular taste percept could be found to depend on a particular receptor, chemical structure, pathway, or cortical structure, the problem of understanding taste perception becomes much simpler. Fortunately, there is some support for the idea that a relationship does exist between perception and physiology.

Adaptation and Cross-Adaptation

If you were to arrange to have a concentrated salt solution, NaCl, flow continuously across your tongue, the initial taste would be strong and salty. After a few seconds, however, the saltiness fades and disappears. The taste, when it has disappeared, is said to have adapted. There is no longer a taste if there is no change in the stimulus. The phenomenon of adaptation is not new to us in our discussion of the sensory systems. We found that the somatosensory system had receptors that adapted. Some receptors, Merkel's discs for example, were slow to adapt whereas others, Meissner's corpuscles, were fast. It is not surprising, then, for you to taste NaCl again, without rinsing your mouth with tasteless water, if the salt concentration is increased so it exceeds the original solution. Keep in mind that this experiment is stimulating many taste buds and, consequently, many taste receptors. The extrapolation from this experiment to the single receptor cell, for example, is tenuous and perhaps not appropriate. Nevertheless, this experiment does lead to interesting results at the behavioral level.

If a different salt, lithium chloride, LiCl, were to flow across the exact same area of your tongue, after you had adapted to NaCl, what would you experience? The answer is that you would not taste LiCl either. This failure to taste one stimulus after being adapted by another, is called **cross-adaptation.** If you had not been adapted to the NaCl, however, you would have immediately tasted the LiCl.

In summary, if you adapt your tongue to the original NaCl stimulus, you will fail to respond to NaCl and LiCl unless they are presented at higher concentrations. When adaptation to one stimulus affects the perception of another stimulus within the same class, cross-adaptation has occurred.

Consider another adaptation study. What would you predict if you were to adapt a participant with the salty taste of NaCl and then stimulate the participant with a sour-tasting substance such as lemon juice? Could the lemon juice and salty taste cross adapt? That is, would the participant's adaptation to salt result in the report of not tasting the sour lemon? The answer is no. The participant would taste the lemon. There is no cross-adaptation between these two taste classifications, salty and sour.

Now consider a different situation. If you were to first adapt your participant to the sour lemon juice and then test for cross-adaptation with another sour taste, say lime juice, would cross-adaptation occur? That is, would your participant taste the sour lime after adapting to the sour lemon? The answer is no. Keep in mind, of course, that you must not activate other unadapted receptors. In addition, these two sour substances are quite complex chemically, so we are making an assumption here that they both belong to the same class regardless of their composition. This assumption, in a gustatory laboratory, is probably not acceptable science. Nevertheless, the point can be made with the example: Cross-adaptation occurs among similar substances or taste qualities. If they are both salty or both sour, then there is cross-adaptation. It appears that most members of a particular taste class can cross-adapt other members of the same class. There is no cross-adaptation, however, between different classes of taste stimuli such as salty and sour.

The phenomenon of cross-adaptation can be generalized at this point to fit the four primary tastes of salty, sour, sweet, and bitter. None of these four classes of taste can cross adapt each another. This failure to cross-adapt, between classes, suggests that there are different physiological mechanisms underlying the processing of these tastes. It also suggests that these four tastes are primaries. They are unique.

There are, however, some difficulties that need to be mentioned. As noted previously, most salt and sour substances cross-adapt within their own taste classification. There are some exceptions. Cross-adaptation does not occur for all the bitter and sweet substances. There are some bitter substances that you can still taste even after adapting to a previous bitter stimulus. This is true for sweet as well. Adapting to a sweet substance does not necessarily mean that your taste for a different sweet stimulus disappears. Thus, at this point it appears that the cross-adaptation studies support a common mechanism for many salt and sour tastes but suggest multiple processes for the sweet and bitter perceptions. Given these cross-adaptation effects, can the data be explained using some of the known physiology of taste? The answer is yes in some ways and maybe in others. Let us look at one possible interpretation. We begin by assuming that the molecules in the salt-adapting solution, Na^+ for example, affect the taste receptor membrane as they enter the cell. That is, the microvilli of the taste cell adapt or change physically because of the entering Na^+. This seems to be a reasonable possibility in view of the known changes that occur at synaptic membranes when they are activated by chemical neurotransmitters. The next step is to assume that the entering Na^+ initiates the normal depolarization of the receptor. Action potentials are then generated in the receptor cell, the neurotransmitter is released, and action potentials are generated in the primary sensory neuron. This also seems to be reasonable. If the stimulus, NaCl, remains at a constant intensity, the receptor membrane quickly begins to change its physical configuration due to the continual interaction with the chemical stimulus. The change in membrane configuration is assumed to close the ion channels that lead to the depolarization of the receptor. The closure effectively increases the receptor's threshold to the stimulus. An increased threshold makes it more difficult for the stimulus to activate the receptor and initiate action potentials. The final assumption is that, if the receptor threshold is raised by the presence of a constant stimulus, it requires a more intense stimulus to exceed the threshold and reinitiate activity in the receptor cell. All of this seems plausible.

Now, consider what happens if another salt, LiCl, having the same strength as the original NaCl, is introduced following adaptation to NaCl. The LiCl cannot initiate receptor activity either, if the new stimulus, LiCl, uses the same receptor channels as the original adapting salt, NaCl. That is, LiCl could not initiate receptor activity because the channels it uses to depolarize the cell have been closed by the previous actions of NaCl. To overcome the channel closure and the increased threshold, a more potent salt stimulus is necessary. On the other hand, if a sweet, bitter, or sour stimulus happened to occur, the closed channels for salt is irrelevant. These other classes of taste use different mechanisms to transduce the chemical stimulus into nervous activity. Thus, the new stimulus activates the taste receptors and causes a new taste percept.

In sum, the data show that most salty and sour-tasting stimuli can cross-adapt within their classifications; this is assumed to occur because they use the same processes for transduction. Stimuli in different classifications do not cross-adapt because they apparently use different transduction processes.

Based on the cross-adaptation studies and the previously discussed mechanisms concerning the methods of transduction, it is possible to conclude that direct entry and channel blockage are involved in the perception of salty and sour. The two transduction processes using second messengers in indirect gating appear to be the most likely candidates for the initiation of the perceptions of sweet and bitter.

Before we continue with other items of interest in taste perception, a few words need be said about the possibility of primary tastes other than these classic four. Over the decades, several candidates have been proposed. Some of these were putrid, acrid, insipid, rough, spirituous, aromatic, starchiness, and even alkaline and metallic. Then, of course, there is the aforementioned umami, which means savoriness. With the exception of umami, the majority of these suggested tastes have lost their appeal as well as their supporting data. We look briefly at the new candidate: umami.

Umami originated from a glutamate derived from seaweed. The chemical substance is commonly known as MSG, monosodium glutamate, and, by itself, has no odor and an unusual taste that is approximated, so they say, by appropriate combinations of the four primary taste qualities. Whether umami is a result of the unique combination of the four tastes or an independent classification of its own is open to debate.

The characteristic use of MSG is to impart a flavor and savoriness to our food. It is similar to other chemicals used as a flavor enhancer. Behavioral experiments on humans and electrophysiological tests with animals have yielded supporting data that the chemical MSG may be unique from the other four primaries. The process by which it generates the action potentials in the receptors and how it is coded within the taste system is unknown.

The research on the chemical compound MSG, and similar derivatives, continues. To give you an idea of the taste of umami, the German word *vollmundigkeit,* meaning "mouthfullness," appears to many humans to communicate the subjective taste of these substances when dissolved in distilled water. The "mouthfullness" reportedly changes after a few moments. Sometimes the perception changes to salty, and other times it may be reported as a light sweetness. If you are not allergic to MSG, you may wish to try this yourself. The substance is readily available at food markets as a food additive and is commonly added to Asian cuisine.

The Tongue as a Taste Map

The location of the papillae and taste buds throughout the oral cavity has been used, in the past, as a means of support for the specificity approach to taste perception. If the four classical tastes could be associated with different and distinct areas of the tongue, for example, then the simple conclusion could be drawn that there was a "labeled-line" system for the sense of taste. Many texts outline the idea of the taste system quite simply. They have shown that the fungiform papillae on the tip of the tongue were most sensitive to sweet, and the foliate and fungiform papillae, along the anterior and posterior sides of the tongue, were most sensitive to salty and sour. Bitter sensitivity was relegated to the rear of the tongue and the circumvallate papillae. If "most sensitive" could be interpreted as "taste restricted to," then this scheme could be interpreted as a labeled-line system. In other words, if the specialized spatial location idea were correct, you could say, for example, that stimulation of the tip of the tongue produces the perception of sweet and the information is carried to the brain by the chorda tympani. The real situation, unfortunately, is not this way. There are no specialized areas where sweet occurs only at the tip, salty and sour only on the sides, and bitter only at the rear. Such a map is incorrect. This latter situation is probably clear to you based on the discussions about receptor transduction. It should be evident that if you were to stimulate the tip with a moderately intense stimulus you could produce any of the four primary tastes. This also holds for the nonlingual areas of the oral cavity. Taste is not spatially mapped within the oral cavity in accordance to the primary tastes. The data showing the tongue map and its sensitivity, however, does appear to be true. The tongue does have the lowest thresholds, highest sensitivity, for specific taste stimuli at particular locations on the tongue—sweet at the tip, and so on. The misinterpretation of these data has led to erroneous statements concerning the taste system in general.

Taste Coding

The taste system does not appear to have strong a database supporting the labeled-line or specificity theory. For example, there are no firm cortical areas for gustation and the taste receptors respond to a variety of different chemicals. If this is the case, how do we actually differentiate one burst of neural activity from another? That is, when the receptors transduce a stimulus and afferent impulses are forwarded centrally, does it mean that the initial stimulus was bitter, sour, salty, or sweet? The reasonable conclusion, at this point, is that there is a pattern of activity sent to the nervous system from the peripheral stimulation. The pattern itself is interpreted as a particular taste perception.

The appeal of the pattern theory comes from several sources. The first, as noted before, is that the receptors themselves appear to be quite willing to transduce a multitude of different stimuli. Their response characteristics, in other words, are quite broad and nonspecific. Second, the usual situation in taste is that stimulation is not restricted to a small portion of the oral cavity. The movement and chewing of food items is very much a part of our everyday experience. This means that the overall pattern and barrage of action potentials received by higher neural centers very likely play a significant role in taste perception. We review, briefly, some of the data supporting the pattern theory of taste perception.

The pattern theory implies that each fiber or neuron responds to the stimulus. Furthermore, if the activity of each neuron were recorded, the pattern (relative spike counts) of activity across the different fibers would vary as a function of the eliciting stimulus. That is, the pattern or relative response magnitude across different neurons is different for KCl and NaCl because they elicit different salty taste perceptions. On the other hand, for the same neurons, the pattern of neural activity is expected to be the same, or highly correlated, when the stimuli are NaCl and LiCl because they elicit similar salty tastes. Similar perceptions should yield, according to the pattern theory, similar neural activity across sensory fibers. Different neural activity patterns mean different perceptions; the same patterns mean similar perceptions.

This type of rationale is supported experimentally by recording the activity pattern from many neurons in the nucleus of the solitary tract and obtaining behavioral taste preferences from the animals. The experiments used taste-avoidance conditioning. Animals trained to avoid LiCl, behaviorally, also avoided NaCl. Furthermore, animals that were trained to avoid KCl did not avoid NaCl. This suggests that the LiCl and NaCl tasted similar and the KCl and NaCl had different tastes. Analysis of the neural patterns produced by these stimuli revealed that the KCl and NaCl patterns were poorly correlated and the LiCl and NaCl patterns were highly correlated. Figure 6.8 reflects the correlation of the neural activity. The NaCl and LiCl stimuli produce highly similar neural patterns, and they produce the same behavioral response. Furthermore, the different neural patterns produced by NaCl and KCl generate different behavioral responses. These data clearly support the pattern theory of taste perception.

Additional data, based on similar electrophysiological experiments and behavioral investigations, show that correlated neural-response patterns produce long reaction times. For example, when animals are required to choose the correct stimulus in a two-alternative forced-choice task, their reaction time is slower when similar neural patterns yield similar tastes. If the two stimuli to be discriminated are not similar, they show different neural-response patterns and the reaction times are fast. The fast reaction times are presumably because the animal can easily differentiate the two stimuli. Finally, taste stimuli that have highly correlated neural patterns also show cross-adaptation.

In sum, the perception of taste appears to be based primarily on the pattern of the neural activity that reaches the central mechanisms. The overall number of impulses and the total barrage of activity create the percept of taste magnitude. This suggests that the more neural activity there is, the sweeter the chocolate cake.

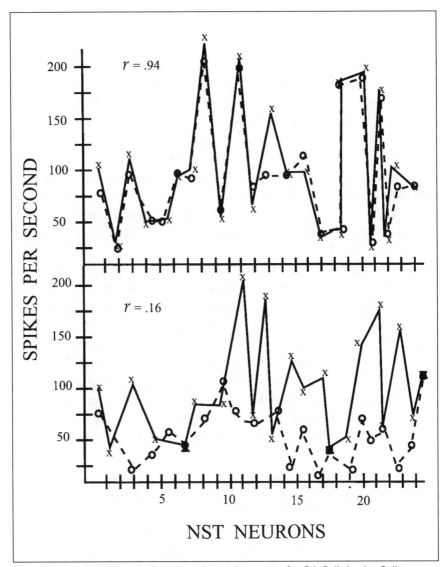

Figure 6.8. Data That Reflect the Neural Response for 24 Cells in the Solitary Nucleus

NOTE: The parameters represent three different salts, LiCl, NaCl, and KCl. The top panel shows a correlation of 0.94 across the pattern of 24 neurons when the stimuli are LiCl and NaCl. The bottom panel reflects a correlation of .16 between the neural patterns when the stimuli are KCl and NaCl. These data, in conjunction with behavioral avoidance conditioning studies, suggest that the perception of taste is dependent on the pattern of neural activity arriving at higher neural centers.

The Hedonics

So, let us get down to answering the question on everyone's mind. Where does the gourmet flavor come from if there are only four or maybe five primary tastes? Do we really combine these primaries to obtain the complex tastes of ravioli, turkey, homemade brews, rhubarb pie, and chocolate cake?

There are things that enter into the flavors we perceive that go beyond the gustatory sense. As you may suspect by now, the dinner prepared by the chef does indeed present an interesting taste dilemma. Not only does the color of the food affect flavor, so does texture, aroma, expectations, temperature, and even your hunger. We briefly touch on a few of these influences on the initial judgment of food flavor.

The color of food is important. There have been a few studies that have investigated the effect of color on savoriness. The most reliable result, when it comes to color, is the idea of visual capture. That is, our taste judgments are very much captured by the visual system. When there is a discrepancy between different sensory modalities, one of the two senses involved usually predominates over the other. This is called **capture.** In this case, we find visual capture occurring most frequently. The taste, and even the smell, is often relegated to secondary status when the colors do not fit the expectations. Individuals complain about the off-flavor, and even feel ill after ingesting something that was "just not right." The complaints are really right on the mark when it comes to ill-colored food.

The texture of the food also has an effect on the flavor and "goodness" of the taste. If you are being served mashed potatoes and there are lumps in it, you notice right away. The texture of the meat, crispness of bacon, celery, carrots, and the smoothness of the grape all enter into your expectations of the taste and the hedonistic evaluation of what you are eating.

Aroma is often the primary role player in the foods we eat (Mozell, Smith, Smith, Sullivan, & Swender, 1969). This is true even though we most often give the credit to our taste receptors. The loss of food taste with the onset of a cold is ample evidence of odor's role in the appreciation of food. Without the sense of smell, we have been told often that we could not differentiate the bite of a crisp apple from that of an onion. This appears to be true rather than false.

Have you ever taken a sip of a cold cup of coffee when you expected it to be warm? Perhaps a hot piece of corn on the cob is better than the one from the refrigerator. The temperature of the food also affects the flavor. The temperature of a steak, hot and right off the grill, differs significantly in taste from a piece of leftover steak.

There is another interesting phenomenon we should consider. Assume, for example, that tomorrow morning at breakfast you take a drink of freshly squeezed orange juice just before you dig into a stack of pancakes with blueberry syrup. After eating a few bites of pancakes, you then pick up your orange juice and take another sip. The orange juice tastes sour this time, not sweet. What happened here? The answer is that the pancakes and blueberry syrup have acted to adapt your taste receptors. So, when you taste the orange juice a second time, the sweetness in the beverage was not potent enough to overcome the raised threshold for sweet. The orange juice is perceived as sour because the "other molecules" in the juice are perceived as sour. The sweetness of the juice is still in the juice, you just cannot perceive it because of the adapted receptors. You taste what is leftover after the sweet is ignored. What is left is sour.

Finally, we consider the way that chemicals are placed in the oral cavity and what happens once they are there. The reason we put something in our mouth, usually, is for its ingestion. This means that it must be chewed, mixed with saliva, and moved around during the process of ingestion. The taste buds, taste receptors, and the trigeminal nerve endings all get into the act. The pattern of activity is affected by the number of receptors involved and the interactions with all our chemical senses—olfactory, trigeminal, somatosensory, pain, and taste—all of which enter into the process we end up calling flavor.

Dysfunctions

The sense of smell can be the most debilitating dysfunction of the three chemical senses, including in this category the trigeminal system. However, the loss of taste can create, in some instances, very distressing situations (Getchell et al., 1991; Miller, 1989; Rozin, 1990). Perhaps one of the most anguishing is that of **dysgeusia**. This is a distortion of the perception of taste that is (a) not really present, that is, a hallucination; or (b) an unpleasant taste that occurs when a pleasant morsel is presented. One possible cause for this distressing condition could be that a substance has entered the bloodstream and, because the gustatory system is in close proximity to blood and interstitial fluids, a taste is generated. Another possible cause of chronic dysgeusia is the result of crushed, stretched, or stimulated cranial nerves serving the gustatory sense. There is, of course, another cause for dysgeusia that is not really a hallucination or caused by stimulation. This is the taste in the mouth caused by infections, abnormal saliva, gingivitis, or poor hygiene.

Viral Infections, Tumors, and Lesions

A number of studies that have indicated that taste can be affected by viral infections. The usual loss is quite small and very likely affects the branch of the VII Cranial Nerve—the chorda tympani. The loss of taste because of otitis media, middle ear infection, has been documented. The loss is very likely due to the infection of the chorda tympani as it passes through the middle ear on its way to the solitary nucleus. If the chorda tympani is affected by the Wallerian degeneration, then there can be a loss of taste perception from the anterior two thirds of the tongue. The recovery of taste is usually incomplete.

A well-known virus, the geniculate herpes zoster, has also been associated with taste dysfunctions. This virus is the common variety that causes chicken pox in childhood. Once the pox has "run its course" and the child recovers, the virus becomes latent and establishes itself within the sensory ganglia. The virus is not gone. Reactivation of the virus, usually in the second half of life, can lead to severe pain, axonal degeneration, and demyelination of the sensory ganglion nerve cells. The nerve fibers themselves appear to act as the conduit for the transport of the virus. The reactivation is called **shingles.** The outbreak is associated with the dermatome of the spinal nerve that held the dormant virus for many years. Chicken pox can now be prevented. An inoculation is usually recommended within the first 18 months of life.

Another well-known source of taste loss is Bell's palsy. The facial nerve, and its branch-serving taste, can be damaged in several ways. The damage can come from virus, neoplasms (tumors), ischemia (obstruction of blood flow), and vasospasm (constriction of a blood vessel). Although well recognized, Bell's palsy has not been investigated extensively regarding taste loss. The usual recovery from the debilitation, however, generally brings with it the return of taste perception associated with the chorda tympani.

Head Trauma

The loss of taste can occur for several unrelated reasons. One is, of course, head trauma. Although not common, it can occur with the destruction of the nerves that innervate the taste buds. The prognosis for recovery usually varies as a function of the extent of the trauma.

Chemical Therapies

A malfunction of the chemical senses usually occurs with the irradiation and chemotherapy associated with cancer. The rapid loss of the taste receptors and the olfactory cells make the loss of olfaction and gustation a likely event during these types of therapies. Associated with the physician's care is the possibility of other types of drugs causing a loss of sensory acuity. Some of the street drugs (cocaine, LSD, etc.) have been implicated but not thoroughly investigated regarding taste sensitivity. The mechanisms involved in taste dysfunction and drugs are not well understood.

Auras

The aura that accompanies epilepsy is often one associated with odor. There are some reported cases, however, when the aura is an extremely bitter taste just before a seizure. These sensory auras are still not understood.

Psychiatric, Hypothyroidism, and Diabetes

Finally, some data show a loss in taste function in some psychiatric disorders, bulimia, hypothyroidism, and diabetes. In bulimia, the primary sensory loss is found in taste receptors on the palate and in the throat because of the purging behavior (Rozin, 1990). There is, of course, the formation of scars and additional damage done to the esophagus because of the stomach acids. Hypothyroidism is associated with the loss of odor and taste. Diabetics often report a loss of taste. In the case of diabetes, the loss begins with the fading of sweetness, then extends to salty, and finally affects the entire range of taste perceptions.

Summary

The neural coding of gustation is, like olfaction, dependent on direct environmental contact with chemical molecules. The pattern of activity initiated by the receptors is received by the higher neural centers to determine, almost instantly, the quality of the environment. The gustatory receptors are even more unique: They conduct action potentials and also release a neurotransmitter at the synapse with the primary sensory neuron. Gustation is a unique sense. In animals other than human, gustation no doubt plays a large role in environmental interactions. The sentries at the gate of nutritional resource are the chemical senses. They play a significant role in our lives.

Suggested Readings

Beauchamp, G. K., & Bartoshuk, L. M. (Eds.). (1997). *Tasting and smelling: Handbook of perception and cognition* (2nd ed.). San Diego, CA: Academic Press.

Finger, T. F., Silver, W. L., & Restrepo, D. (2000). *The neurobiology of taste and smell* (2nd ed.). New York: Wiley-Liss.

Getchell, T. V., Doty, R. L., Bartoshuk, L. M., & Snow, J. B., Jr. (Eds.). (1991). *Smell and taste in health and disease.* New York: Raven Press.

Halpern, B. P. (1999). Taste. In R. A. Wilson & F. Keil (Eds.), *The MIT encyclopedia of the cognitive sciences* (pp. 826-828). Cambridge, MA: Bradford Books.

McLauglin, S., & Margolskee, R. F. (1994). The sense of taste. *American Scientist, 82,* pp. 538-545.

Rozin, P. (1990). Social and moral aspects of food and eating. In I. Rock (Ed.), *The legacy of Solomon Asch: Essays in cognition and social psychology.* Hillsdale, NJ: Lawrence Erlbaum.

CHAPTER 7

The Vestibular System

A little nausea and dizziness often occurs in the modern world. A day at the lake sailing in your friend's new boat sounds like a great idea. Sometimes, however, an adventure becomes a misadventure. State and county fairs have their unique place in this respect. The amusement rides are called, for obvious reasons, by unique monikers—for example, The Hammer, The Whip, The Octopus, The Belly-Snapper, and of course, The Roller Coaster— are named appropriately. Whether or not you are among the thousands of people who get thrills and surges of euphoria on these stimulating rides is your concern. Without any doubt, the rides have to be classified as exciting. It just depends on how excited you want to get. What is important here is that our everyday living involves the silent vestibular system.

Introduction

Whether you have experienced carnival rides or not, you can imagine the nausea that could occur with these activities. The cause of the queasy feelings that some people get, however, are examined more fully as we examine the vestibular sense, sometimes referred to as the sense of balance. It is important to note, incidentally, that to refer to the vestibular sense as the sense of balance is restrictive. The vestibular sense extends beyond just postural balance. It is a complex system intimately related to eye movements, postural reflexes, head motion, and gravitational balance.

Unlike the other sensory systems we have discussed, the vestibular activity does not usually enter prominently in consciousness unless a disruption occurs in its smooth operation. Consider, for example, the intricate coordination required when you look at the wall clock as you are leaving the classroom. A stable visual perception requires that you automatically coordinate head and eye movement while simultaneously maintaining your balance and posture without stumbling, leaning, tilting precariously, or falling flat on your face. This type of behavior is simple, automatic, and unconsciously accomplished every moment of our waking day. We usually are unaware, and have little concern about, how it occurs unless it is disrupted. A disruption can lead to falls from ladders, stumbling, nausea, hearing loss, dizziness, visual distortions, and in some cases, chronic disability.

The chapter is partitioned in three sections. The first portion is dedicated to the organization and function of the peripheral mechanisms within the inner ear. This includes the otoliths, semicircular canals, receptor cells, and supporting structures. The second section outlines central mechanisms, neural structures, and conductive paths concerned with the vestibulo-ocular and postural reflexes. The chapter concludes with a discussion of some vestibular dysfunctions and their perceptual and behavioral effects.

Vestibular Periphery

Where does the vestibular sensory organ reside, and how many of them are there? The answer is—on each side of the head. There are two peripheral vestibular organs carved in the **petrous** (from the Latin, *petrosa,* for "stony") portion of our temporal bones. The next question is, where is the petrous portion of the temporal bone? To locate your temporal bone, put your index finger in your ear canal as a reference, then move your thumb directly behind your ear and pinch your ear. The bone you feel next to your thumb is the temporal bone. Within this part of the skull is the **inner ear** or the **labyrinth,** where both the vestibular and auditory peripheral mechanisms are found. The labyrinth contains chambers intricately sculpted within the bone. The chambers and ducts are filled with fluids, membranes, receptors, supporting structures, active metabolic processes, and the synapses for primary sensory neurons. The axons from the primary sensory neurons form the **VIII cranial nerve.** It conducts afferent activity from the vestibular and auditory peripheral mechanisms to higher central regions and is, therefore, called the **vestibulocochlear nerve.** Figure 7.1 indicates the location of this intriguing part the skull.

The inner ear, as stated previously, contains the peripheral structures for both the auditory and vestibular senses (Dallos, 1992). The external and middle ear are associated only with audition and are discussed more thoroughly

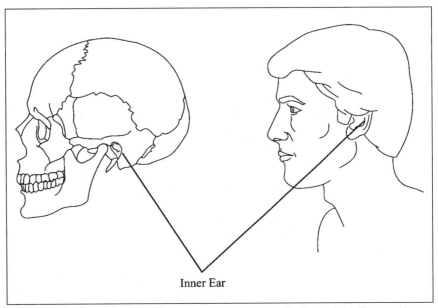

Inner Ear

Figure 7.1. Location of the Inner Ear in the Petrous Portion of the Temporal Bone

in Chapter 9. For completeness, however, Figure 7.2 includes the external and middle ear and the cochlea of the inner ear.

The external ear includes the **pinna** (where earrings are usually located), **external auditory meatus** (ear canal), and the **tympanic membrane** (ear drum). The latter membrane physically separates the external and middle ear. The middle ear is an air-filled chamber containing three small bones (the **ossicles: malleus, incus,** and **stapes**), two muscles (**stapedius** and **tensor tympani**), and a narrow tube that leads to the throat (**eustachian tube**). As noted in the chapter on gustation, a branch of the VII facial nerve, the chorda tympani, passes through the middle ear on its way to the brain stem. The vestibular portion of the inner ear consists of three **semicircular canals** (**horizontal, superior,** and **posterior**), and the **otolith organs** (**utricle** and **saccule**). The remaining division of the inner ear is dedicated to the auditory sense (the spiral-shaped cochlea). The VIII cranial nerve enters the brain stem through a passageway in the petrous bone known as the **internal auditory meatus.** The VIII cranial nerve contains axons from both the auditory and vestibular portions of the inner ear. Accompanying the VIII cranial nerve through the internal auditory meatus is the branch of the VII cranial nerve, the chorda tympani.

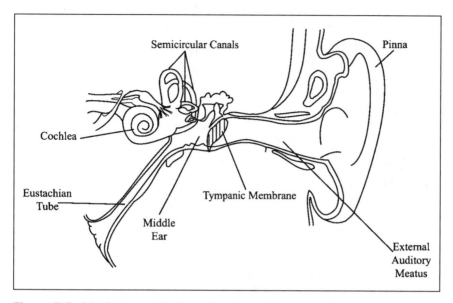

Figure 7.2. Vestibular and Auditory Structures of the Inner Ear

Figure 7.3 shows a more detailed picture of the vestibular structures of the inner ear, including the labyrinth after the surrounding petrous bone has been removed. An important point to note is that the three semicircular canals are perpendicular, at right angles, to each another. Because of this approximate 90° spatial orientation, every angular movement of the head changes the neural activity in at least one pair of the semicircular canals. Every time your head moves, or stops moving, either voluntarily or involuntarily, the neural activity from the semicircular canals, on both sides of your head, changes. The neural activity sent to the brain is used to monitor the three-dimensional **angular rate of acceleration** (movement) of the head. It is important to note here that the semicircular canals respond to the rate of movement. In response to turning or nodding your head, the semicircular canals change their **tonic** (steady or constant) activity. The spontaneous or tonic rate of activity is about 100 action potential per second from the primary sensory neurons. The neural activity is initiated within the **ampulla** associated with the semicircular canal. The ampulla, as shown in Figure 7.3, is the enlargement near the end of each canal where it joins the utricle. It is within this dilation that the specialized receptors for sensory transduction are located. The ampulla is examined more thoroughly after we briefly discuss the otolith organs.

Figure 7.3 shows the enlarged circular-shaped portion of the labyrinth that contains the otolith organs, the utricle and saccule. The otolith systems

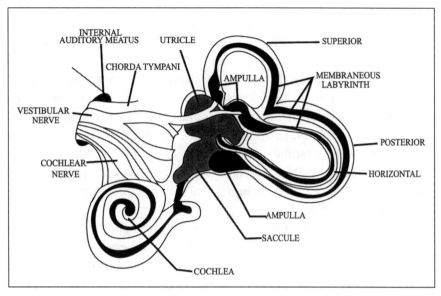

Figure 7.3. Vestibular Structures: Semicircular Canals, Cochlea, Ampulla, Membraneous Labyrinth, Utricle, Saccule, Internal Auditory Meatus

are located near the **vestibule,** the middle portion of the labyrinth, between the semicircular canals and the cochlea. The otoliths respond to gravitational forces and the head-body orientation relative to gravity. In this latter case, the otolith organs respond to **linear acceleration.** The exact receptive mechanisms are discussed shortly. Two examples suffice for now.

When you get in a car and rapidly speed down the road, you clearly notice the linear acceleration of the machine as long as the speed continues to increase. The perception of acceleration is primarily associated with the utricle and saccule mechanisms. If you are sitting upright in the car, the utricle and saccule are the primary informants for the perception of linear motion. This is because of the orientation of the receptor cells within this vestibular system. This does not mean, of course, that the semicircular canals fail to note any changes. Your head does move backward during the acceleration. The semicircular canals are not likely to remain passive.

Assume, in another example, you are blindfolded and strapped in a psychophysicist's rotating chair in the vestibular laboratory. Your head and body are secured, and you are, effectively, part of the chair. The chair can be rotated at various speeds. In this experiment, the chair begins to move and continues to increase in speed until a constant rate of rotation is attained. Your normally operating vestibular system allows you to perceive the initial angular and linear acceleration as the chair begins to rotate. You continue to notice the rotation rate increase until the chair reaches a constant maximum speed. Once the chair reaches a stable and constant rate of rotation, the semi-circular canals fail to inform you that the chair was moving. At this point, lacking other sensory cues, you are unaware that you were spinning. This is because the vestibular system responds to change. Once the speed of rotation is attained, there is no further increase or decrease in motion. The vestibular system returns to its normal spontaneous rate of activity and indicates to you that you are not spinning. As noted previously, this effect depends on the other senses not being stimulated—you have a blindfold on and you do not see the room spinning. The vestibular system responds to changes in head and body motion; if there are no changes, there are no sensory inputs to inform you of the movement.

These examples are analogous to a common situation that occurs in air travel. When an aircraft begins its takeoff down the runway, you always notice the linear acceleration as the plane seeks its flying speed. Once the critical speed is attained, the plane becomes airborne and climbs to its cruising altitude. When you finally reach cruising altitude, you are, for example, moving at 500 mph. You may notice that you do not feel the plane's movement without other sensory cues coming in play (such as the visual cues of the ground or clouds). The vestibular system has adapted. Nothing is abnormal as far as the vestibular system is concerned. The vestibular system, in sum, responds to changes in motion. How these neural changes are activated within the vestibular system is the topic of the following sections.

Vestibular Labyrinth

We should more fully describe the inner ear of the vestibular system before we continue with the transduction mechanisms of the system. Figure 7.3 shows the **bony labyrinth** or outer shell of the inner ear after the majority of the temporal bone has been surgically removed. Figure 7.3 also shows the outline of an internal labyrinth. The labyrinth within the bony labyrinth, the shaded area in Figure 7.3, is the **membranous labyrinth.** The membranous labyrinth is also called membranous ducts. The membranous labyrinth contains a fluid, specialized receptors, supporting cells, membranes, and structures for the vestibular sense. An analogy may be helpful here. A tractor tire is constructed in two parts: the external tire that meets the ground and an inner tube that contains the air. The tire is, in the analogy, the bony labyrinth and the inner tube is the membranous labyrinth. An important difference in the analogy needs to be emphasized. Although there is no space between the tire and the inner tube, there is a duct or space between the bony labyrinth and the membranous labyrinth. This space is filled with a fluid called **perilymph.** The membranous labyrinth, in a manner of speaking, "floats" in the perilymph of the intricately sculpted caverns of our temporal bone. The membranous ducts are also filled with a fluid. This fluid is **endolymph.** The fluid surrounding the membranous labyrinth, perilymph, is ionically similar to cerebrospinal fluid. In contrast, the endolymph has an ionic content that is similar to neurons—high in K^+ and low in Na^+. The K^+ is intimately associated with the depolarization of the true receptors located within the membranous ducts of the labyrinth.

Ampulla

The ampulla is an enlargement near one end of each semicircular canal. The membranous labyrinth in the ampulla contains specialized structures that permit us to detect angular velocity. This apparatus consists of **hair cell** receptors, the **crista** holding the hair cells, and the **cupula,** a gelatinous mass that lies over the hair cells. The thin membrane of the cupula extends from the crista to the roof of the ampulla. Each hair cell has on its upper surface a special arrangement of cilia consisting of a single **kinocilium** and approximately 60 to 70 **stereocilia.** These cilia are embedded in the overlying cupula. Figure 7.4 shows the organization of these structures within the ampulla.

Figure 7.5 shows an enlarged view of some hair cells in the ampulla. The orientation of the cilia is shown in Figure 7.5(a). The drawing shows the gra-

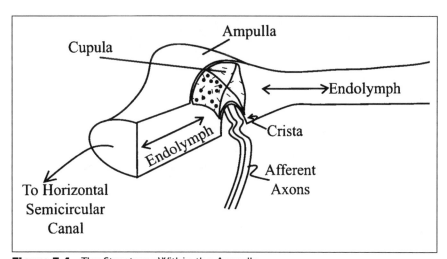

Figure 7.4. The Structures Within the Ampulla

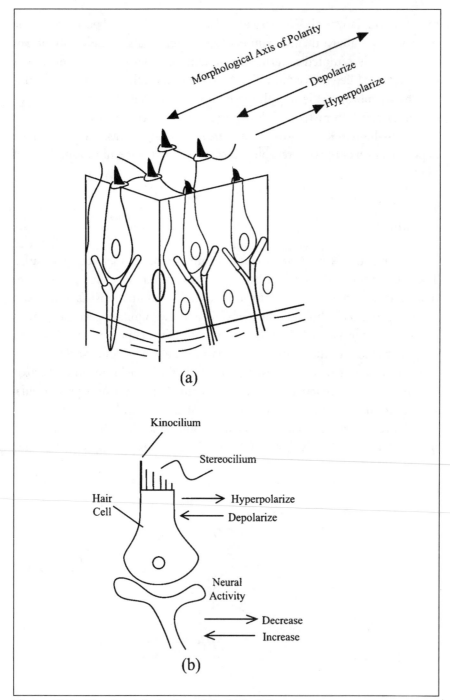

Figure 7.5. Directional Activation of the Hair Cell

NOTE: (a) morphological axis of polarity in the ampulla and (b) hyperpolarization and depolarization of the hair cell

dations of the stereocilia, from tallest to shortest, with a single tall kinocilium always located next to the tallest group of stereocilia. This systematic organization provides a **morphological axis of polarity** that intimately affects the response of the hair cell. When the stereocilia are bent or displaced toward the taller kinocilium, the hair cell depolarizes. When the stereocilia are bent away from the kinocilium, the hair cell hyperpolarizes. Movement of the cilia perpendicular to this morphological axis does not affect the hair cell potential.

Because the membranous duct of the semicircular canal is completely filled with endolymph and the thin cupula stretches across the opening within the ampulla, any movement of endolymph necessarily has to move the cupula. The movement of the cupula, by the endolymph, is the basis of the hydromechanical modulation of the hair cell receptor potential. When the head is turned, the endolymphatic fluid within the membranous labyrinth lags slightly behind the head movement. This lingering of the fluid, relative to the movement of the head, displaces the cupula. The displaced cupula, because of its direct linkage to the kinocilium and stereocilia, bends the cilia. If the movement of the head causes the stereocilia to bend toward the kinocilium, the hair cell depolarizes and an increase in neural activity results. If the head movement is in the opposite direction, the stereocilia bend away from the kinocilium, the hair cell hyperpolarizes, and neural activity decreases. Figure 7.6 demonstrates how a head turn, to the left, affects the neural activity within the horizontal semicircular canals. Keep in mind that the morphological axis of polarity in the horizontal canals determines the change in hair cell activity.

In summary, movement of the head in the horizontal plane (when you are standing erect and you turn your head left or right) causes the bilateral horizontal semicircular ducts to work together—one side is inhibited while the other side is excited. In the example shown in Figure 7.6, the neural response is excitatory in the left duct and inhibitory in the right. The operation of the superior and posterior ducts is similar to that of the horizontal ducts. There are two caveats, however. First, the superior duct on one side of the head is in the same plane as the posterior duct on the other side; these two canals operate as functional pairs. Second, unlike the horizontal canals, the morphological axis of the hair cells within the superior and posterior ducts is away from the utricle rather than toward the utricle. Nevertheless, like the horizontal pair of ducts, the superior-posterior pair work in the same bilateral inhibitory-excitatory manner; namely, movement of the fluids in the plane of the superior-posterior ducts results in excitation in one duct and inhibition in the other.

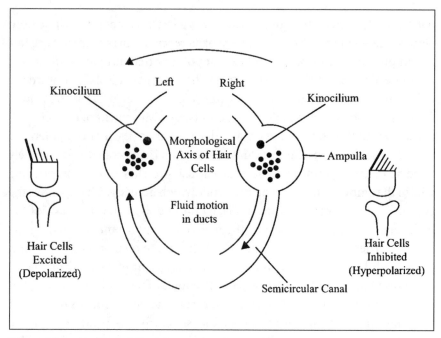

Figure 7.6. Horizontal Semicircular Activity as a Result of a Left Head Turn

NOTE: The receptors in the left ampulla are excitatory; those in the right are inhibitory.

Otolith Organs

The utricle and saccule are the otolith organs. They contain hair cell receptors like those in the semicircular canals. The utricle and saccule can be mentally visualized as a fluid-filled pouch containing a specialized receptor area.

This specialized area is called the **macula.** *Macula* is Latin for "spot." The macula is, then, the spot where the receptors are located. The orientation of the macula differs, however, for the two organs. When you are standing erect, the macula is in the horizontal plane in the utricle. In the saccule, however, the macula is in a vertical position on the medial side of the pouch. On top of each macula is a gelatinous membrane analogous to the cupula. This thin membrane is like frosting on a cake. Below the frosting is the macula containing the hair cells. The hair cells within each macula have their cilia firmly attached to the overlying membrane. Finally, the membranes overlying each macula are weighted by **otoliths** (Greek *lithos* for "stone," *oto* for "ear"). These otolith stones are also referred to as **otoconia.** These stones, made of calcium carbonate, provide the necessary mass to move the cilia of the hair cells when the head or body is tilted.

The orientation of the macula in the two otolith organs provides the means for judging bodily position relative to gravity. If the head or body is tilted in any direction, the weighted membrane (frosting) slides and moves as a function of gravity. The movement of the membrane bends the cilia of the receptors within the utricle and saccule. The bending of the cilia leads to changes in the receptor and to changes in the neural activity leaving the otolith organs. Because of the unique morphological axis of polarity within the utricle and saccule, any directional change of the head or body, relative to gravity, results in receptor depolarization or hyperpolarization.

Figure 7.7 summarizes the neural activity of the semicircular canals and the utricle and saccule when the head is moved. The figure depicts an increase in the sustained neural activity as a function of movement.

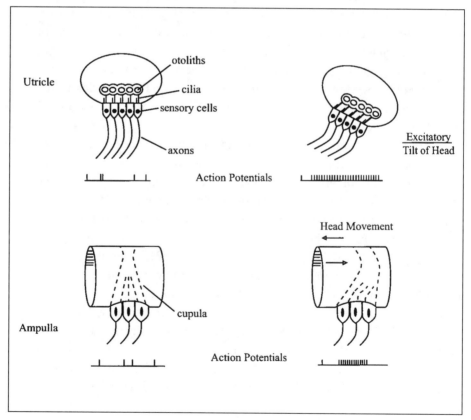

Figure 7.7. Changes in the Ampulla and Utricle as a Function of Head Movement

Receptor Transduction

We have reached the point in our discussion when the question becomes: What causes the receptor hair cell to depolarize and hyperpolarize? We know that the cell depolarizes with the deflection of cilia toward the kinocilium and hyperpolarizes when the deflection is away from the kinocilium (Hudspeth, 1982, 1985, 1989; Meyer, Furness, Zenner, Hackney, & Gummer, 1998; Pickles & Corey, 1992). The question remains, however, what is occurring within the cell to cause the modulation of the synaptic neurotransmitter and the activation or inhibition of action potentials? We begin this discussion by looking closely at a hair cell. Figure 7.8 shows a diagrammatic close-up of this true receptor and its functional operation.

Figure 7.8(a) shows a side view of a hair cell. In this particular perspective, the large kinocilium and the smaller stereocilia are shown with important connections between stereocilia within the different rows. The connections between the stereocilia are the **tip links** (Pickles, Comis, & Osborne, 1984). The tip links, fine strands of connective tissue, attach the tip of one smaller stereocilium to the shaft of a larger stereocilium in an adjacent row. There are no connective tip links between stereocilia within rows. Figure 7.8(a) shows the side view so the row-to-row tip links are clearly displayed. The tip links are critical areas of activity in receptor transduction and neural modulation.

Figure 7.8(b) shows a hypothesized model for the hair cell transduction. The mechanical deflection of the hair cell bundles, on the apex of each receptor, results in the opening and closing of ionic gates at the tips of the stereocilia. When there is no stimulation, approximately 10 to 20% of these gates are open at any one time. This normal random oscillation of the gates, opening and closing, results in a small continuous release of neurotransmitter. As discussed shortly, the positive ions that incessantly enter the cell cause it to be perpetually active. The sustained random generation of approximately 100 impulses per second permits the receptor to signal both an increase (excitation) and a decrease (inhibition) in neural activity. This tonic neural activity may be viewed as a background against which increases and decreases in stimulation are judged. When a stimulus occurs to deflect the cilia, by moving the cupula or the otolith membrane, additional channels are opened or closed and the neural activity varies accordingly (Hudspeth, 1982, 1989).

The tip links and the gates are assumed to be under some tension and are shown in the model as springs. Thus, when the cilia move toward the

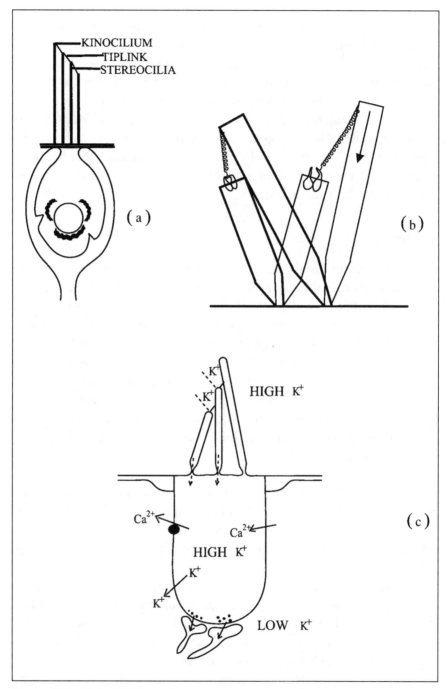

Figure 7.8. Hair Cell Transduction

NOTE: (a) side view of hair cell showing tip links between stereocilia, (b) hypothesized spring-loaded tip link gates that open and shut as a function of hydormechanical movement, and (c) ionic exchange leading to depolarization and hyperpolarization kinocilium and depolarization occurs, the tip link (spring) is stretched and the gate is opened. Figure 7.8(b) shows this as movement to the right. The stretching of the link by the deflection of the cilia causes the distal attachment of the link to slide down the stem of the longer stereocilia. This reduces the tension. When the deflection is in the other direction, to the left in Figure 7.8(b), the tension is relaxed and the gate closes. In this latter case, with the deflection to the left, the tip link attachment, after a momentary gate closure, slowly climbs upward on the long stereocilia until a slight tension is re-established. Once the tension is reinstituted, the gate is partially open and the tonic neural activity resumes.

Receptor Depolarization

A depolarization of the receptor occurs with an influx of K^+ through the open gates located at the tips of the stereocilia. The receptor potential, caused by the influx of positive ions, releases the neurotransmitter at the base of the cell. The opening and closing of the gates can occur within 40 microseconds.

Because of the relatively high concentration of K^+ in the endolymph, you might assume that the influx of K^+ is the result of the concentration gradient between the endolymph and the hair cell. This, however, is probably not the case. The contents of the hair cell are very much like the cytoplasm of a typical neuron. That is, like the endolymph, the concentration of K^+ is high and the concentration of Na^+ is low. Thus, if ionic channels were to open, the concentration gradient is not likely the reason for K^+ influx into the cell. This is because the concentration gradient across the apex of the hair cell is near zero. In other words, the number of K^+ ions in the endolymph and hair cell are nearly the same, so there is negligible ion flow as a result of differences in concentrations. The K^+ is drawn into the hair cell for a different reason. The reason for the influx of K^+ is because of the potential gradient between the receptor and the endolymph.

The electrical potential within the hair cell is between −45 and −70 mv at its resting state. This potential is the K^+ equilibrium value—the value at which the cell is at rest. The endolymph that bathes the cilia, on the other hand, is near +80 mv. This results in a potential difference of 125 to 150 mv across the apical portion of the hair cell. The consequence of this electrical difference, positive in the endolymph and negative in the inner hair cell at the apex, is a strong attraction for positive ions to enter the cell when the channels or gates are opened. This potential gradient causes the rapid flow of K^+ into the cell. The initial swift depolarization is explained by an influx of K^+.

In sum, the direct gating of the channels by the movement of the cupula or otolith membranes yields an essentially instantaneous hair cell depolarization by the influx of K^+. The flow of K^+, however, does not just initiate the depolarization of the cell. The K^+ also opens voltage-gated Ca^{2+} channels that lie on the lateral surface of the hair cell. When the Ca^{2+} gates are opened and Ca^{2+} enters the cell, there is an amplification of the depolarization originally begun by the K^+.

The next question is, what happens to the K^+ and the Ca^{2+} when they enter the cell? Do they continue to accumulate within the cell or are they removed by some kind of metabolic pump? Do they just slowly leak out? The answer for the Ca^{2+} is straightforward. There is a Ca^{2+} pump that removes the Ca^{2+}. The K^+, on the other hand, leaves the cell almost as rapidly as it enters. The reason for its rapid departure is twofold. First, unlike the cilia at the apical portion of the hair cell, the base of the hair cell is not surrounded by endolymph. The base of the cell is immersed in perilymph. This detail has an important consequence on hair cell operation. The distribution of ions in the perilymph and hair cells differ significantly. The difference is that the perilymph is high in Na^+ and low in K^+. The perilymph is similar to extracellular and cerebrospinal fluid. The difference between the internal status of the cell and the perilymph produces a strong concentration gradient to draw K^+ out at the base of the hair cell. Secondly, the entering K^+ has opened the voltage-gated Ca^{2+} channels. The entering Ca^{2+} ions have two effects. First, they amplify the depolarization of the cell. Second, they open more K^+ channels at the base of the hair cell for the efflux of the K^+. Thus, what happens to the K^+ as it enters the cell at the apex? It depolarizes the cell and then leaves almost as fast as it enters (in about 40 microseconds). The efflux of the K^+ at the base of the hair cell results in the cell's rapid return to a stable resting condition. Figure 7.8(c) shows this depolarization sequence and is summarized in the following list.

1. Movement of the cupula or otoliths deflects the stereocilia toward the kinocilium and opens the gates.
2. K^+, drawn in by potential gradient, enters the cell.
3. K^+ influx depolarizes the cell and opens voltage-gated Ca^{2+} channels.
4. C^{2+} influx increases depolarization begun by the K^+ and opens additional K^+ channels at the hair cell base.

5. The K^+ channels, opened at the apex by the mechanical movement, close.

6. The K^+ leaves through the gates at the base of the cell because of the high concentration gradient and an electrical gradient that rejects the positive K^+. The cell, consequently, returns to its original tonic condition of 80 to 100 action potentials per second.

7. Ca^{2+} is removed by an ionic pump.

Receptor Hyperpolarization

The hyperpolarization of the hair cell, and the consequent decline in action potentials, occurs when the apical K^+ gates close. The gate closure is due to the deflection of the cilia away from the kinocilium by the cupula or the otoliths. The K^+ ions, however, continue to leave the hair cell through basal-lateral K^+ channels that remain open for a brief period. The loss of the positively charged K^+ results in a cellular hyperpolarization and a brief cessation of neurotransmitter release at the synapse. The failure to release the neurotransmitter, of course, results in the cessation of action potentials in the afferent neuron.

Vestibular Central Pathways

Everything we have discussed thus far has involved peripheral mechanisms within the inner ear. The next step is to look at the pathways and central mechanisms involved in processing these peripheral signals. The starting place is the vestibular branch of the vestibulocochlear nerve, the VIII cranial nerve. This nerve, as its name implies, contains the afferent paths from two separate sensory systems. Our attention is on the 20,000 myelinated bipolar neurons forming the vestibular branch of the nerve. The cell bodies for these primary sensory neurons lie in **Scarpa's vestibular ganglion** near the internal auditory meatus.

The axons that compose the vestibular branch, once they pass through the internal auditory meatus, immediately enter the brain stem and make synaptic connections within the **vestibular nuclear complex** in the medulla. The vestibular nuclear complex is, as the latter word suggests, complex. It has four morphologically distinct nuclei with equally well-defined functions. These structural areas are called the superior, inferior, lateral, and medial nuclei. The primary function of these nuclei is to integrate and relay the sensory information from the receptors located in the semicircular canals, utricle, and saccule. Although there are four separate nuclei in the vestibular complex, they make connections with only three systems in the central nervous system. The vestibular nuclei project to the extraocular eye motoneurons (vestibulo-ocular system), postural motoneurons (vestibulo-spinal system), and the cerebellum (vestibulo-cerebellar system).

Vestibulo-Ocular System

Assume for a moment that you and your friend are engaged in a leisure drive down a gravel country road in your pickup. You have your video camera to shoot any moose you happen to see. You spot a herd of moose and ask your friend to take your cheap video camera and get some pictures of them as you drive by. Later that evening you put the tape into your VCR to see the day's events. Is the video as clear and crisp on the monitor? Not likely.

The images on the screen jump, rock, and vibrate with every bump in the road. The image on the TV screen is unstable and nearly always out of focus. The reason is, of course, that the visual image formed on the tape during filming was not adjusted for camera bounces. The image you and your friend saw from the truck, however, was stable and vividly clear. Your visual image differs from the camera's recording of the same scene because the vestibular system was adjusting your visual image according to the bumps in the road. In other words, the vestibular system told your brain that it was your head and body that were moving, not the moose seen through the visual system. The visual system, moreover, was being adjusted as you focused on the moose. In this case, your brain was told that your eyes are moving, your head is moving, and the world is stable. The camera and the TV set, unfortunately, do not have this miraculous **vestibulo-ocular reflex (VR)** between the vestibular system and the visual (ocular) motor system. We briefly examine the vestibulo-ocular reflex and its automatic operation..

The movement of each eye is under the control of three cranial motor nerves—the oculomotor (III), the abducens (IV), and the trochlear (VI). These nerves control the contraction and relaxation of six muscles, four rectus muscles (superior, inferior, medial, and lateral), and two oblique muscles (superior and inferior). Figure 7.9 shows these muscles, and their innervations. The very idea that 25% of all the cranial nerves are associated with eye movement indicates the importance of such a system. The vestibular system interacts with each of these motor nerves and, subsequently, affects the six eye muscles.

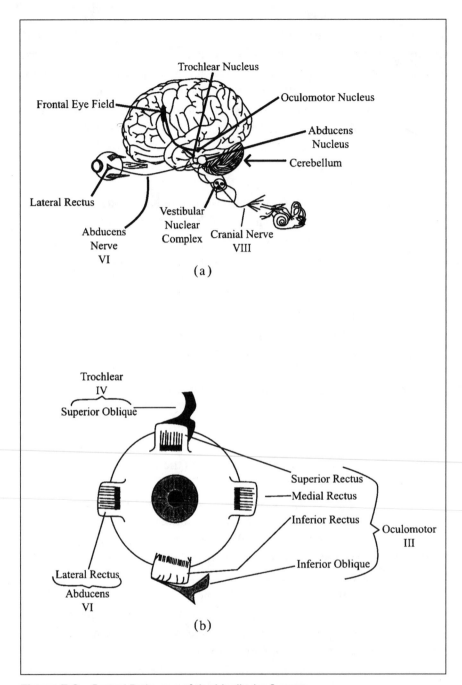

Figure 7.9. Central Pathways of the Vestibular System

NOTE: (a) projections to the vestibular nuclear complex and the Vestibulo-ocular reflex and (b) The muscles of the eye and the three cranial nerves that control them.

There are two kinds of eye movements we need to consider. First is the voluntary **conjugate movements.** This type of eye movement is occurring right now as you read this page. Your eyes, controlled by the **frontal eye field** located in your motor cortex, is directing your eye to make small **saccadic** movements (jumps) along these horizontal typed lines. This eye movement is not involved with the vestibulo-ocular reflex. The second kind of eye movement, directly involved with the vestibular system, is **compensatory movements.** The name of this movement reflects its function: Eye movements are made to compensate for head movements.

The compensatory eye movements are the direct result of the vestibulo-ocular reflex. The movement occurred when you watched the moose herd. Specifically, as your head rotated in the horizontal plane, your eyes moved to maintain a steady visual image. The eye movement was reflexive and automatic. Every time you visually focus on an object in the world and then move your head while maintaining your focus, your vestibulo-ocular reflex is engaged. The visual image remains stable because your eyes move to maintain the focused impression. This did not happen when the camera took the picture. For the camera, no compensations were made for the bumps in the road.

The compensatory eye movements in this example are relatively simple. The primary eye muscles involved with the horizontal head movement are the lateral and medial rectus of each eye. As the lateral rectus of the left eye contracted, the medial rectus of the same eye relaxed. In the right eye, the lateral rectus relaxed while the medial rectus contracted. The reflex is relatively simple for a horizontal head movement.

Consider, however, the vestibulo-ocular reflex activity that occurs when you visually maintain a steady focus on an object in the world and then move your head in rotational or circular motion. In this case, your perception is that your head is moving in a circular motion and the visual world is steady—all automatically accomplished and unconscious.

What part of the central nervous system is involved in the reflex? The ampulla in the semicircular canals and, perhaps, the utricle send their inputs to the medial and superior portions of the vestibular nuclear complex. The cells in the medial and superior vestibular nuclei project their axons to the motor nuclei of the three cranial nerves controlling eye movement: the oculomotor nucleus, the abducens nucleus, and the trochlear nucleus. These nuclei, in turn, project to the six muscles of each eye. Figure 7.9(a) shows the pathway for one of the eye muscles, the lateral rectus muscle of the left eye.

Vestibulo-Spinal System

The vestibulo-spinal system has as its goal the maintenance of posture and the precise adjustment of body orientation relative to gravity. This is partially accomplished by the lateral and medial portions of the vestibular nuclear complex. These portions of the vestibular nuclei receive their inputs from the semicircular canals and both otolith organs. The projections from the vestibular nuclei are sent to the neck, trunk, and limb motoneurons. The motoneurons, of course, adjust the muscular system to help us remain erect.

Bodily adjustments, relative to gravity, and the associated neck reflexes are automatically initiated. This can be observed easily everyday. You usually stand on two feet. If, however, you decide to stand on one foot, you can. It is generally a simple task because you usually keep your eyes open. The visual inputs help orient you regarding what is up. It becomes more difficult, however, when you close your eyes and stand on one foot. In this situation, you are almost entirely dependent on the vestibular system and the **postural reflex.** Generally speaking, you cannot stand on one foot, with your eyes closed, without exerting significantly more effort. The task is much more difficult when you are barefoot and standing on a thick carpet. Notice when you do stand on one foot, with your eyes closed, that you focus on your entire body and limb position. Can you stand on one foot, eyes closed, easier if your arms are straight down beside you or if your arms are held out parallel to the floor?

Finally, it is important to understand that the vestibular or postural reflex (also called the "neck reflex" and the "righting reflex") follows a sequential plan to keep us erect and informed about any possible body tilt relative to gravity. The sequence is quite logical. The vestibular labyrinth is in the head; the head is connected to the neck; the neck is connected to the trunk; the trunk is connected to the limbs. Because the head is mobile and pivots on the neck, the neck becomes a critical link in the orientation of our head relative to our body. Our loss of balance, relative to gravity and our body position, is noted first by a tilt or movement of our head; the postural reflex is almost immediately initiated when the body position begins to follow an unwanted movement away from an erect stance.

Vestibulo-Cerebellar System

The input to the inferior vestibular nuclei comes from the semicircular canals and both otolith organs. The inferior vestibular nuclei, in turn, project to the cerebellum. The cerebellum, in turn has efferent fibers returning to the vestibular nuclei. The smooth control of movement and coordination, as hypothesized, is modulated by the vestibular system through the cerebellum.

Dysfunctions

The first thing that comes to mind when you think of a vestibular disorder is dizziness. There are, of course, different amounts and kinds of dizziness. Some dizziness is fun, like the carnival rides: fun and not seriously disorienting at all. Others kinds of dizziness, such as getting up too rapidly, bending over to get that quarter on the floor, or feeling dizzy from looking down from a cliff, can be briefly disorienting and only slightly worrisome. More serious dizziness can also occur (Barber & Sharpe, 1988). Some individuals report **vertigo** in which they feel the sensation of spinning or where the surroundings appear to be spinning out of control. In these cases, once high blood pressure, heart arrhythmia, and visual disease are ruled out, it is usually a problem with the vestibular system in the inner ear. In addition to the dizziness, there is sometimes a hearing disorder.

A well-known cause of vertigo is Menière's disease, first identified by a French physician in 1861. It is thought to be caused by an increase in endolymph with an accompanying increase in endolymphatic pressure in the semicircular canals and the vestibule. Because the vestibular and auditory membranous labyrinth are continuous, it is not uncommon for the individual to have hearing loss and **tinnitus** associated with the vertigo. Tinnitus refers to a continuous ringing or noise within the ear.

Vestibular neuronitis is another common vestibular disorder. It is not associated with hearing loss, and the first experience is usually an acute attack of severe vertigo lasting for hours or days. Sometimes a loss of balance lasts for weeks or months and persists for months or years. The cause is usually associated with a viral illness that many believe to be the cause of the infected nerve.

There is also a group of antibiotics that cause severe and sometimes permanent destruction of the inner ear. The drugs, usually only prescribed for life-threatening bacterial infections, belong to the mycin family. Streptomycin is a commonly prescribed drug that often, with only short treatments, causes severe damage to the inner ear, particularly if the patient also has impaired kidneys. Stopping the drug usually halts further damage although, as noted previously, life-threatening diseases may preclude the cessation of the drug. Dizziness, permanent hearing loss, and loss of balance are the usual results in this family of drugs.

A stroke may also be the cause of dizziness. A "small stroke," transient ischemic attack, often occurs in the brain stem. The transient ischemic attack is the result of a temporary lack of blood supply to the brain and may cause transient numbness, tingling, or weakness in a limb. Other signs may include temporary blindness and difficulty with speech.

Acoustic neurinoma is a central cause of dizziness. A tumor that usually occurs in the internal auditory meatus, presses on the nerve and causes false signals to be sent to the brain. The tumor usually is found in the Schwann cells of the vestibular nerve. Hearing can also be affected.

The treatment for dizziness and vertigo varies according to the signs and symptoms. One sign of an impaired vestibular system is the occurrence of an irregular **nystagmus.** Nystagmus is rapid and uncontrollable horizontal back-and-forth movements of the eyes. The nystagmus often accompanies a vestibular problem. One common vestibular examination is the **caloric test** (Stockwell, 1988). It involves the monitoring of eye movement while one ear at a time is irrigated, alternately, with warm and cool water. Sometimes warm and cold air is used instead of the water. Because of the proximity of the horizontal semicircular canal to the external auditory meatus, it is believed that the heat and cold create a convection current within the endolymph of the membranous labyrinth. The endolymph generates a recognizable pattern of eye movements. By recording the eye movements, you can evaluate the functional status of the vestibular semicircular canals. Another approach to evaluation is computed tomography and brain stem auditory-evoked potentials. These tests can reveal abnormal growths, such as acoustic neurinomas, within the brain stem. Treatment for dizziness is usually accomplished by using drugs, surgery, and occasionally psychotherapy. In this latter case, the dizziness may be due to extreme anxiety and hyperventilation. Counseling can often help an individual gain control of the anxiety attacks and avoid the hyperventilation.

Summary

The vestibular system is a silent partner in our daily activities of turning, starting, stopping, jumping, walking, and bending. The sensory apparatus carved out of the temporal bone is an intricate mechanism that initiates the signals for our posture, visual coordination, and smooth coordinated movement. The semicircular canals and otolith organs, the utricle and saccule, are located in the membranous labyrinth of the inner ear. The transduction is accomplished by a true receptor, the hair cell that responds to angular velocity, linear movements, and gravity. The vestibulo-ocular reflex operates automatically and provides us with a stable visual image. The postural reflex is part of the vestibulo-spinal system and enables us to correct our posture and position, relative to gravity.

Suggested Readings

Barber, H. O., & Sharpe, J. A. (1988). *Vestibular disorders.* Chicago: Year Book Medical Publishers.

Hudspeth, A. J. (1989). How the ears work. *Nature, 341,* 397-404.

Stockwell, C. W. (1988). Conventional bithermal caloric tests. In H. O. Barber & J. A. Sharpe (Eds.). *Vestibular disorders.* Chicago: Year Book Medical Publishers.

CHAPTER 8

Auditory Stimuli

Introduction

The goal of this chapter is to discuss the physical stimuli that produce auditory perceptions. This is no mean task. The stimuli range from simple laboratory tones to vastly complex sounds of music and speech. In addition, there is an array of other environmental sounds that have meaning for us, such as dog barks, cat purrs, bird songs, car horns, train whistles, sizzling bacon, toilet flushes, slamming doors, breaking glass, thunder, and so on.

We examine auditory stimuli from three perspectives: (a) frequency and phase, (b) complexity, and (c) intensity. This approach allows us to get a grasp on the stimuli that energize our auditory system and provide us with our perceptions. There are several books on the topic of sound that may be of interest. A few have been included in the Suggested Readings section at the end of this chapter.

Frequency and Phase

As just noted, auditory stimuli vary from simple to complex. We begin with an example of the simple tone. Following the simple tone description, we combine several simple tones and compose a **complex waveform.**

Figure 8.1 shows five images of a cork boat floating on a small pond. In 8.1(a), the pond is quiescent as it awaits the impact of a falling marble. In 8.1(b), the marble has made its initial contact with the surface of the water. This collision has forced the water to rise around the source of the disturbance. This rise in the water, labeled 1, is the first simple wave in a ripple of

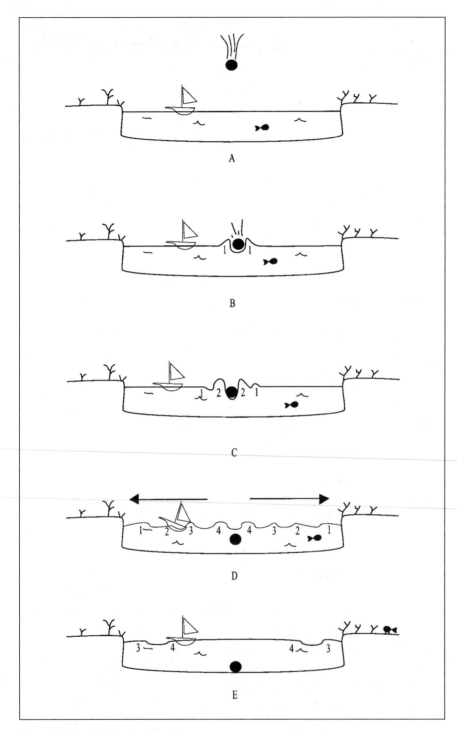

Figure 8.1. Ripples in a Pond

waves that results from the impact. In Figure 8.1(c), the marble has sunk deeper in the water, and the surface has begun to undulate and show the second wave in the cyclic ripple. Wave 1 has moved toward the shore and lost some of its initial size, and Wave 2 has been formed. It should be noted here, that the further a wave moves from its origin, in this case the impact, the smaller the wave becomes. Waves lose energy as they move away from the source.

The next depiction, 8.1(d), shows four waves that have moved away from the source of impact. The wave furthest from the source, Wave 1, has continued to decline in magnitude until it has almost disappeared. The last diagram, 8.1(e), shows the pond returning to its normal calm state. The last two simple waves in the ripple are just arriving at the distant shore. They have also diminished in size. This relatively unsophisticated example provides some basic concepts for our discussion of sound.

First, the ripples in the pond were generated by a source of energy. In the case of the pond, the source of the ripple was the marble disturbing the water. Sound is similar because it always has an origin or a source. Something in the environment must make a disturbance if a sound is to be generated.

Second, a sound, like the ripples in the pond, must have a medium in which to travel. In the pond example, water is the medium. In normal everyday auditory events, air acts as the conducting medium for sound. More viscous or dense materials such as water, steel, and the bone of our skull, however, can conduct sound.

Third, the ripples in the pond, once produced, decay in magnitude as a function of distance from the source. Sound operates in a similar manner. The further sound travels through its normal medium, air and objects in the environment, the weaker it becomes. An interesting aspect of sound is that the high-frequency stimuli that produce perceptually high pitches tend to lose their energy faster than do sounds that produce low pitches. The reason for this is that high-frequency stimuli are absorbed and reflected more readily off objects in the environment. The lower-frequency sounds "bend" and "flow" around the objects and continue. The loss of high frequencies is why thunder is perceived to have a sharp crisp high-pitched "crack" when it is right above your head, yet is heard as a low-pitched rumble when heard a few miles away from the source. The low-pitched sounds do not fade as fast as the high-pitched sounds. An analogy can be found in the large slow-moving waves of the ocean. As waves roll in and meet the supporting pillars of a pier, they just move around the pillars and keep on going. The waves of the ocean are low in frequency and simply wrap themselves around the obstacle in the environment. This is similar to the low-frequency stimuli.

Fourth, it is clear that the little cork boat floating on the surface of the pond did not move to the shore during the disturbance. The boat stayed at the same location within the pond. This is because the water particles on which the boat was floating were not moved to the shore; the water was simply the medium used to transmit the disturbance. The boat, of course, moved up and down as the waves passed underneath. The pressure changes caused by the impact were transmitted through the medium. The molecules of water were pressed together to form an increase in the height of the water surface, a peak, and then the water molecules were dispersed to form a trough. Just like the surface of the pond, molecules are compressed and dispersed in the air to form sound waves.

The fifth point to note is the speed of the waves as they travel through the medium. The speed of sound varies as a function of the temperature and density of the medium. If the temperature is near 20° Centigrade (68° Fahrenheit) the speed of sound through the air is approximately 767 mph. In our pond, with the water at the same temperature, the sound travels about 3,284 mph. The speed increases dramatically when the medium becomes dense. The speed of sound in a piece of steel at the same temperature approaches 13,332 mph. The only place where sound is not conducted is in a vacuum. In this case, there is no medium through which the sound is propagated.

Finally, all complex sounds can be analyzed into simple sounds. What this means, in regard to the pond example, is that ripples produced by one marble can be made more complex by dropping a second marble into the water before the waves from the first marble have disappeared. The waves made by dropping the two marbles results in a complex wave, or a **complex waveform.** The ripples from one marble, when algebraically added to the ripples from the second marble, result in a complex ripple. The waveform is complex because it consists of several simple waves added together.

One important aspect of complex waveforms is that they form the acoustical environment. There are no simple auditory stimuli in our environment; it is all complex. Part of the task of the auditory system is to analyze these complex sounds. We hear complex waves and automatically analyze them.

A mathematical process known as **Fourier analysis** can accomplish the analysis of complex waveforms in sine wave components. Although Fourier mathematics are beyond our scope, it is important to understand that the environment generates sounds that are, exclusively, complex. The auditory system is confronted, consequently, with an enormous task. It must decipher the waveforms into simpler components analogous to the mathematical process of Fourier analysis.

When the auditory system analyzes complex sounds into component frequencies the process is known as **Ohm's acoustic law.** As we learn, the hearing mechanism cannot do this perfectly, but it does an admirable job. Frequency analysis is the first step in auditory perception.

The stage is now set for a discussion of simple and complex waveforms. We begin with frequency. **Frequency** is measured in Hertz (Hz). Hertz refers to the number of complete cycles or oscillations that occur in a 1 second interval of time. Figure 8.2 illustrates this idea.

Figure 8.2 shows some simple stimuli, called **sine waves** or **sinusoids.** The sine wave terminology comes from trigonometry and indicates that waves in this example, when first turned on, begin at zero **phase.** This is noted in the figure as a phase of $0°$. Simple waves can have starting points anywhere from $0°$ to $360°$. Sinusoids begin at $0°$. A zero starting phase is often referred to as "sine phase" and a stimulus that is initiated at sign phase is a "sine wave."

Each of the six sinusoids has a different frequency. The figure shows the variations in pressure for each sinusoid as a function of time. This is how a sinusoid appears if it is viewed on an oscilloscope. An oscilloscope has an electron beam that sweeps rapidly across the surface of the screen of a cathode ray tube from left to right. As it sweeps across the face of the tube, the waveform of the sinusoidal oscillations is traced on the screen. The oscilloscope is one way to examine a waveform; it shows how the stimulus amplitude varies as a function of time. The sinusoids look like those in Figure 8.2.

The six sinusoids in Figure 8.2 decrease in frequency, from top to bottom, as they increase in amplitude. Sinusoid 1, at the top, has 12 complete cycles within a 1-msec interval. A millisecond is one thousandth of a second. So, with 12 complete cycles in a millisecond, the frequency is 12,000 Hz. Sinusoid 6, the bottom sinusoid, on the other hand, has 2 complete cycles in the same time frame. Thus, Sinusoid 6 has a frequency of 2,000 Hz; there are 2,000 complete cycles in a second.

Stimuli can be viewed from a different perspective. Instead of amplitude being shown as a function of time, it can be exhibited as a function of frequency. In the latter mode of presentation, the amplitude of the stimulus is represented by the height of a vertical line plotted as a function of frequency. In other words, the amplitude is plotted on the vertical axis and the frequency is on the horizontal axis. This display is called a **line spectrum.** Figure 8.3 shows the line spectrum for the stimuli displayed in Figure 8.2. There are six vertical lines, one for each stimulus. Stimulus 6, which is 2,000 Hz, has the largest vertical line, indicating it is more intense than the others.

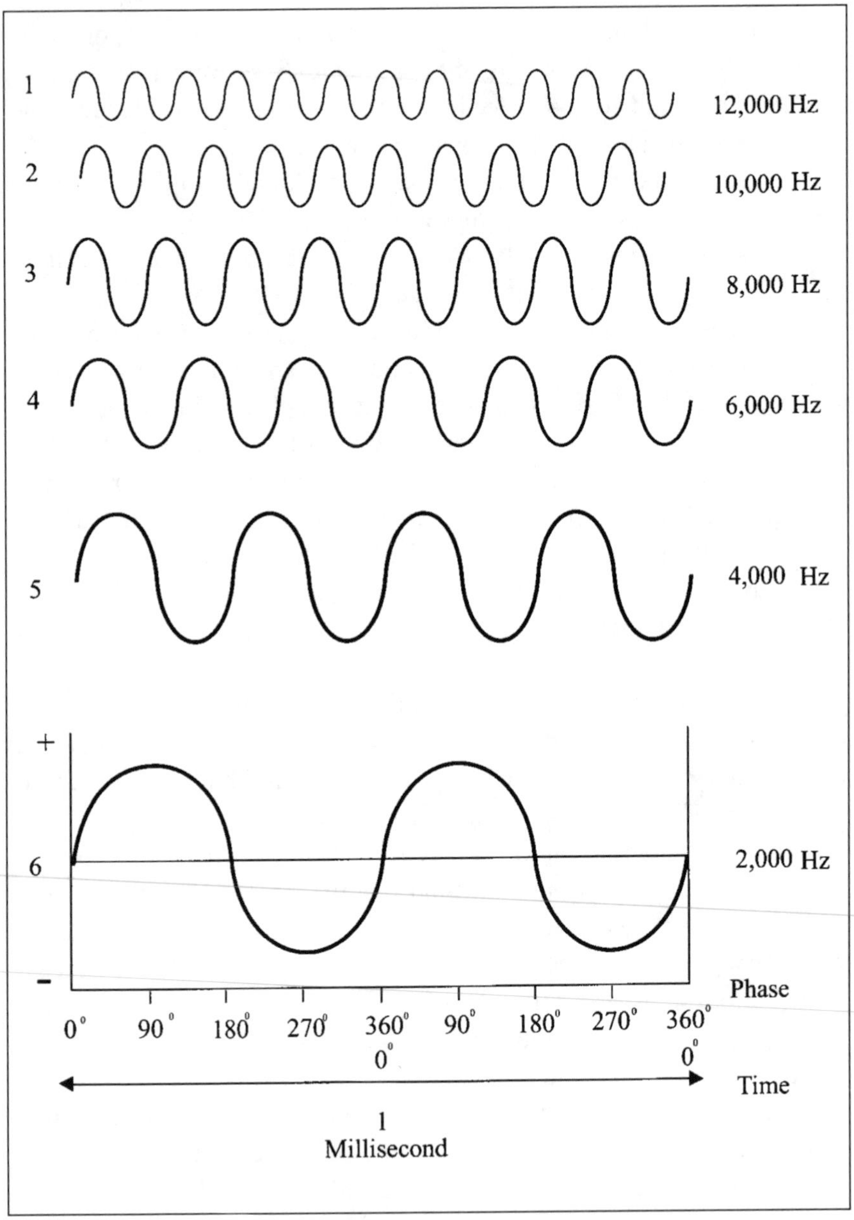

Figure 8.2. Six Sinusoids Displayed in the Time Domain

Complexity

A complex stimulus is, for our purposes, easily defined. Any auditory stimulus composed of more than one frequency is complex. Figure 8.4 shows

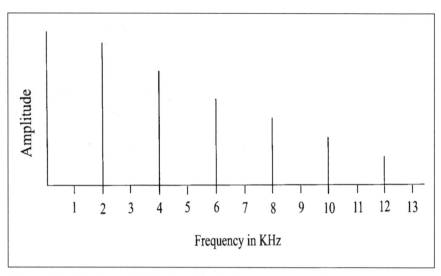

Figure 8.3. *Six Sinusoids Displayed in the Frequency Domain*

an example of a complex wave. Figure 8.4(a) shows two simple sinusoids, A and B. Sinusoid A is 3,000 Hz and Sinusoid B is 1,000 Hz. The amplitude of the two stimuli is represented by the vertical axis, labeled Pressure in dB. In Figure 8.4(b) the two sinusoids, A and B have been algebraically summed. This results in the complex waveform, labeled A + B. The algebraic addition of the amplitudes at each moment in time, yields a complex waveform. The waveform in this example contains the two frequencies, 1,000 Hz and 3,000 Hz.

Consider now a different stimulus. It is also complex. It is so complex, in fact, that it contains all the frequencies we can hear plus a few more we cannot. The lowest frequency in the complex is 1 Hz and the highest is 20,000 Hz. All the 20,000 frequencies are added together to form the complex waveform, and every frequency has the same average amplitude. This waveform has a special name: **white noise.** What does white noise look like in the time and frequency domains? Figure 8.5 shows the line spectrum and a representative time waveform for white noise.

Consider first the line spectrum. As we know, the line spectrum displays every frequency in the complex as a vertical line; thus, there are 20,000 individual vertical lines—one for each frequency. Furthermore, the height of the each line represents the average amplitude of each frequency. Thus, all vertical lines are the same height. Figure 8.5(a) shows the resulting line spectrum for this white noise. When the line spectrum for the white noise is compared

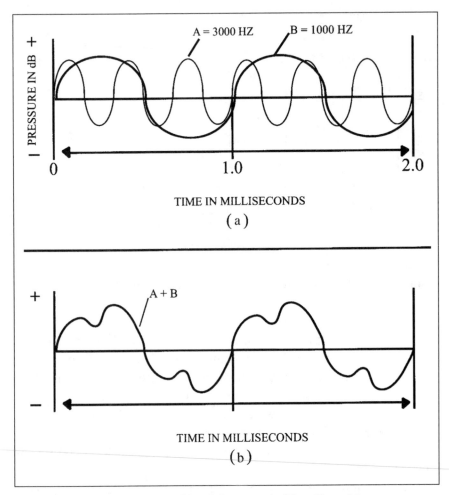

Figure 8.4. Complex Auditory Stimuli Composed of Two Sinusoids

with the line spectrum for the complex waveform discussed previously (Figure 8.3), there is an immediate noticeable difference. The white noise line spectrum in Figure 8.5 has no vertical lines. This is simply because every frequency in the **noise** is present. If a vertical line were plotted for every frequency, the result is a solid rectangle because all the lines are side by side and touching. So, it is easier to just plot a horizontal line and let the line represent the average amplitude of all the frequencies in the noise.

Figure 8.5(b) shows the waveform for white noise, as a function of time. There are significant differences between the waveform for the noise and for the complex waveform shown in Figure 8.4(b). Aside from the number of frequencies composing noise, the noise is clearly nonperiodic. The amplitude of

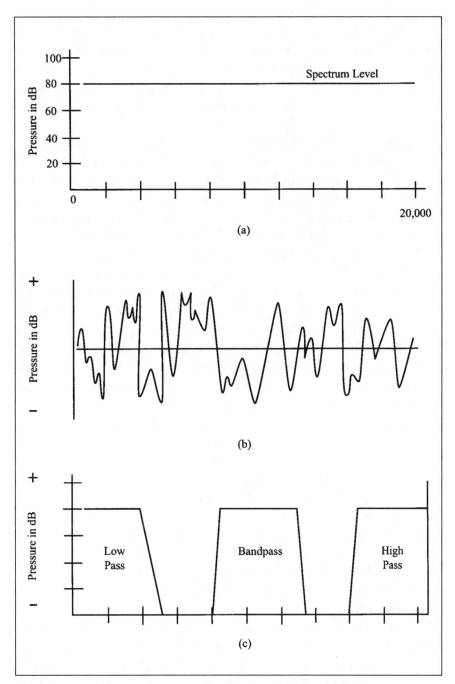

Figure 8.5.   Line Spectrum and Time Waveform for White Noise

NOTE: (a) White noise is displayed in the frequency domain as a line spectrum, (b) the white noise diplayed in the time domain, and (c) the white noise shaped to have low-pass, bandpass, or high-pass characteristics.

the noise waveform varies randomly and shows no periodicity. By periodicity, we mean that by knowing what the amplitude is at any one point in time, we know what the amplitude is at some future time. The waveform repeats itself and is therefore predictable. In Figure 8.5(b), there is no systematic periodicity in the white noise waveform. White noise varies randomly and does not repeat itself.

Before we continue, it is necessary to briefly discuss a technique used to "shape" and "form" a noise spectrum. By experimentally manipulating the shape and form of the noise, investigations can be done that yield information regarding how sounds are processed. Scientists manipulate a noise by passing it through electronic filters. A filter selectively removes particular frequencies of the noise so that the output is "shaped." By passing noise through a filter, investigators can obtain a **low-pass noise,** a **high-pass noise,** or a **bandpass noise.** Low-pass noise is exactly what the term suggests. Only low frequencies in the noise, below a particular frequency, pass through the filter and are present at the output. Frequencies above the cutoff are filtered out and removed by the filter. A high-pass noise does the opposite. All frequencies above the cutoff frequency pass through the filter; the low frequencies are filtered out and removed. A bandpass noise has two cutoff frequencies—a low cutoff and a high cutoff—so that the filter passes those frequencies between the two cutoff points—hence, *bandpass* Figure 8.5(c) diagrammatically demonstrates these three concepts. The cutoff frequencies, of course, can be manipulated so that noise characteristics such as low-pass, high-pass, or bandpass noise can become a variable of interest.

Between the single sinusoid and the white noise lies the vast majority of complex sounds that form the auditory environment. One additional example of such complex sounds is shown in Figure 8.6, which depicts different aspects of the same musical note, A above middle C.

Figure 8.6(a) shows an example of a complex waveform produced by synthesizing (adding) the four frequencies displayed in 8.6(b). These four frequencies have a special link to one another: They are harmonically related. A **harmonic** is an exact multiple of the lowest frequency in the complex. The lowest frequency in a complex is called the **fundamental frequency.** The fundamental, therefore, is also the first harmonic (1×440 Hz). The second harmonic is 880 Hz and the second multiple of the fundamental (2×440 Hz). The third harmonic is 1,320 Hz (3×440 Hz) and the fourth harmonic is 1,760 Hz (4×440 Hz). If you are following this logic, then you should realize that the fifth harmonic has a frequency of 2,200 Hz (5×440) and the ninth harmonic is 3,960 Hz. Only the lower four harmonics are shown in Figure 8.6.

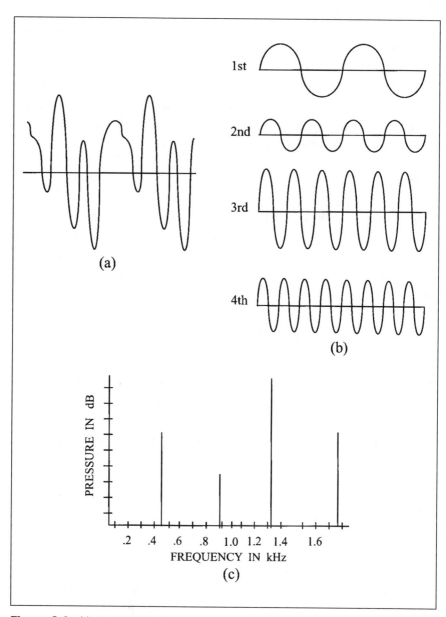

Figure 8.6. Harmonic Waveforms

NOTE: (a) A complex harmonic waveform composed of the four first four harmonics of a 440 Hz fundamental, (b) first four harmonics of the 440 Hz fundamental, and (c) spectrum analysis of the complex waveform shown in (a).

When harmonic sinusoids are summed, the result is a **periodic wave-form.** The periodicity can be seen in Figure 8.6(a) because the waveform re-peats itself. When a waveform is composed of nonharmonic sinusoids, on the other hand, the result is a nonperiodic complex.

Figure 8.6(c) shows the complex waveform in the frequency domain as a line spectrum. In this perspective, the waveform has been Fourier analyzed in its component frequencies and displayed graphically.

Intensity

Consider a relatively common event. Practically everyone has heard a persistent mosquito and the rumble of thunder. An interesting point about these sounds is the difference in magnitude. The drone of a mosquito, irritat-ing as it may be, is relatively feeble when compared to the penetrating crack of thunder overhead. These two disturbances illustrate a range of intensities that the auditory system must quickly and proficiently manage every day.

In our world, there are many soft, almost imperceptible sounds. The rus-tle of leaves or the gentle sigh of a pet sleeping at our feet are two examples. On the other hand, there are intense sounds in our environment: screeching si-rens, roaring jet aircraft, pulsating hard rock music, cracking thunder, and gas-powered lawn mowers and snow blowers. The **intensity** of sounds you encounter clearly ranges from subthreshold to the painful and physiologi-cally damaging. The enormous range to which the auditory system responds requires the use the **decibel (dB),** as a metric. The use of the decibel enables us to handle more easily this vast range of intensities. Table 8.1 on page 223 shows pressure changes, in dB, that range from just detectable to pressures that yield physical damage and pain.

The decibel is used to quantify the physical magnitude of a sound. By us-ing decibels, investigators can transform the range of stimulus intensities to a manageable size. You should also keep in mind that what we are attempting to measure is the amplitude or size of the waveforms shown in the previous fig-ures. Although somewhat imprecise, *intensity* and *amplitude* are used inter-changeably in this discussion. Our goal is to get an idea about the magnitude of sounds and how they are measured.

The Decibel

The goal of this section is to define a decibel and quantify the magnitude of the auditory stimulus. One method of quantifying auditory stimuli is to measure the **power** of the sound. The unit of power we are concerned with is the watt per square centimeter, **watt/cm**^{2}. When power is the unit used to quantify the sound, the range of perceptible intensity from weakest to most intense is enormous. The auditory system can respond to power that can increase by a hundred million million. This is 10 raised to an exponent of 14, 10^{14}, which equals 100,000,000,000,000.

There is a problem, however, in using the watt/cm^2 as the metric for quantifying sound. The problem is the extremely small values of power that we can hear. In air, the medium in which most sounds are perceived, the weakest perceptible power we can detect (the absolute threshold) is near 10^{-16} watt/cm^2. That is a very small number. At the other extreme, where pain occurs because of the intensity, the power is still quite small, near 10^{-3} watt/cm^2. The watt/cm^2 puts us at a disadvantage; we are working with extremely small numbers. The way around this is the use of logarithms and the incorporation of a reasonable reference value. What we do is form a ratio of the sound we want to know about with a reasonable reference. That is, we put the observed sound power in the numerator (S_o) and the reference value in denominator (S_r). This forms the ratio S_o/S_r. Scientists have chosen, as the reasonable reference value, the power near the absolute threshold of human hearing, 10^{-16} watt/cm^2, at 2,000 Hz. They then take the logarithm of this ratio and multiply it by 10. This yields the decibel using power at absolute threshold as the reference. The formula is:

$$dB = C \log_{10} \left(\frac{S_o}{S_r} \right)$$

The constants for the dB formula are C = 10, and $S_r = 10^{-16}$ watt/cm^2. The formula then becomes:

$$dB = 10 \log_{10} \left(\frac{S_o}{10^{-16} \; watt \, / \, cm^2} \right)$$

All that remains is to measure the power of the stimulus of interest, S_o, and solve the equation. Here is an example when S_o is equal to 10^{-6} watt/cm^2.

$$dB = 10 \log_{10} \left(\frac{10^{-6}}{10^{-16}} \right)$$

$$dB = 10 \log_{10} (10,000,000,000)$$

$$dB = 10(10) \dots \text{so, the answer is 100 dB}$$

You should remember when you solve this equation that you divide the ratio by subtracting exponents. This means that $10^{-6}/10^{-16}$ becomes $(10^{-6}-10^{-16})$. Because both exponents are negative, you use the simple "change the sign and add" rule you learned in the grade school, $(-6)+(+16)=10$. We take the logarithm of 10^{10}, ten billion, 10,000,000,000. The $\log_{10}$ of 10^{10} is 10.

When the stimulus is measured in watt/cm^2 with a reference value of 10^{-16} watt/cm^2, the decibel is expressed as **intensity level** (IL). If an investigator uses a different reference, the use of *intensity level* is not appropriate. Intensity level is restricted to those situations in which the reference, S_p, is 10^{-16} watt/cm^2. As a reminder, the value of 10^{-16} watt/cm^2 is an arbitrary value chosen because it is near the absolute threshold of a 2,000-Hz sinusoid for human hearing.

A final example is probably useful. See if you can calculate the IL if the observed stimulus, S_o, had a power equal to 10^{-12}. The answer is 40 dB. If you had trouble with this calculation, you should review the previous few paragraphs until you feel comfortable with the topic. You can practice and check your answers by using the data in Table 8.1. This table shows the dB for different values of S_o with 10^{-16} watt/cm^2 as the reference. It also shows examples of everyday sounds for particular dB levels, and there is a column that indicates the dB when pressure measurements are the metric of interest. Pressure measurements are our next topic.

Sound Pressure Level

A more common means of measuring sound in air is **sound pressure level** (SPL). Even with sound pressure level, however, the perceptible magnitude of sounds is still large. The range, in pressure units, from the least perceptible to the most intense, is about ten million, 10^7.

The unit of sound pressure can be stipulated in different metric units. The pressure unit can be in pascals, newtons, or dynes. We restrict ourselves to a single unit, the dyne per square centimeter, dyne/cm^2. For completeness, however, note that 0.0002 dyne/cm^2 is equal to 20 μPascal and 20 μNewton/m^2. The decibel using the SPL reference is:

$$dB = 20 \log_{10}\left(\frac{S_o}{.0002\,dyne/cm^2}\right)$$

Two changes occur in the equation when sound pressure is the metric. The constant, C, becomes 20 and the denominator in the ratio, S_p, becomes

TABLE 8.1 Power and Pressure Measurements, Decibels, and Environmental Sounds

dB	Observed Power in watt/cm$_2$	Observed Pressure in dyne/cm^2	Examples of Environmental Sounds
0	10-16	0.0002	Absolute Threshold
20	10-14	0.002	Soft Whisper
40	10-12	0.02	Very Quiet Room
60	10-10	0.2	Normal Conversation
80	10-8	2.0	Average City Street
100	10-6	20.0	Rock Band at 20 feet
120	10-4	200.0	Very Loud Thunder
140	10-2	2000.0	Physiological Damage

NOTE: All measures are in reference to 10^{-16} watt/cm^2 or 0.0002 dyne/cm^2.

0.0002 dyne/cm^2. The reference value, once again, is the absolute threshold of human hearing at 2,000 Hz.

An example of the dB calculation is given next in which the observed pressure, S_o, is 20.

$$dB = 20 \log_{10} \left(\frac{20}{.0002} \right)$$
$$dB = 20 \log_{10} (100{,}000)$$
$$dB = 20 (5)$$
$$dB = 100$$

This relatively brief discussion of the decibel has left out a few points that are considered important in a more advanced course on acoustics. For our purposes, however, we have covered the major characteristics of sound magnitude. The few aspects that need to be kept in mind are briefly summarized here.

First, it should be clear that the decibel notation is dependent on a reference. With no reference, there is ambiguity and uncertainty concerning the actual magnitude of the sound. It is similar to saying that you are 33 inches taller than your dog. This may be useful information, but you still do not know exactly how tall you are until the height of the reference is known, in this case the dog. If the dog is only 8 inches tall, then you are just over 3 feet tall, 41 inches. If the dog is 27 inches tall, then you are 5 feet tall, 60 inches. It all depends on the reference. This is the case in decibels. You must know the reference value if the decibel scale is to make any sense. The usual situation is to assume that the reference is 0.0002 dyne/cm^2 when the reference is not explicitly mentioned. When you are told that the stimulus is 40 dB, you presume, unless told otherwise, that the reference is the absolute threshold of human hearing stipulated in SPL, 0.0002 dyne/cm^2.

Second, Table 8.1 shows a clear relationship between the two references: power and pressure. Acoustic power is proportional to pressure squared. As the table shows, a 100-fold increase in acoustic power is equivalent to a 10-fold increase in pressure. A 100-fold increase in power or a 10-fold increase in pressure equals, in both cases, a 20 dB increase. This is seen in the table by considering the 100-fold increase in acoustic powers of (10^{-12} to 10^{-10}) and the 10-fold increase in pressure (0.02 to 0.2). The increase is from 40 to 60 dB.

Finally, the dB notation using pressure units is of practical use in laboratory research and in the clinic when evaluating hearing loss. In most of these situations, the auditory stimuli are conveniently presented to an individual over an earphone. The earphone acts as a transducer to change electrical voltage to sound pressure. The movement of the earphone diaphragm caused by voltage fluctuations results in corresponding pressure changes in the air that surrounds the earphone. The known sound pressure variations at the earphone are then used to evaluate the auditory system. A research participant, or client having a hearing test, has the earphone placed next to the ear and perceives, or does not perceive, the sound pressure variations transduced by the earphone. By systematically varying frequency and intensity, you obtain the absolute threshold of hearing. The absolute threshold is the weakest stimulus intensity that can be perceived. The result is an **audiogram** that can reveal hearing losses at particular frequencies relative to a population norm.

A final note should be made regarding a reference value often used in the quantification of sound. This reference is **sensation level (SL)**. Sensation level is the intensity of a sound, in dB SPL, above the absolute threshold. For example, if the absolute threshold for an individual were 60 dB SPL at 2,000 Hz, a 40 dB SL stimulus is equivalent to 100 dB SPL (40 dB above the 60 dB SPL absolute threshold). This is a very loud sound for anyone with normal hearing. However, it is just 40 dB to an individual with a 60 dB loss at 2,000 Hz.

Finally, sounds have a sequence of occurrence in time. This temporal aspect of sound is clearly important in auditory perception. For example, if a stimulus is too brief, it may not be detected or, if one sound follows another too rapidly in time, a previous sound may be covered or masked by a subsequent sound. These temporal considerations are important in language comprehension and animal communication as well as everyday interactions with the world.

Summary

The auditory stimulus is measured in decibels (amplitude), Hertz (frequency), and degrees (phase). Sound travels through a medium at various speeds with the speed depending on temperature and density of the medium. The level or intensity of a sound is measured in decibels for a given reference. Usually the reference is intensity level or sound pressure level. Our environmental sounds are always complex.

Suggested Readings

Evans, E. F. (1982). Basic physics and psychophysics of sound. In H. B. Barlow & J. D. Mollon (Eds.), *The senses*. New York: Cambridge University Press.

Gelfand, S. A. (1990). *Hearing: An introduction to psychological and physiological acoustics* (2nd ed.). New York: Marcel Dekker.

von Bergeijk, W. A., Pierce, J. R., & David, E. E., Jr. (1960). *Waves and the ear*. Garden City, NY: Doubleday.

CHAPTER 9

Audition

They support eyeglasses, are frequently the sites of self-inflicted wounds, and are the most unusual pieces of cartilage on our head. The appendages I refer to are attached to the side of the head and are called the **pinna,** Latin for "wing," or **auricle,** Latin for "ear." They are what most people refer to as the ears. The ears are unique because they are provided with musculature that allows some animals to move their pinna as an aid in locating the source of a sound. In fact, many animals depend on this ability for their existence. As intriguing as this may be, the musculature of the pinna has a negligible function in the human species.

Although you have already been introduced to the external ear in Chapter 7, we reexamine it in this chapter and provide more information relative to its function in auditory perception. Figure 9.1 shows the **external** and **middle ear** with some labeled components.

External and Middle Ear

We begin with the pinna. There are six landmarks of importance to us. First, there is the **lobule.** This is part of the ear that is usually referred to simply as the earlobe. It is one of the less useful portions of our auditory system. There are two ridges: One begins at the top of the pinna that runs around the outer edge—the **helix;** the other ridge, the **antihelix,** makes an approximate half-circle below the helix. Above the antihelix and below the superior portion of the helix is a small depression called the triangular *fossa,* Latin for "ditch." The fifth aspect of the pinna is a landmark of some importance: It is the relatively deep depression at the opening of the external auditory meatus.

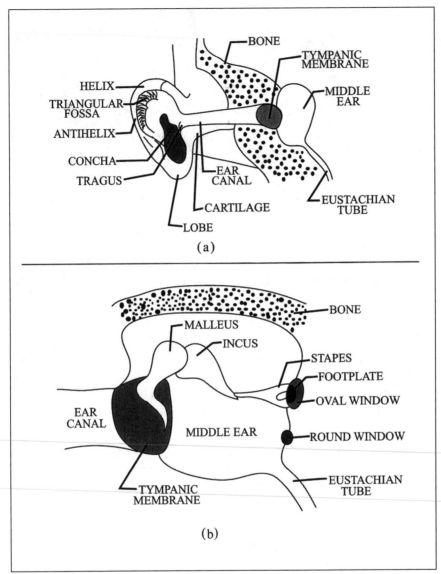

Figure 9.1. The External and Middle Ear

This depression is the **concha.** Finally, near the mouth of the concha, toward the anterior portion of the pinna, is a little flap called the **tragus.** These contours and depressions are important in "modifying and shaping" the environmental sounds that enter the external auditory meatus (the ear canal). The shape of the pinna is uniquely involved in sound localization. Each of us has our own uniquely formed pinna (Batteau, 1967). The external auditory meatus is carved in the temporal bone and sealed at the end by the tympanic membrane, commonly referred to as the eardrum.

The inner portion of the canal has the distinction of producing the earwax—cerumen that provides protection and moisture for the delicate tissues in the canal.

The middle ear, as shown in Figure 9.1(b), is an air filled cavity located just beyond the tympanic membrane. The middle ear contains the three smallest bones in the human body, the malleus, incus, and stapes. These three bones, as a group, are called the ossicles. The ossicles provide the means for the airborne sound to reach the sensitive receptors within the inner ear. The three bones are linked together and form the **ossicular chain.** The first bone in the series is malleus. One end of the malleus is attached to the inside of the tympanic membrane and the other end is connected to the second bone in the sequence, the incus. The incus is connected to the stirrup-shaped stapes. The last connection is the binding of the stapes footplate to a thin membrane that separates the middle and inner ear. This latter membrane is the **oval window.** On the medial side of the oval window is the inner ear filled with a noncompressible fluid, perilymph. It should be mentioned at this point that the ossicles do not dangle unsupported within the middle ear. They are suspended by ligaments and by two muscles. The muscles are involved in a protective reflex and are discussed more fully in the following paragraphs.

Two other important structures need to be mentioned before we continue. The first is the eustachian tube leading from the middle ear to the throat. It is through this conduit that the pressure within the middle ear is kept at an equilibrium with the atmospheric pressure on the other side of the tympanic membrane. When you drive up in the mountains, the change in altitude causes a change in the atmospheric pressure surrounding you. You nearly always notice a change in the surrounding atmospheric pressure because of an uncomfortable feeling in the ear. This is the difference in pressures on each side of the tympanic membrane. To relieve this uncomfortable pressure difference, you usually "pop" the ear by swallowing, yawning, or moving the jaw. These movements briefly open the eustachian tube and permit the influx of air from the throat into the middle ear. This influx of air equalizes the pressure on both sides of the tympanic membrane. The popping sound is the tympanic membrane snapping back to its original position. Having an unequal pressure between the middle ear and the outer environment results in a loss of hearing. This occurs because the eardrum is drawn tight by the pressure difference and the conduction of sound through the middle ear is impeded.

The second item of importance concerns the smallest muscles in the body. These are the middle ear muscles previously noted (Borg & Counter, 1989). These muscles are the tensor tympani and the stapedius. The names of these two muscles clearly suggest where they attach. The stapedius muscle is attached at one end, as is the tensor tympani, to the bone within a crevice of the middle ear. The other end of the stapedius is attached to the stapes. The contraction of the stapedius muscle causes the footplate of the stapes to be drawn into the middle ear. Because the oval window and the footplate are physically attached, the contraction draws the oval window toward the middle ear. The total effect of an active stapedius is to reduce movement of the stapes and the oval window membrane. In an analogous manner, the tensor tympani, which is attached to the tympanic membrane, draws the eardrum inward making it taut. The simultaneous contraction of these two muscles draws the flexible membranes inward and makes the ossicular chain rigid. This reduces the conduction of high-frequency sound through the middle ear and protects the receptors within the inner ear from intense sounds (Reger, 1960).

Function of the Middle Ear

A question often occurs at this point. Why are there bones in our ears? There is a membrane at each end of the ossicular chain. Why place bones between two membranes? A more efficient design might be to leave the whole middle ear out of the system and have one membrane at the end of the canal. The cochlea would then be immediately on the other side of the tympanic membrane and sound could move the membrane directly. The ossicular chain is not necessary. This "design" would, however, cause a mismatch between air and fluid.

Recall what happens when a rock is thrown in a flat trajectory across the surface of a pond. When the rock first strikes the water, it does not immediately sink. The rock skips and does not sink because water is denser than air. The rock flew through the thin air, struck a more rigid surface of the water, and skipped. Each time the rock strikes the water, it loses speed and energy. Finally, when the rock has been slowed enough by the impacts, it sinks to the bottom of the pond.

The answer to why we have bones in our ears is related to the reason why the rock does not sink into the pond on the first impact. There is a mismatch between the air and fluid. The air is thin and easily disturbed but the fluid is not. This is called an **impedance mismatch.** At the point of interface between the two mediums, air and fluid, there is a loss of energy. If something is not done to improve the transmission of energy between the air in the environment and the fluid within the inner ear, there is a loss of acoustic energy. The loss of energy causes a decline in auditory perception. The receptors in the fluid of the cochlea are not stimulated. The bones in the middle ear function to help correct the impedance mismatch. The impedance mismatch yields a loss in energy of about 30 dB. The way to recover from this handicap is to implement three mechanisms: resonance within the ear canal, mechanical leverage by the ossicles, and a tympanic membrane that is larger than the oval window (Fischler, Frei, Spira, & Rubenstein, 1967; Wever & Lawrence, 1954). Let us look briefly at each mechanism.

The first mechanism is the ear canal. It is basically a tube with one end closed by the tympanic membrane. Because of this closed-tube characteristic, the ear canal has a resonance that selectively amplifies particular frequencies. The selective amplification occurs because a periodic force, the sound wave from the environment, is amplified when it is applied to a structure or body that naturally resonates and matches the periodic frequency of the applied force. In other words, the frequencies in the environment near 2.5 kHz match the natural resonance of the external auditory meatus. This match results in an amplification of the sound by 5 to 10 dB and a partial recovery of some of the energy lost by the impedance mismatch.

The mechanical leverage of the ossicles is the second set of mechanisms used to preserve energy. This leverage idea can be understood by considering a problem. Assume that a 300-pound boulder is in the road and you cannot move it no matter how hard you try. It is too massive. If, however, you get a large, strong pole and a few cement blocks you can get leverage and move the boulder. You simply wedge the pole under the boulder and over the stack of cement blocks to form a fulcrum. You then pull down on the long end of the pole. The boulder is likely to move because the leverage system adds force to your attempt to move the unyielding object. This is, by analogy, what the ossicles do in the middle ear to recover energy loss.

In addition to this lever system, the middle ear uses a size factor to help overcome the mismatch. The size of the tympanic membrane at the end of the ear canal, in contrast to the size of the oval window, results in an amplification of the sound. The force placed on the larger tympanic membrane by the environmental pressures must be the same as the force placed on the much smaller oval window by the stapes. This size mismatch between the larger eardrum and the smaller oval window results in a pressure increase at the inner ear. This leads to another source of recovery of energy due to the mismatch.

The total pressure increase by the three mechanisms of the middle ear approaches 25 dB. Thus, the external and middle ear design amplifies the sound at the inner ear by an amount that almost equals what is otherwise lost by the impedance mismatch.

Finally, it should be emphasized again that the smallest muscles in the body, the stapedius and tensor tympani, have an important function as well. They act as protective devices. When an environmental sound occurs with a pressure so intense that inner ear mechanisms can be severely damaged, the muscles contract bilaterally. This reflexive contraction occurs when the sound is near 80 dB SPL and protects the sensitive receptors within the inner ear. The muscular reflex does require, however, some time to respond. The latency is approximately 10 msec for a quick, intense sound. Because of this relatively slow action of the muscles, an impulsive blast, such as a rifle shot near the ear, reaches the sensitive receptors of the inner ear before the muscles can react. The intense sound , particularly if it occurs often, causes permanent hearing impairment. In fact, a continuous long exposure to noise having an overall level above 80 dB SPL results in permanent hearing impairment. The insidious aspect of this situation is that you can go deaf without knowing it until it is too late to protect yourself. With the exception of intense blasts, there is rarely any pain involved with noise **induced hearing loss.** The "Walkman era" is likely to become the hearing-impaired generation.

The Inner Ear

Panel (a) of Figure 9.2 shows the middle ear and the two thin membranes that divide it from the **inner ear.** One membrane, the oval window, has already been introduced. The other membrane, the **round window,** is equally important for the function of hearing. On the medial side of the two windows is the inner ear filled with perilymph. The windows are in direct contact with the perilymph within the coiled structure called the **cochlea.** The cochlea is the auditory portion of the inner ear. The other portions consist of the semicircular canals, saccule, and utricle and are associated with the vestibular sense. The cochlea derives its name, not surprisingly, from its snail shape and coiled appearance. The cochlea, like the rest of the inner ear, is carved out of the temporal bone. It makes about $2\frac{3}{4}$ turns as it spirals from its base, near the oval and round windows, to its apex.

Panel (a) of Figure 9.2 also shows the cochlea stretched out to show the three scalae or canals (also called ducts). The inner scala, the **scala media,** is filled with endolymph and is a continuation of the membranous labyrinth of

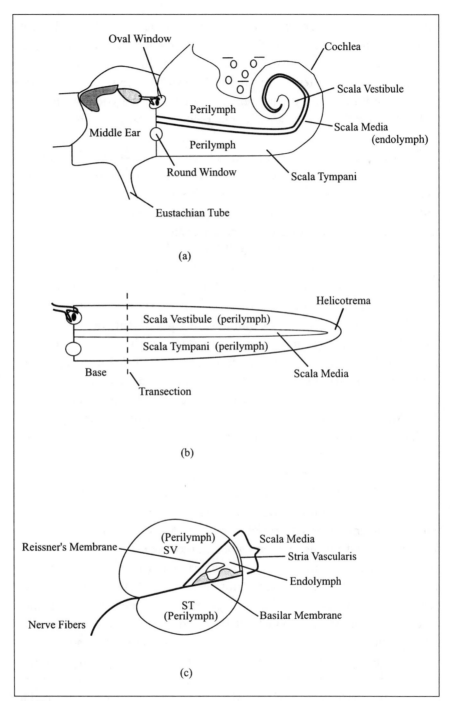

Figure 9.2. Auditory Portion of the Inner Ear

NOTE: (a) cochlea, (b) cochlea unrolled, (c) cross sectional view of the cochlea.

the vestibular system. The other two scalae, the **scala vestibuli** and the **scala tympani,** communicate with each other at the apex of the cochlea through an opening called the **helicotrema.** These latter two scalae are also connected with the vestibular system. Thus, the scala vestibuli and the scala tympani contain the same fluid, perilymph. At the base of the cochlea, the scala vestibuli and scala tympani are in contact with the oval and round window, respectively.

To discuss the cochlea in a meaningful way it is necessary to take some liberties with the anatomical structure. It is, of course, impossible to unwind a cochlea formed from the temporal bone. Nevertheless, in this computer age and with our visual capabilities, we can pretend to unroll the cochlea and even cut it in half to look into the three scalae. If we were to do this, the result is similar to that shown in Figure 9.2(b) and (c).

These panels show the cochlea unrolled and cut in half (a transection). Panel (b) shows the base of the cochlea with the oval and round window to the left and the helicotrema and apex to the right. The scala media is shown in this lateral view as a very narrow tube running the length of the cochlea and ending at the apex. A transection of the cochlea is made at the vertical dashed line and the cochlea is rotated to provide the cross-sectional view looking into the cochlea from the basal end. This latter view, shown in Panel (c), depicts the three scala in cross section. The scala vestibuli is separated from the scala media by Reissner's membrane. The scala tympani is partitioned from the scala media by the osseous spiral lamina and basilar membrane. An enlarged view of the scala media is portrayed in Figure 9.3.

Within the scala media is the **organ of Corti.** The organ of Corti consists of several different cells and tissues that operate together to produce action potentials for the sense of hearing. The organ of Corti consists of the **outer hair cells, inner hair cells, tectorial membrane**, the **arch (or tunnel) of Corti** formed by the **pillar cells,** and the supporting cells of Henson and Deiter. The organ of Corti rests on the basilar membrane and is outlined within the square of Figure 9.3. The basilar membrane is located between the outer wall of the scala media, attached to the wall by the **spiral ligament,** and a bony shelf called the **osseous spiral lamina** located toward the **modiolus.** The modiolus is located in the center of the cochlea where nerve fibers enter and exit.

There are approximately 3,500 inner hair cells forming a single column on the basilar membrane. The column runs the length of the basilar membrane, from base to apex. The cilia on the inner hair cells are not attached to any other structure but are totally immersed within the endolymph of the

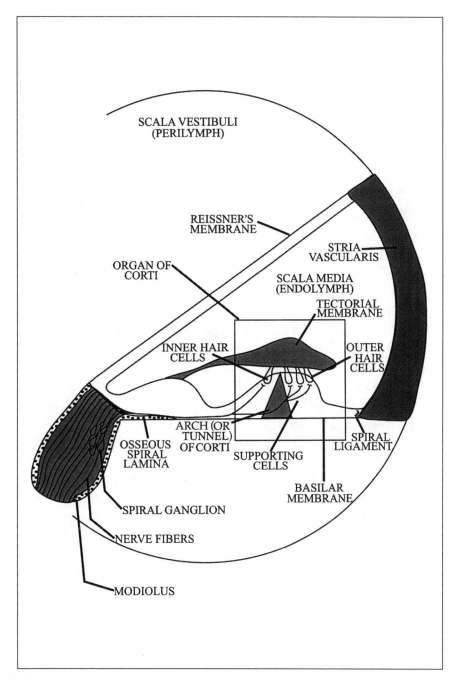

Figure 9.3. Cross Section of the Cochlea Showing the Scala Media, Organ of Corti, and Supporting Structures

scala media under the tectorial membrane. This means that any flow, eddy, or movement of endolymph beneath the tectorial membrane affects the cilia of the inner hair cells. The estimated 12,000 outer hair cells, on the other hand, are arranged in three rows (four or five rows near the apex) with the tallest cilia firmly attached to the overhanging tectorial membrane. Thus, there is a mechanical linkage between the outer hair cells and the tectorial membrane. The rows of outer hair cells also extend the length of the basilar membrane. The arch of Corti is the structural marker that divides the two types of hair cells. The hair cells and their orientation on the basilar membrane are shown in Figure 9.4. Keep in mind that the transduction mechanisms for these cells are the same as the hair cells within the vestibular system (Chapter 7). That is, the movement of the cilia causes a depolarization or hyperpolarization. The depolarization releases a neurotransmitter at the synapse with the primary sensory neuron.

There are approximately 30,000 primary sensory neurons whose axons compose the afferent acoustic branch of the VIII cranial nerve, the vestibulocochlear nerve. The arrangement of these nerve fibers is interesting because 90 to 95% of them (about 28,000) are connected to the inner hair cells. This means that there are, on the average, about eight to nine afferent fibers attached to each inner hair cell. Some inner hair cells actually have many more. In contrast, a single fiber is attached to a minimum of 4 outer hair cells and may be attached to over 10 separate outer hair cells. As we learn, this arrangement of afferent innervation has functional significance in the way the auditory system performs its task.

In addition to the afferent fibers leaving the cochlea, there are about 1,800 efferent neurons that enter the cochlea. A little over one half of these efferents synapse directly onto the inner hair cell afferent fibers (axoaxonic connections). The remainder of the efferents make synapses directly on the outer hair cells. This arrangement has a meaningful effect on the function of the cochlear activity. The efferent or centrifugal axons originate in a brain stem nuclear complex called the **superior olive.**

Finally, we arrive at a physiological structure located on the outer wall of the scala media, the **stria vascularis.** The stria vascularis is composed of secretory cells as well as cells that function as active energy-consuming ionic pumps. The activity of the stria vascularis results in the production of endolymph within the cochlea (and the vestibular system). The +80 millivolt endolymphatic potential within the scala media is generated by the active transport of ions. The ionic concentration of Na^+ and K^+ within the endolymph is believed to result from an active Na^+/K^+ ionic pump in the stria

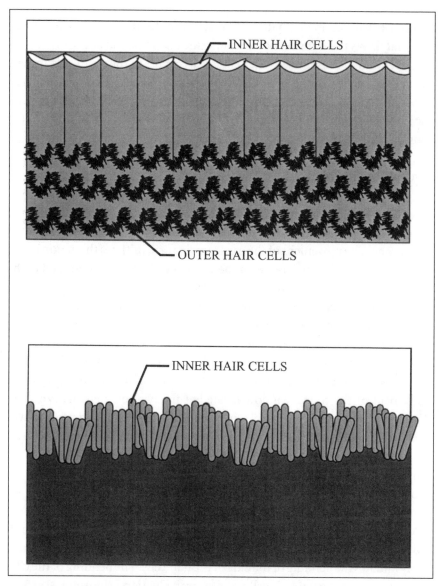

Figure 9.4. Outer and Inner Hair Cells Showing Their Orientation and Configuration

vascularis. The importance of the positive **endolymphatic potential** was discussed in Chapter 7 (Gulick, Geshcheider, & Frisina, 1989; Hudspeth, 1982, 1985, 1989; Pickles, Comis, & Osborne, 1984; Pickles & Corey, 1992) In Chapter 7, the receptor potential of the hair cell and the modulation of the neurotransmitter substance at its base was shown to be dependent on the positive +80 mv endolymphatic potential. The potential acts as a kind of battery that drives the transduction of hair cells. The same transduction process that occurs in the vestibular-system hair cells occurs in the cochlea to initiate the neural activity for the sense of hearing. A complete discussion of the hair cell transduction process was provided in Chapter 7. For now, we focus on some issues concerning the hydromechanical events that initiate the transduction process.

Hydromechanical Events of the Cochlea

We begin by considering a small predicament. When a sound from the environment is conducted through the ear canal, it moves the tympanic membrane. The movement of the eardrum, in turn, initiates the action of the ossicles. Because the final ossicle in the sequence, the stapes, is bonded to the oval window, it attempts to move the oval window as a function of the sound stimulus. The dilemma is that there is perilymph within the cochlea. The perilymph is a noncompressible fluid. For the stapes to move the oval window, the perilymph within the cochlea must be displaced. Either the perilymph must flow or something within the cochlea has to yield, bend, or flex so the oval window can move freely. The solution to this quandary is the movement of the round window located at the base of the scala tympani. When the stapes presses the oval window inward, the round window moves outward in the middle ear by an equal amount. Conversely, when the oval window is drawn outward by the stapes, the round window is displaced inward. The final solution, then, is that the movements of the oval and round windows are reciprocal and the perilymph is displaced as a function of the activity of the stapes. The stapes, of course, is driven by the environmental sound conducted through the external and middle ear system. The perilymph movement is important because it is the movement of this fluid that indirectly initiates the bending of the cilia of the hair cells. The bending of the cilia is, of course, the start of hair cell receptor transduction (Hudspeth, 1985).

The next question concerns the movement of the perilymph itself. How does the perilymph flow from the scala vestibuli to scala tympani so the round window moves and relieves the pressure? There are two answers to this question. The first answer begins with our recollection that the perilymph is continuous throughout the two scala. That is, the perilymph can flow back and forth through the helicotrema at the apex of the cochlea and displace the round window. Although the perilymph does indeed flow through the helicotrema, you must keep in mind that the helicotrema is an extremely small opening. It is, in fact, too small to handle rapid movements of perilymph caused by environmental sounds. Consequently, a second mode of perilymph movement handles normal sound-pressure fluctuations. The second method of perilymph movement is the flexing and bending of the scala media and the internal elements within the scala media. When the oval window oscillates because of a complex acoustic stimulus, the perilymph displaces the entire scala media. The movement of the scala media flexes the basilar membrane and concomitantly activates the hair cells. An inward movement of the oval window, for example, displaces perilymph and the basilar membrane downward in the scala tympani so the round window moves outward to relieve the pressure. When the stapes pulls the oval window outward, toward the middle ear, the scala media and basilar membrane holding the receptors are drawn upward in the scala vestibuli and the round window moves inward. As we see shortly, the activation of the receptors and our analysis of the acoustic environment are intimately tied to the basilar membrane movement. Because Reissner's membrane is only two cell layers thick, it is a nonparticipant in this dynamic activity. That is, Reissner's membrane bends as easily and simply as a single strand of hair in a summer breeze. It adds no resistance, and its main function is the separation of the endolymph from the perilymph. This division of the two fluids is, of course, critical to the function of the auditory system.

The perilymph displacement depends on the physical characteristics of the basilar membrane. The basilar membrane varies in width from the base to the apex of the cochlea. Even though the cochlea narrows as it curves toward the apex, the basilar membrane widens. The change in width results in a decline in stiffness as the membrane approaches the apex. The combination of these two basilar membrane characteristics, width and stiffness, provide the mechanical means of producing a **traveling wave** within the cochlea.

Traveling Waves in the Cochlea

Figure 9.5 displays a diagrammatic view of the basilar membrane with the organ of Corti and Reissner's membrane removed. The top panel (a) shows an unstimulated membrane increasing in width from the base to the apex. Panel (b) shows an instantaneous view of the basilar membrane after it has been stimulated by a sinusoidal tone. The shape of the basilar membrane reflects the traveling wave that develops in the perilymph. The traveling wave in this example has three important characteristics. First, it always begins at the base and moves or travels toward the apex. Second, as the wave travels toward the apex of the cochlea it releases its energy by depressing the basilar membrane until it reaches a final place of maximum amplitude. Third, once the maximum amplitude is reached, the wave dissipates and stops. Keep in mind as you view Panel (b) that the organ of Corti is "riding" on this membrane. The traveling wave and the movement of the basilar membrane results in a movement of the tectorial membrane and the endolymph within the scala media.

The endolymph, in the space between the tectorial membrane and the surface of the inner hair cells, is driven or displaced by the traveling wave. The tectorial-membrane-driven endolymph is believed to affect the stereocilia bundles and activate the inner hair cells. In addition, there is a mechanical bending of the stereocilia of the outer hair cells because they are physically attached to the tectorial membrane. Finally, it should be clear from looking at Panel (b) that the maximum inner hair cells and outer hair cells transduction is initiated at the point where the maximum basilar membrane displacement occurs. The point of maximum hydromechanical activity or displacement is shown in Figure 9.5(b).

Panel (c) shows the traveling wave from a different perspective. It shows a side view of the basilar membrane when a tonal stimulus is presented. Two images of the basilar membrane displacement are shown. The images are at two different instances of time, labeled Time A and Time B. If you were to obtain many different views at many different points in time, an "envelope" could be drawn that encompasses the maximum displacement of the basilar membrane along its length. The dotted line in Panel (c) represents such an envelope. The envelope reflects the maximum displacement of the basilar membrane as a function of distance from the base. For the moment, we need only keep in mind that the traveling waves are rather broad. That is, they do not in this particular view come to sharp points or peaks at their maximal point of displacement. These traveling waves represent the Nobel-prize-winning work of Georg von Békésy's observations and are discussed in more detail later in the chapter (von Békésy, 1947, 1960).

In summary, the shape and displacement of the basilar membrane, when stimulated by an auditory stimulus, depends on a traveling wave that develops within the perilymphatic fluids of the cochlea. The traveling wave produced by a single frequency displaces the basilar membrane maximally at a particular location along the membrane. The place of maximum displacement depends on the frequency of the simple tone. The point of maximum displacement results in maximal receptor transduction.

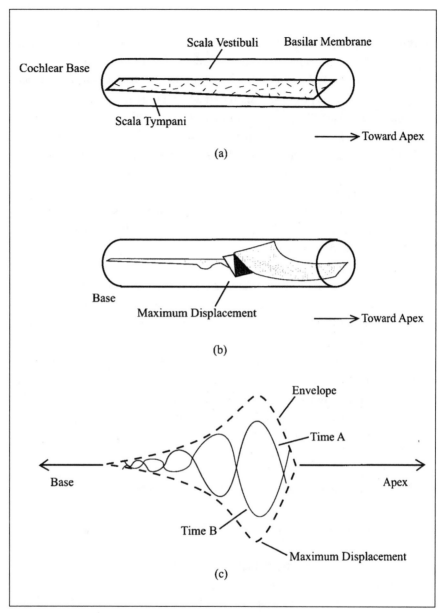

Figure 9.5. The Basilar Membrane and the Traveling Wave

NOTE: (a) the basilar membrane widening from base to apex, (b) a traveling wave display-ing a maximum displacement at a particular place on the basilar membrane, and (c) a cross section of the basilar membrane showing the envelope of the traveling wave.

A question often arises at this point. Why does the traveling wave always start at the base of the oval window and travel to some maximum point before dying out? The answer is rather simple. As was mentioned previously, the traveling wave depends on the physical characteristics of the basilar membrane. The two most relevant characteristics are (a) the width of the membrane and (b) the decline in stiffness as the membrane widens. Given these two parameters, it is a physical truism that when a pressure builds on a flexible boundary, such as the basilar membrane, a wave is set in motion that always begins at the region of highest stiffness (at the base of the basilar membrane) and propagates toward the area with the least resistance (toward the apex). The wave has a speed of travel that depends on the characteristics of the medium. The speed or velocity of movement is directly related to the stiffness of the flexible boundary, the basilar membrane. Because the stiffness of the basilar membrane decreases as the wave moves up the cochlea, the speed of the traveling wave also decreases.

As the speed of the traveling wave decreases, the amplitude or displacement of the basilar membrane increases. Thus, as the traveling wave moves down the cochlea from the base toward the apex, it slows down and simultaneously increases the displacement of the membrane. The point at which the propagation of the wave stops, the velocity obviously is zero. The energy of the wave then becomes focused at this particular stopping place on the membrane. The basilar membrane movement at this particular place is at its maximum. If the frequency of the stimulus changes, the place of maximum displacement also changes. The high frequencies have a maximum displacement near the base. The low frequencies propagate further along the membrane before they reach the place of maximum displacement. High frequencies displace and activate receptors at the base of the cochlea, and low frequencies activate receptors near the apex.

A Little Auditory Theory

Before we go too much further, it is wise that we consider a little history and some of the intellectual thoughts that have preceded us (Wever, 1949). A brief look at the past permits us to gain a fuller appreciation of the traveling wave and the basilar membrane activity.

The historical theories of hearing have been concerned mostly with our ability to perceive music. In fact, most theories dealt primarily with this concern. As the Greek philosophers searched for knowledge and how our five senses worked, they too were concerned with the perception of music. One of their views was that the inner world was a mirror of the external world; that is, "like is perceived by like." In hearing, what that meant was that the musical sound waves in the environment (the air) were replicated or matched to the air within our ear. We heard because the airwaves in the environment came in contact with the air in the middle ear. There was contact between the external sound and the internal sound of the perceiver. For hearing, the sound in the external air was matched with a sound in the air of the ear. Thus, the eardrum was the place of contact for sound and the air in the middle ear was "special." It was assumed to be implanted during gestation. In this theory (which lasted almost 2,000 years), it was the special "implanted air" that provided us with the ability to hear. We heard a high pitch because the physical stimulus matched the implanted air and generated a high pitch.

The discovery of the eustachian tube in the 16th century caused some concern with the implanted air theory. The air was not pure. The air in the middle ear was the same as the air outside in the real world. What this did, for several decades, was to cause theorists to modify the theory so that the implanted air was not in the middle ear; rather, it was shifted to the cochlea. Here is where the implanted air theory stayed until the 18th century. At that time, it was finally demonstrated, and accepted, that the cochlea was filled with fluid and could not be part of the implanted air theory. Once the cochlea had been fully examined and the anatomical facts became secure, theory and thought began to move toward current concepts.

Resonance and Place

Although there were many individuals who suggested, hypothesized, and theorized about perception and hearing, it was not until the 19th century that a more modern theory came to dominate the field. The theory was proposed by **Hermann Ludwig Ferdinan von Helmholtz**—a genius who was a physiologist, physicist, and only incidentally, a psychologist. His mind and scientific contributions rank von Helmholtz, in the eyes of many, to be among the greatest of scientists. One of his books, *Die Lehre von den Tonemphfindungen als physiologische Grundlege für die Theorie der Musik,* or *On the sensations of tone as a physiological basis for the theory of music,* was published in 1863 and is still referenced by investigators (von Helmholtz, H. L. F., 1863/1954). His theory was not the first "resonance" theory but, because of his eminent status, intellectual analysis, and writing skills, his **resonance theory of pitch** came to dominate the field.

Von Helmholtz's theory was based on his knowledge of physiology, physics, and music. Like his theory of color vision, which we explore in the next chapter, the theory was based on the scientific evidence available at the time and was well constructed. Von Helmholtz was constantly revising his theory so that it blended with newly discovered auditory anatomy and physiology. He incorporated an extension of Müller's doctrine of specific nerve energies and Ohm's acoustic law with his knowledge of music and the concept of resonance.

The theory set forth by von Helmholtz was designed to explain how we respond to biologically relevant sounds. Complex environmental sounds are composed of many frequencies, each of which varies continuously in amplitude and time. The cochlear mechanism has an enormous task. It must analyze the time-varying stimulus in its component parts, Ohm's acoustic law, and represent the sound in a pattern of neural discharges. To do this, von Helmholtz hypothesized that there was a series of resonating elements within the cochlea. Each resonator responded to a specific frequency. The resonators were initially hypothesized to be the pillars that formed the arch of Corti. He later changed the source of the resonation to other structures. One structure was the transverse fibers that appeared to cross the basilar membrane. However, the basic theme of his theory was maintained; namely, different frequencies activated different resonators within the cochlea. The resonators, once they are activated by the stimulus, elicit specific nerve fibers for the perception of pitch. In this manner, each resonator was associated with a specific fiber (the extension of Müller's doctrine). The resonators were tonotopically arranged along the basilar membrane, from base to apex—high frequencies at the base and low frequencies near the apex. By extension of this rationale, von Helmholtz argued that the basilar membrane could analyze a complex sound into its separate components. When a complex stimulus occurs in the environment, the ear acts as a Fourier analysis device. That is, those resonators that match the frequencies in the complex become active. For example, if a complex stimulus contains 400, 600, 800, and 1,200 Hz, then the four resonators in the ear that match these frequencies respond. The brain, therefore, receives information in the pattern of neural activity coming from these four "places." The theory, then, juxtaposed the physical frequency of the stimulus with the psychological perception of pitch. According to the theory, pitch depended on the frequency in the stimulus. Furthermore, because the resonators were located at different places on the basilar membrane, von Helmholtz's theory came to be known as the **place theory of pitch.**

As the 20th century dawned, the place theory of pitch was well known. The specific resonating structures or fibers, however, had not been discovered. It was during this period, 1920 to 1930, that **Georg von Békésy** began to work on the problem. His approach was to visually look within the cochlea to observe its activity. While observing the basilar membrane and its structures through a microscope, he presented a well-controlled stimulus to the system. His observations, using cochleae from human and animal cadavers, revealed that the details of von Helmholtz's theory were incorrect. There were no resonators. What von Békésy noted was that the traveling wave moved from the base toward the apex. As the wave moved on the basilar membrane, it steadily increased in its activity until it reached a maximum. Then it rapidly dissipated. What von Békésy observed was the traveling wave we have already discussed.

The place theory of pitch was, because of von Békésy's work, revised. Pitch, in this view, was still associated with the frequency of the stimulus. However, pitch was now dependent on the place where the traveling wave displaced the basilar membrane maximally rather than the result of resonating fibers or structures within the cochlea. This version of the place theory of pitch is viable today. Although it has been modified by recent discoveries, the concept of a traveling wave is firmly established. For his endeavors, von Békésy was awarded the Nobel Prize in 1961.

Problems and Solutions: The Traveling Wave

One expects that there are few, if any, problems associated with the traveling wave concept because it is well established. The traveling wave can be seen, it exists, and it flows in the manner we just described. What kind of problems can there be?

One difficulty occurred when investigators measured our ability to differentiate one frequency from another. We can differentiate between two frequencies quite well. In other words, we can tell the difference between 1,000 and 1,003 Hz. The difference between these two frequencies is the difference threshold. In general, we can differentiate two frequencies if they differ by approximately 0.3%. This means that if the standard frequency were 1,000 Hz, the majority of us can differentiate this 1,000 Hz from a comparison frequency of 1,003 Hz. If the standard frequency were 2,000 Hz, the majority of us could differentiate it from a comparison of 2,006 Hz. This acuity raised some significant questions when it was contrasted with the observed shape of the traveling waves for sinusoidal stimuli. The traveling wave, observed by von Békésy and others after him, was broadly tuned. The question was, how could a broadly tuned traveling wave provide the information necessary to differentiate frequencies that were so close together? If a 1,000 Hz traveling wave is so broad and the traveling wave for 1,003 Hz is also broad, they must overlap significantly. How does the cochlea process such broad, overlapping traveling waves and give us this discriminative ability?

The broad tuning of the traveling wave was mentioned earlier and was shown in Figure 9.5. Figure 9.6 shows a different view of traveling waves using four different frequencies. It displays the envelopes for the separate frequencies. Traveling Wave A is for frequency of 8,000 Hz. Traveling Wave B is representative of a frequency of 1,003 Hz. Traveling Wave C (the dashed envelope) is for a frequency of 1,000 Hz, and Traveling Wave D is 400 Hz.

Given these four traveling waves it should be apparent that A and D can be easily discriminated. They activate different portions of the basilar membrane and do not overlap. Even if the two stimuli, 8,000 Hz and 400 Hz, were presented simultaneously, the cochlear analyzer, the basilar membrane, easily differentiates the two. The problem arises, however, when we view the two traveling waves labeled B and C. These two traveling waves overlap significantly. How can the cochlear analyzer process a broad spectrum with many frequencies? The overlapping traveling waves make the information necessary for us to detect a 3-Hertz difference impossible, but we can do it. How do we do it? That is the problem. It makes no difference whether the two tones are presented sequentially, 1,000 Hz then 1,003 Hz, or simultaneously. The auditory system detects a difference. In fact, when the two tones, 1,000 and 1,003 Hz, are presented simultaneously, they interact and produce perceptual beats or interactions that help us detect when a single tone is present in contrast with both tones (Moore, 1997). Clearly there is something missing in our place theory of pitch. The theory cannot be completely correct if it does not account for our obvious perceptions. How do we reconcile this? What is the cochlea doing?

Frequency Tuning Curves

One method of investigating the problem just outlined is to consider the possibility that the waves formed in cadaver cochleae are different from those that travel the basilar membrane in noncadaver ears. Because of the difficulty of directly observing the traveling wave in a living organism, the task had to be postponed until technology and methods could be developed. Meanwhile, investigators were recording the activity of the afferent primary sensory neurons coming from the cochlea. These neurons, 90 to 95% of which were coming from the inner hair cells, were instrumental in the search for an answer to the problem. The investigations yielded the "receptive field" idea for the auditory system—the **frequency tuning curve.**

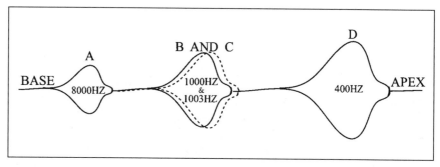

Figure 9.6. Traveling Wave Envelopes for Four Different Sinusoidal Stimuli

The frequency-tuning curve came from the recording of a single afferent nerve fiber while varying the frequency and intensity of the stimulus. The easiest way to get a feeling for this important concept is to consider the procedure used to plot a frequency-tuning curve.

First, a live normal-functioning neuron is found in the anesthetized experimental animal. The cell has a natural spontaneous rate of firing without any stimulus being present. The goal is to determine the stimulus frequency and intensity required to increase the firing rate above the spontaneous value. With this in mind, the investigators turns on a low-level sinusoid and presents it to the animal while sweeping the frequency back and forth across the spectrum. For example, they may begin by setting the intensity at a fixed level, say at 10 dB SPL, and then varying the frequency systematically from low to high and high to low while observing the neural activity of the cell. If no increase in activity is observed, the next step in the investigation is to increase the intensity—from 10 to 15 dB—and repeat the frequency sweeps. The investigators continue in this manner until an increase in neural activity is noted. Once an increase occurs, they record the stimulus intensity and frequency.

By repeatedly increasing the intensity and sweeping the frequency from low to high and high to low, the investigators can plot the results in the manner described—plot the intensity of stimulation that initiates the increase in neural activity as a function of the frequency where it first occurs. This yields the tuning curve. A group of frequency tuning curves for different neurons is shown in Figure 9.7.

It is clear from Figure 9.7 that the primary sensory neurons are sharply tuned. That is, each neuron has a **characteristic frequency** or **best frequency** of response. The idea of an *adequate stimulus* should come to mind here. The characteristic frequency is the frequency with the lowest intensity that increases the firing rate. Frequencies, other than the best or characteristic frequency, may increase the firing rate of the neuron, but they require more

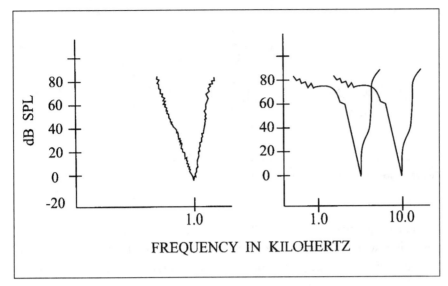

Figure 9.7. Frequency Tuning Curves

intensity if they are to do so. This kind of response indicates that the neuron, and possibly the inner hair cell to which it is attached, is selectively tuned to respond to a particular frequency. The neuron responds best and most readily when its characteristic frequency is present in the stimulus.

The sharpness of the frequency tuning curves when contrasted to the traveling waves seen in the cochlea reaffirmed the idea that there was something happening between the traveling wave and the neural output (Khanna & Leonard, 1982; Narayan, Temchin, Relco, & Ruggero, 1998). How could the untuned shape of the traveling wave yield such narrow bands of neural output? The shape of the frequency tuning curves suggested that there was a critical element missing between the hydromechanical traveling wave and the neural output of the cochlea. The search for the mechanism that allows us to analyze the complex waveforms of our environment has led to amazing revelations. One of the first discoveries was the significant difference between the traveling wave observed in a cadaver ear and traveling wave seen in a noncadaver undamaged cochlea.

Tuning the Cochlea

The technological endeavors of the last few decades have allowed scientists to observe the traveling wave in vivo. The results of investigations using noncadaver ears revealed that the traveling wave is incredibly sharper in the living animal than it is after death. The changes that occur within the cochlea immediately after death clearly affect the manner in which the wave is formed. In addition, the intensity of the stimulus required to see the traveling wave in a cadaver cochlea was problematic. To see the traveling wave, von Békésy had to have a stimulus level in the range of 120 to 140 dB. It was suspected, and later confirmed, that high intensities were part of the problem. The basilar membrane was overstimulated and led to a linear appearance. By linear we mean that the traveling wave was the same shape at all frequencies and all intensities. When lower intensities are used and noncadaver cochleae are observed, the sharper traveling wave varies as a function of the intensity of the stimulus. When the stimulus level is high, like von Békésy's, the traveling wave is broadly shaped. However, when the intensity of the stimulus is decreased to levels more appropriate for normal functioning, the traveling wave changes shape significantly. It becomes pointed and finely tuned. This means that the shape of the traveling wave changes as a function of the stimulus level. The traveling wave hydromechanics is nonlinear. At stimulus levels up to approximately 40 to 50 dB above threshold, the shape of the traveling wave in the noncadaver ear closely matches the frequency-tuning curve observed in individual neurons. The correspondence between the frequency tuning curve and the basilar membrane traveling wave is shown in Figure 9.8.

Outer Hair Cells

Even after it was confirmed that the traveling wave and the frequency-tuning curve were both narrowly tuned up to approximately 40 to 50 dB above threshold, the question did not go away. The question merely took another form: What improved the sharpness of the traveling wave in the noncadaver cochlea? The answer to this question came from one of the most unexpected places. The outer hair cells sharpen the traveling wave (Dallos, 1992; Dallos & Harris (1978).

The current understanding of the hydromechanical events within the cochlea is that the traveling wave is initially formed because of the basilar membrane characteristics: stiffness and width. This traveling wave provides the basis of our ability to analyze complex waveforms. That is, the first step in frequency analysis, Ohm's acoustic law, is the formation of the traveling wave (Licklider, 1956). The next step in the process is the sharpening of the traveling wave at the point of maximal displacement. An active outer hair cell feedback process accomplishes the wave enhancement. The outer hair cell response to a traveling wave is to selectively amplify the basilar membrane

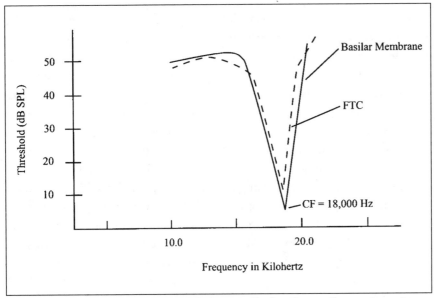

Figure 9.8. Basilar Membrane and Frequency Tuning Curves Comparison at 18 Kilohertz

motion by adding its own energy to the system at the point of maximum basilar membrane displacement. This active enhancement sharpens or fine-tunes the passive hydromechanical movement and the analysis capability of the cochlea. It is the added boost of mechanical energy that helps provide us with our ability to differentiate and detect separate frequencies occurring in our complex environment. The entire ability to discriminate certainly does not depend only on the frequency tuning curves, but it is the start of a remarkable auditory capability.

Figure 9.9 diagrammatically displays the enhancement of a passive traveling wave. The enhancement is accomplished by an "active region" of outer hair cells.

The outer hair cells undergo significant changes in their length and shape as the shearing movement between the cilia and the tectorial membrane mechanically bends the cilia. When the traveling wave moves the basilar membrane, it deflects the outer hair cell cilia and produces a receptor potential within the cell. A deflection of the basilar membrane upward by the traveling wave depolarizes the cell. The depolarization, in turn, results in a physical contraction of the outer hair cells. A hyperpolarization of the cell occurs when the traveling wave causes the basilar membrane to be depressed in the scala tympani. When the downward deflection occurs, the hyperpolarization

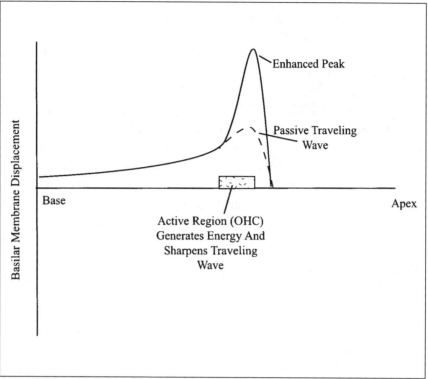

Figure 9.9. Enhancement of a Traveling Wave by the Active Region of the Outer Hair Cells

of the receptor potential causes the outer hair cells to elongate and become physically longer. The cyclic changes in outer hair cells' length, contraction and elongation, alter the movement of the basilar membrane by feeding energy back in the system. This energy amplifies and causes a sharp "peak" in the traveling wave at the particular point or place where the outer hair cell is located. The energy necessary to peak and sharpen the traveling wave is generated by the outer hair cells in the "active region" just basal to the characteristic frequency.

Inner Hair Cells

Because the stereocilia of the outer hair cells are directly attached to the tectorial membrane, the changes in outer hair cell length cause significant vibratory energy to be transmitted to the tectorial membrane itself. The transmission of the energy to the tectorial membrane, it is hypothesized, initiates cyclic vibratory movement of the endolymph in the space below the tectorial membrane. The vibratory cyclic movements of the endolymph between the tectorial membrane and the surface of the inner hair cells, result in the fine-tuning of the inner hair cells. For frequencies above approximately 4,000 Hz, the inner hair cells located at the "place" of maximum basilar membrane displacement are easily activated. They are activated because the outer hair cells actively sharpen the hydromechanics of the basilar membrane. In other words, the peaking of the traveling wave occurs because of the active involvement of outer hair cells. This improves the sensitivity and frequency selectivity of the inner hair cells. This improvement is important because the inner hair cells, not the outer hair cells, are the auditory receptors sending impulses to the higher centers. The inner hair cells are, you recall, innervated by 90 to 95% of the afferent fibers that form the auditory branch of the VIII cranial nerve.

One of the final products in this sequence of events is a cochlea that is uniquely sensitive to environmental pressure changes and is excellent at performing the frequency analysis task. There is, however, an important alternative to the place theory of hearing. The other option is **volley theory** (Wever, 1949; Wever & Bray, 1937). The development of this theory, and the supporting data, is our next topic.

An Alternative to Place Theory

The eminence of the place theory in the 1800s did not stop scientists from postulating different mechanisms to account for our ability to perceive pitch. One popular approach was that proposed by William Rutherford (1886) near the close of the 19th century. During this period, the phonograph and the telephone were just coming into existence. Rutherford's theory was, in some respects, modeled after the electronics of the day. His theory was initially called the frequency or telephone theory. His theory was quite simple. He proposed that the cochlea did not have resonators as von Helmholtz suggested. Rutherford believed that the whole basilar membrane, instead of having individual fibers or cochlear elements for each frequency in the stimulus, vibrated according to the frequencies in the stimulus. The neural elements or receptors simply responded to each frequency in the stimulus. The basilar membrane translated the sound, complex as it was, into nerve vibrations that had the same frequency, amplitude, and waveform as the stimulus. The receptors were not resonators nor were they tuned to a single frequency. The basilar membrane moved as a function of the frequency of the stimulation and initiated impulses in the nerve fibers that equaled the frequency or frequencies in the stimulus.

The basilar membrane acted like the telephone or speaker of the phonograph player. Vibrations in the air vibrated the basilar membrane and neural elements mirrored the frequencies in the stimulus.

The telephone theory, then, pushed the analysis capability, championed by von Helmholtz and the place theorists, out of the cochlea and into higher brain centers. The brain became the analyzer of the neural impulses sent to it by the cochlea. The basilar membrane was merely a high-fidelity speaker that transduced the sound to a neural pattern that matched the stimulus. If the frequency were 500 Hz, the nerve fibers fired 500 times a second and send this message to the brain. If the stimulus were 5,000 Hz, each fiber sent 5,000 impulses to the brain. It was the brain that determined our analysis ability, discrimination, and overall hearing capability.

Keep in mind that the characteristics of nerve fibers were not well known at the time Rutherford was proposing his theory. Although the speed of nerve conduction was known and had been measured by von Helmholtz (even though Müller had been emphatic in his statement that it was too fast to be measured), the refractory period of the neuron had not been quantified. The lack of physiological knowledge, therefore, was not a hindrance. Nerve fibers were assumed to be capable of responding fast enough to follow the frequency of the stimulus.

In 1900, there was little problem in believing that a neuron could respond 10,000 or 20,000 times per second. This belief, however, was short lived. As you probably remember from previous chapters, an action potential is only a millisecond in duration (0.001 of a second). This means that a neuron can only fire, under ideal conditions, 1,000 times a second. The problem then becomes clear. Neurons cannot signal a frequency that is greater than its absolute refractory period. It is a physical impossibility. In fact, it is a rare neuron that can respond 1,000 times a second. Most neurons can react only 300 to 400 times per second when initially stimulated, and this initial rate of activity is not maintained. After the first burst, a neuron nearly always adapts, and the spike tempo declines to less than its initial burst rate.

In summary, Rutherford's telephone theory could not be maintained as he initially proposed it. The physiological restrictions on the response rate required a modification. The modification came when **Glenn Wever,** a scientist working at Princeton University, suggested a volley principle based on

physiological evidence associated with nerve fibers. The volley principle became the volley theory.

The Volley Theory

The idea outlined by Wever, briefly, was that neural fibers have a limited
rate of firing. This limit is, at the maximum, near 1,000 spikes a second. This
restriction, however, did not hinder the idea that the number of impulses
per second may code the frequency of the stimulus. To send a barrage of 1,000
neural impulses to the brain did not mean each neuron had to fire 1,000
times. Instead, a pattern of 1,000 impulses could be generated by several neurons if they fired (a) at the same point in the cycle and (b) on different cycles
of the stimulus. The diagram in Figure 9.10 shows this idea. Each fiber responds to the stimulus at the peak of the cycle (90°) and on every sixth cycle.
Fiber A fires on the first and sixth cycle, Fiber B on the second and seventh cycle, Fiber C on the third and eighth, and so forth. The result of this sequence of
neural firing is a continuous volley of neural activity shown at the bottom of
Figure 9.10. Although each fiber only produces, for example, 200 impulses
per second, the combination or sum of all five fibers is 1,000 impulses per second. In other words, if each fiber has its impulse initiated at the same "point"
in the cycle (90°) but not on every cycle, then the result is a synchronized volley of 1,000 impulses. The total volley of neural output "follows" the frequency of the stimulus. The 1,000 impulses per second comes from a combination of several fibers rather than 1,000 from each fiber.

The question now is how does the theory work in practice? What exactly
is happening to the inner hair cells to provide a neural output that follows the
frequency of the stimulus? The answer lies in the activation of the inner hair
cells and the idea of **phase locking.** This is the next step in the story.

Phase Locking

Because of viscous drag of the endolymph surrounding the stereocilia of
the inner hair cells, the inner hair cells respond more to the velocity (speed of
movement) of the basilar membrane than they do to the actual displacement.
This is particularly true when the frequency of the stimulus is lower than
about 400 Hz. When the frequency increases above 400 Hz, however, the velocity of the movement plays less of a role, and displacement of the basilar
membrane becomes more important. What this means for the activity being

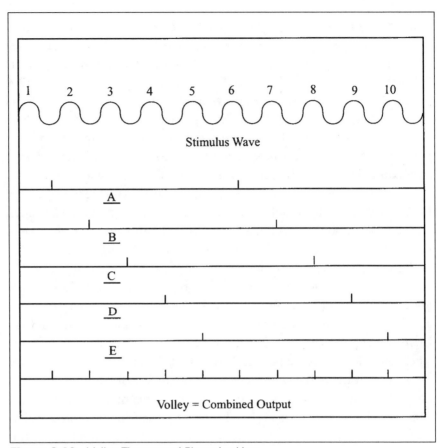

Figure 9.10. Volley Theory and Phase Locking

sent to higher brain centers is that inner hair cells are **phase locked** at the lower frequencies but not at high frequencies.

Phase locking is the terminology used to indicate that bursts of activity from neural fibers "follow" the frequency of the stimulus. That is, the neuron becomes active near the same point in each cycle of the stimulus. For example, if the frequency of the stimulus were 200 Hz, the inner hair cells would depolarize and hyperpolarize once each cycle by the velocity of the endolymphatic movement. The inner hair cell depolarizes and hyperpolarizes 200 times in a second and generates 200 bursts of activity. There are bursts of activity occurring at the same place in the cycle (at same phase angle) so the onset of cell activity is locked in phase. The inner hair cells, and the afferent fibers attached to them, are activated when the movement is toward the tectorial membrane. At that point, when the inner hair cell moves upward and causes shearing of hairs in one direction, the neural response is generated. The activity is initiated, then, at a particular phase angle in each stimulus cycle. Thus, the inner hair cell and the neural fiber are phase locked to the stimulus. They are "locked in" and respond once for each cycle of the stimulus. The result is 200 bursts of neural activity for a 200 Hz signal, 300 bursts for a 300 Hz signal, and so forth. When the stimulus frequency is greater than approximately 300 to 400 Hz, the volley principle comes in play. The volley principle permits the pattern of neural activity to be synchronized with stimulus frequencies up to approximately 4,000 Hz by being phase locked, but not to every cycle.

In summary, for the low frequencies (less than 400 Hz) the inner hair cell is depolarized and hyperpolarized once during each cycle of the stimulus. Each depolarization yields a burst of activity in the afferent nerve fiber. Thus, the frequency of the stimulus reported to the brain is coded using the number of impulses per second as well as the interval of time between the spikes. The temporal or telephone theory suggests that, because there is phase locking at low frequencies, our perception of pitch depends on the periodicity of neural activity sent to the brain, not the stimulation of a particular place on the basilar membrane. When the frequency of the stimulus increases to the point where phase locking is not possible, the volley principle comes in play. Many fibers are activated at the same phase angle, but they do not respond on every cycle. Thus, synchronized neural firing can be maintained up to about 4,000 Hz. This means that the volley theory can explain how we perceive pitch for frequencies below 4,000 Hz. At frequencies above 4,000 Hz, phase locking cannot be accomplished so the bursts of neural activity become unsynchronized (nonperiodic). In this latter case, where the frequency is above 4,000 Hz, the place of maximum basilar membrane displacement, the place theory, becomes a dominant means of explaining how we perceive pitch. Between about 1,000 Hz and 4,000 Hz, it is assumed that both place and volley play a role. Interestingly, this portion of the spectrum, 1,000 to 4,000 Hz, is the most sensitive and yields the lowest absolute threshold.

The perception of pitch appears, at this point, to be easily explained. When the frequency of the sinusoid is low, phase locking and periodicity occurs, and we detect pitch based on the number of neural impulses arriving at higher auditory centers. The telephone theory and volley theory are the explanatory devices for the low frequencies. If, on the other hand, the frequency is high, above about 4,000 Hz, the pitch may be determined by the place on the basilar membrane that has the maximum stimulation. Place theory is invoked. If the frequency of the stimulus is in the 1,000 to 4,000 Hz range, then both place theory and volley theory are called on to explain our pitch perceptions.

Although this seems simple enough, there are questions that quickly come to mind. First, what happens to the pitch if the stimulus is not a single frequency but is instead a complex composed of several frequencies? For example, the musical note A above middle C, when played by a musical instrument, is not a pure tone; it is a complex sound consisting of multiple harmonics with a fundamental frequency of 440 Hz. We do not hear each harmonic as an individual pitch. We perceive a single pitch of 440 Hz. Second, why do we hear a pitch of 440 Hz in situations when the fundamental frequency, 440 Hz, is not part of the stimulus? Under such conditions, when the fundamental is missing, we still hear a 440 Hz pitch. This conundrum is called the case of the missing fundamental (Schouten, Ritsma, & Cardoza, 1962). We perceive a sound that is not in the stimulus. It is an illusion.

An Interesting Illusion

We begin our discussion of illusions with a definition. An **illusion** is a misinterpretation or false perception of an existing sensory stimulus. An illusion differs from a **hallucination** because a hallucination is not a misinterpretation of anything existing in the real world; rather, a hallucination is a perception with no precipitating environmental stimulation. With a hallucination, you hear voices, smell odors, and see visions (e.g., of angels or extraterrestrials) when they do not exist in the physical world. Illusions and hallucinations are, clearly, not the same. We restrict ourselves to illusions.

One explanation of the missing fundamental was based on the idea of nonlinearity. A nonlinear system is a system that distorts an input in such a way that the output contains elements (frequencies in the present case) that were not part of the original input. An example is a poorly designed amplifier that distorts the human voice and music. What went into the amplifier is not what came out.

The Case of the Missing Fundamental

Although there is no completely satisfactory answer about how the brain accomplishes the task of synthesizing the missing fundamental, it appears that higher auditory centers do this amazing task by using the pattern of activity produced by the complex activity of the basilar membrane. Thus, even though the basilar membrane does not provide specific information about the fundamental, enough information is sent to the brain via the neural pattern in the VIII cranial nerve to produce the missing low-frequency component. The information contained in the neural temporal pattern is integrated or combined to produce the perceived pitch. A periodicity is assumed to occur because the complex waveform contains high harmonics that are maintained in the VIII cranial nerve. The pitch that is perceived has been appropriately called **periodicity pitch. Residue pitch** is also often used to describe the pitch of a complex waveform. The "residue" in this case refers to a complex without the fundamental frequency. A common illusion is discussed in the next paragraph. It is not usually recognized as an illusion, but it is.

The phone rings and you pick it up. You immediately recognize your friend's voice. This is not an unusual occurrence. You see his face and recognize your friend everyday. You know who is on the phone almost instantly. The friend's voice is not high pitched or "tinny." It sounds full, modulated, and is easily comprehended and identified. There is, however, an interesting fact about telephone communication. The phone acts as a bandpass filter. The phone passes frequencies between approximately 300 and 3,000 Hz and filters out all the rest. What is transmitted is not the full resonant voice as the speaker produces it. The phone removes the lower frequencies. In fact, every phone conversation contains an illusion. The auditory system replaces the missing fundamental extracted by the inexpensive telephone. The stimulus that arrives at your receiver lacks the fundamental. You listen to the voice and fill in the missing parts. You are not even aware that it is being done. We can understand and identify people easily when the phone company uses a narrow bandwidth. This suits the phone company fine and us too. The fundamental frequency for speech, incidentally, is in the neighborhood of 150 to 200 Hz for females and 75 to 125 Hz for males.

Sounds From Our Ears

What would happen if a scientist decided to insert a miniature microphone and speaker in your auditory canal? You know what could be done? Once the speaker and microphone were tightly sealed in your ear, the speaker could be turned on and the microphone could be used to listen for echoes. This suggestion may sound odd, but the experiment has been done (Kemp, 1978). Figure 9.11 shows the experimental configuration that is used to conduct such investigations. The sound source produces a signal and a microphone records the echo. The investigation was based on theoretical considerations suggested 30 years before the experiment. The measurement of sounds from the inner ear, by systems like the one shown in Figure 9.11(a), have become almost routine today. In fact, since the discovery of the echoes, there have been over 800 publications on the subject. The sounds were initially called "Kemp's Echoes," after the investigator who first reported them. They have since been relabeled by the more scientific name of **otoacoustic emissions.** Figure 9.11(b) shows a representative schematic of an otoacoustic emission that follows an evoking stimulus.

Research in the last few years, although still not completely confirmed, indicates that the otoacoustic emissions are by-products of a normal-functioning cochlea. If the cochlea is damaged or nonfunctional in some way, the emissions are distorted or missing in the damaged part of the cochlea. The otoacoustic emissions are always missing if disease, ototoxic drugs, or loud noises destroy outer hair cells. The loss of otoacoustic emissions when outer hair cells are missing or destroyed suggests that the emissions arise from the outer hair cells. During the traveling wave amplification process, the outer hair cells may produce minute waves within the cochlea. The physical contractions and elongations by the outer hair cells are assumed to generate movements in the fluid-filled environment. The tiny waves generate acoustic signals in the cochlea. The otoacoustic emissions are, therefore, weak signals transmitted from the inner ear, through the middle ear, to the tympanic membrane, and then in the ear canal. Once the sound reaches the ear canal, the sensitive speaker records it.

There are two types of otoacoustic emissions. There is the **spontaneous otoacoustic emission** that occurs in approximately 40 to 60% of all normal hearing adult ears. These emissions are measured or detected in the ear canal in the absence of any external signal. They are indeed "spontaneous." In contrast, there is the **evoked otoacoustic emission (EOAE)** like the one used to introduce this topic. The evoked otoacoustic emissions are emissions that occur following the presentation of various types of stimuli. These evoked otoacoustic emissions occur in nearly 100% of all normal ears. If an individual has a hearing loss greater than 40 dB at any one frequency, the evoked otoacoustic emissions are missing at that frequency.

Otoacoustic emissions are now used to investigate hearing in neonates, infants, and children as well as adults. The idea is to use a noninvasive miniature speaker and microphone to provide an objective means of detecting cochlear hearing loss. For example, investigations thus far have shown that the

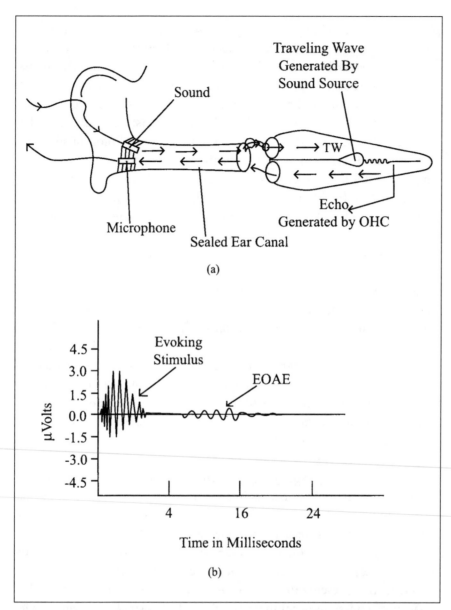

Figure 9.11. Diagram of the Experimental Configuration Used to Evoke and Record Otoacoustic Emissions

NOTE: OHC = outer hair cell; EOAE = evoked otoacoustic emissions.

evoked otoacoustic emissions vary in amplitude as a function of age. Young infants and children have large evoked otoacoustic emissions that decline with age.

The Real World

This chapter has used several figures and diagrams to display the mammalian peripheral auditory mechanisms. These figures are necessary if you are to obtain even a small insight about this most remarkable sensory system. I feel, however, that it would be negligent of me if I did not put the system in proper perspective. To do this, I suggest that you draw one basilar membrane, top view, as close to its actual size as you can. The basilar membrane is 0.08 mm at the base, 0.5 mm wide at the apex, and 35mm in length. You can draw it close to these dimensions by using an ink pen. Draw it underneath the following heading:

BASILAR MEMBRANE

When you look at the line you have drawn, remember that lying on top of that line are 15,500 hair cells with 30,000 afferent neurons making synapses beneath it. In addition, you should know that the figure displaying the traveling wave (Figure 9.5) is grossly exaggerated. The displacement of the basilar membrane at absolute threshold is subatomic in dimension. The estimate is that for hearing to occur the basilar membrane displacement must be 10^{-10} to 10^{-11} m (0.0000000001 to 0.00000000001 of a meter). The normal auditory mechanism detects a sound when the basilar membrane is displaced by the diameter of a hydrogen atom.

Auditory Pathways

There have been many aspects of peripheral auditory processing presented in this chapter. You may have wondered, however, just how the system can be so versatile. Language, music, laughter, thunder, mosquito buzzes, dog barks, cat purrs, car horns, and the wind in the trees are all discriminated and interpreted because of the output from only 30,000 nerve fibers from each cochlea. How such a small number of axons can yield such a complex world brings to mind a Winston Churchill quote: "Never have so many owed so much to so few."

It is the task for the remaining parts of the chapter to present neural processing beyond the cochlea. We do this by examining the auditory pathway from the cochlea to the cortex. As we proceed, it becomes apparent that there is more than one auditory path. Each path, so it appears, accomplishes a special function or interpretation of the auditory stimuli surrounding us. The auditory pathway, shown in Figure 9.12, is our starting point. We consider, in sequence, each neural processing station within the path. The first stop is the cochlear nucleus.

The Cochlear Nucleus

The cochlear nucleus is located in the brain stem immediately beyond the cochlea. There is, of course, a cochlear nucleus for each cochlea. For the sake

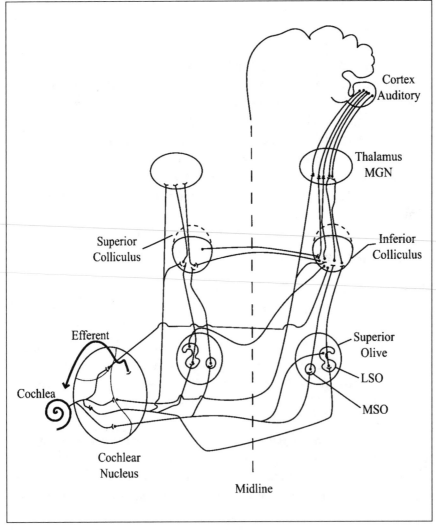

Figure 9.12. Central Pathways of the Auditory System

of clarity, only one half of the pathways in the system are shown in Figure 9.12. The figure displays one afferent axon entering the left cochlear nucleus. The axon does what every other axon does when it enters the cochlear nucleus: It diverges in many terminal branches. The result is that each axon makes synaptic connections to many different cells in different locations within the cochlear nucleus. This divergence and synaptic connection to different cells has led to the conclusion that there are several parallel paths to higher neural centers. Moreover, each path appears to have a different function. Each function is dependent on the kind of synapse, type of receptive cell, and the cellular interactions that occur within the cochlear nucleus. Each group of cells extracts specific kinds of information from the cochlear fiber input.

An interesting point here is that the activity in each cochlear nerve fiber contains all the information necessary to produce the parallel paths having different functions. For example, there is a path that uses the "on" response of the cochlear fiber as an aid in localizing the source of the sound in the environment. There is a different path that uses the same cochlear nerve activity to produce complex auditory perception (e.g., music, language, as well as localization). There are several **tonotopic maps** within the cochlear nucleus. A tonotopic map is a map of the basilar membrane activity in the frequency domain. The basilar membrane, from base to apex, is laid down in the cochlear nucleus in several locations. The tonotopic maps are also found in each of the higher neural centers shown in Figure 9.12. The cochlear nucleus is partitioned in distinct areas according to their location within the nucleus. These areas are the dorsal cochlear nucleus (DCN), posteriorventral cochlear nucleus (PVCN), and the anteriorventral cochlear nucleus (AVCN). Figure 9.12 shows these areas and the associated ascending pathways to higher neural centers as well as an efferent branch that leaves the cochlear nucleus and joins the **olivocochlear bundle.**

The olivocochlear bundle originates from the ipsilateral and contralateral superior olive and is the efferent path leading to the hair cells within the cochlea. This efferent path was noted previously and is discussed more thoroughly later in the chapter.

The cochlear nucleus is complex. Not only are there numerous afferent fibers ascending to higher centers, but there are also interactions within the cochlear nucleus that apparently shape, form, and in many ways "smooth" the neural activity prior its ascent to higher centers. Both the PVCN and the AVCN, for example, send fibers to the superior olive. Within the superior olive, there are two other nuclear centers, the medial superior olive (MSO) and the lateral superior olive (LSO). There are also pathways that bypass the superior olive and make synaptic connections in the ipsilateral and contralateral inferior colliculus on the way to their final destination, the medial geniculate nucleus (MGN) of the thalamus. There is, finally, a fiber group that leaves the cochlear nucleus and goes directly to the contralateral inferior colliculus. This brief description of the afferent paths from the cochlear nucleus, as complex as it sounds, is in reality an overview and a simplification. The system really is much more complex. Our goal now is to examine the next set of nuclei in the system, the nuclei of the superior olive.

The Superior Olive

The primary areas of interest within the superior olive, as noted previously, are the medial superior olive (MSO) and lateral superior olive (LSO). The MSO and LSO receive fibers from both the ipsilateral and the contralateral cochlear nucleus. This means that the MSO and LSO almost immediately begin to process interactions that occur from the two ears. It is well known that the sounds that arrive at the two ears are nearly always different. The difference in stimuli at the two ears is referred to as an interaural difference. Sometimes a sound arrives at one ear before it arrives at the other, and sometimes the intensity differs at the two ears. Given this situation, there are two interaural differences. There is the interaural intensity difference and an interaural temporal difference. Because sounds in the environment bombard us continually and we have to interact with the perpetual sound chaos, the neural input needs to be processed quickly and accurately. Knowing where the sound originates in the surrounding environment is one of the primary activities of the system. This process is known as spatial localization. The LSO and MSO accomplish spatial localization.

Consider first a normal auditory system and a sound source that is more intense on the right side than on the left. Because the sound is more intense on the right side, the auditory system initiates more activity from the right side. This is a normal occurrence and is an example of the intensity-frequency principle. As the intensity increases, the frequency or number of neural impulses increases. In addition, a more intense stimulus activates more large-diameter axons. Keep this idea in mind for later.

Consider now a sound that is complex with many frequencies. If the complex stimulus reaches the right side of the head first, the low frequencies flow around the head. This is a simple physical phenomenon. Low frequencies bend and flow around small solid objects, whereas high frequencies are deflected. The low-frequency flow around the head results in a phase difference at each ear. The phase difference is, of course, a time difference. Because a low-frequency wave flows around the head, it stimulates the right ear at one time (phase angle) and the left ear at a different time (phase angle). This difference in the timing at the ears is the cue used to determine the direction and location of the low-frequency sound source. The high frequencies in the complex stimulus do not flow around the head. Rather, high frequencies are deflected and cause a **sound shadow** on the opposite side of the head. A sound shadow reflects the fact that the high frequencies do not flow around the object in the environment, the head in this case. The sound in the sound shadow is less intense. The high frequencies are deflected, and an intensity difference occurs. The object (head) causes an intensity difference between the ears. Figure 9.13 displays a simple but useful model of how the MSO and LSO perform this localization task.

Both the MSO and LSO are assumed to employ coincidence detector neurons. A coincidence neuron is a cell that is activated (or inhibited) by the simultaneous occurrence of synaptic activity from two sources. As Figure 9.13 shows, for a coincidence detector to become active (or inhibited), action potentials must arrive at the coincidence cell from the left and right at the same time. If, for example, activity arrives from one side too early (or too late) to coincide with activity at another synapse, then the coincidence detector does not change its activity state. Spatial localization is determined by changing the state of different groups of coincidence detectors. In other words, localization cues are initiated when groups of coincidence detectors change their normal status. Which group of coincidence detectors changes status determines the spatial localization of the sound.

Given this information, we have some questions regarding sound localization. Where are these coincidence detectors located and how are they specialized relative to the intensity and temporal cues in the stimulus? Are the two pinna involved in our ability to localize sounds? Localization is not restricted to a stationary head. We move our heads (some animals move their ears) and constantly shift our vision. How important and useful are these eye and head movements? Do the auditory and visual systems interact, and, if so, how? In addition, do animals other than humans have different neural capabilities for localization (Heffner & Masterton, 1990; Masterton, 1992).

The answer to the first question, based on investigations with recording electrodes, is that the MSO is acutely sensitive to temporal difference in the arrival of sound sources. In other words, the MSO uses the temporal cues in the stimulus for sound localization. The LSO, on the other hand, uses the differences in intensity at the two ears to determine the location of a sound in the environment. The information from both nuclei, MSO and LSO, is processed

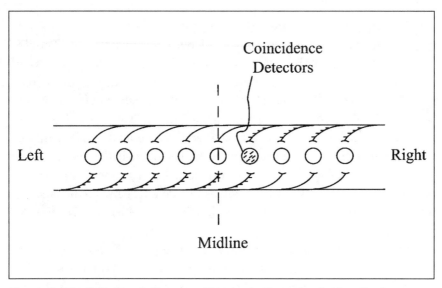

Figure 9.13. Coincidence Detectors That Are in Operation for Localization

by the higher centers in the effort to identify and interpret the sound environment. For example, the crack of a twig heard by a rabbit may be interpreted as a fox or another rabbit. Once the sound is detected, it is important to orient the head and see what it is.

The second question is one that is often not considered. If you were to take a moment and look at the pinna of several different individuals, you would find, not unexpectedly, that they all differ in their structure. The pinna is bigger, smaller, longer, deeper, curved, molded, and shaped differently for nearly everyone. Do these differences help or hinder in our ability to detect sounds and locate their source? The shape of the pinna is important in determining which frequencies enter the external auditory meatus. Investigations using insert microphones placed near the tympanic membrane show that the spectra of the sound at the eardrum varies as a function of the angle in which the sound reaches the head. Every turn of the head changes the spectra arriving at the eardrum. These changes based on the shape of the pinna are important cues to the location of sound in the environment. The sound spectrum at the eardrum changes as a function of the location of the sound and angle of incidence when it reaches the head. The pinna changes the spectrum of the sound as a function of its shape (Batteau 1967; Wightman & Kistler, 1989). Does this mean that if your pinna were exchanged with someone else, you would have difficulty locating a sound in space? The answer is no. Experiments have shown that we adapt quite well when provided with the spectrum of a sound that has been "processed" by someone else's pinna. The important aspect of this discussion is that the spectrum at the eardrum varies as a function of the pinna and the angle at which the sound reaches the side of the head. Our ability to adjust to the continually changing environment by turning our heads and adjusting the spectrum of the sound is remarkable.

This ability leads us to the third question regarding how head movement and the visual interaction help us in our investigation of the environment. This question is addressed by considering the inferior colliculus.

The Inferior Colliculus

Figure 9.12 shows the paths that project to the inferior colliculus. The inferior colliculus receives inputs from both the ipsilateral and contralateral superior olives as well as inputs from the contralateral cochlear nucleus. To visualize this in Figure 9.12, it is helpful to keep in mind that only one half the afferent pathways are displayed.

The inferior colliculus has generally been assigned two tasks in the auditory modality. First, it is a relay station for the ascending fibers to the thalamus and cortex. Second, and for our purposes more interesting, the inferior colliculus is a reflex center. As noted previously, the inferior colliculus receives input from both superior olives. This suggests, and the evidence supports it, that the inferior colliculus is involved in combining or synthesizing the activity rather than just acting as a relay to the higher centers. Indeed, the data suggest that the inferior colliculus is in contact with the neural centers just above or superior to it—the superior colliculus. This latter set of neural elements are directly associated with the visual modality. This suggests even further that the inferior colliculus processes the localization information from the MSO and LSO and sends it on to the visual system. The information received by the superior colliculus is used to almost immediately direct the eyes to the place where the sound was localized. In addition to the movement of the eyes in the direction of the spatially localized sound, there is another activity that aids in the orientation and processing of spatial sounds. The head turns in the same direction as the eyes. The motor activities associated with the head turn and eye movement are often called a visual-auditory reflex.

A final interesting aspect of the inferior colliculus is its intimate association with the auditory startle response. The auditory startle response is the sudden behavioral "jerk" or "jump" that occurs in nearly every normal-hearing organism when a loud unexpected sound occurs. Because the inferior colliculus is intimately associated with the reticular activating system, the motor response is quickly initiated by a loud intense sound. The response is unlearned.

The Thalamus

The thalamus, as noted in previous chapters, is a major relay center in the brain. This idea of a relay center only is a serious understatement of the thalamus. Nearly all sensory inputs pass through this important nucleus, but there is significant processing that occurs before the information is forwarded to higher centers. In the case of audition, the medial geniculate nucleus is the structural area involved.

The medial geniculate nucleus receives its inputs from two sources. First is the ipsilateral inferior colliculus. This nucleus, as we know from the previous discussion, does a significant amount of processing associated with localization and reflexes. These processes are a major part of the operation of the medial geniculate nucleus. This is not an unexpected phenomenon when you examine the fibers that converge on this higher center. The majority of the inputs arise from the ipsilateral inferior colliculus. You have to note, however, that there are interactions between the ipsilateral and contralateral inferior colliculus before ascent to the medial geniculate. This clearly indicates that many of the neurons in the medial geniculate are binaurally sensitive. The geniculate is sensitive to interaural intensity and timing cues passed on from the inferior colliculus. Therefore, not only does this higher center act as a relay to the auditory cortex, it is also involved in the processing of the interaural cues for localization.

The second input to the thalamus, shown in Figure 9.12, is a direct pathway from the contralateral cochlear nucleus. Although the function of this input is still debated by investigators, it appears that a rapid input from the contralateral ear, with an almost immediate relay to the auditory cortex, is related to an instant cortical attention process. In other words, although hypothetical, it is likely that the rapid input to the thalamus and the cortex is a cue that an environmental event has occurred. This cue instantly initiates a cortical analysis of incoming activity and a search for its identification. What is it?

The Auditory Cortex

The cortex is often assumed to be the "place" where the real auditory processing occurs. As we have seen, however, there are significant neural events occurring in the lower centers of the auditory pathway. The cortex, however, is significant. The inputs to the auditory cortex ascend from the ipsilateral thalamus. The thalamus, in turn, has received the majority of its inputs from the contralateral inferior colliculus. The configuration of ascending paths shown in Figure 9.12 indicates that the contralateral cortex processes sounds activating each cochlea. This does not mean that the input from the ipsilateral ear is ignored nor that the activity fails to reach the ipsilateral cortex. This means that there is a crossover of the pathways. An estimated 60% of the ascending fibers arrive at the contralateral side of the cortex.

The cortical location of the auditory inputs is shown diagrammatically in Figure 9.14. The primary cortical area is labeled A1 and lies within the Sylvian fissure (lateral fissure) of the temporal lobe. The A1 area is also known as Heschl's gyrus. Just posterior to A1 is a secondary area known as the planum temporale. The planum temporale in the left hemisphere is also called Wernicke's area.

The cortex for the auditory system is further organized in the usual columns and layers. The columns are assessed with microelectrodes and reveal once again the tonotopic maps (Roe, Pallas, Hahm, & Sur, 1990). Each column of cells, approximately 0.3 mm in width, responds to a narrow range of frequencies. As an example, one tonotopic map has high frequencies in the anterior portion of the A1 and the lower frequencies are located progressively toward the posterior. The tonotopic map flows, in this example, from anterior to posterior. There are other tonotopic maps with different orientations.

The function of the auditory cortex is often considered from the human perspective. That is, how does the primary and secondary auditory cortex process our most important auditory signals—language and speech? The answer appears to be that the planum temporale, Wernicke's area, in the left hemisphere is significantly involved with speech perception. This statement, however, needs to be tempered because speech perception does not always occur in the left hemisphere. Some individuals process speech in the right hemisphere.

The perceptions of nonspeech sounds are also of importance. The perception of music is one that almost immediately comes to mind. The data appear to support the possibility that music and rhythmic sounds are processed in the right hemisphere in Heschl's gyrus. Heschl's gyrus is larger in the right hemisphere than the left. This conclusion, therefore, appears to be relatively obvious and straightforward. There is, however, a caveat. Musicians with perfect pitch (identifying the pitch of a musical note without an external reference) tend to have more activity (as determined by fMRI [functional

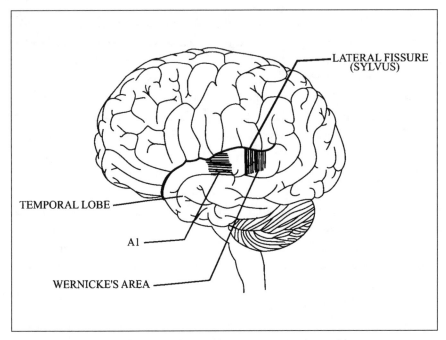

LATERAL FISSURE (SYLVUS)

TEMPORAL LOBE

A1

WERNICKE'S AREA

Figure 9.14. Cortical Representation of the Primary Auditory Cortex

Magnetic Resonance Image]) in the left planum temporale than do nonmusicians or musicians who do not have perfect pitch. This interesting result casts a cloud over the possibility that musical ability is firmly entrenched in the right hemisphere (Deutsch, 1992).

In addition to the processing of speech and music, the role that the cortex plays in sound localization and identification should be considered. Sound localization is improved with a normal-functioning auditory cortex. The interesting thing about cortical processing in this case is that the bilateral removal of the cortex in animals (monkeys) does not entirely destroy sound localization. There is a loss, naturally, but it is not complete. The monkey can respond, when trained, to discriminate and locate sounds in the left and right auditory space. It appears that a bilateral loss of primary auditory cortex in a human most likely results in a similar deficit. There has not been a human volunteer for such a research project. The data on humans comes from autopsies, and such anatomical data cannot definitively support the idea that humans with bilateral auditory cortex damage still have localization abilities. However, there appears to be a high probability that humans with bilateral auditory cortex damage still have some sound localization capabilities. A complete bilateral removal of the auditory cortex could very likely destroy speech comprehension and musical appreciation.

Dysfunctions

The auditory system is vulnerable. Problems can develop because of environmental effects (noise), medical intervention (drugs), infections, tumors, miscellaneous accidents, and aging. These problems are outlined under three different headings: **conductive hearing loss, sensorineural hearing loss,** and **noise-induced hearing loss.** The latter is, in fact, a subset of sensorineural hearing loss. We briefly look at these three categories as well as speech deficits that occur with cortical accidents.

Conductive Hearing Loss

This type of hearing impairment is limited to the conduction apparatus of the external and middle ear. The title, conductive hearing loss, is quite descriptive and defines the problem. Soft or moderately intense environmental sounds cannot be perceived because they never reach the inner ear through the ear canal and ossicular chain. There are numerous problems that lead to conductive hearing loss: a plugged ear canal due to an accumulation of cerumen, a punctured eardrum, an infection in the middle ear (**otitis media**), ossification (bone growth) that restricts the movement of the stapes and the oval window (**otosclerosis**), ossicles not joined (damaged), and pressure difference across the tympanic membrane because of a plugged eustachian tube. Anything that prevents the sound from reaching the inner ear through the normal air conduction mechanisms is considered a conductive loss. The loss is fairly constant across frequency. Conductive hearing loss can be compensated for by hearing aids. In some cases, the problem can be treated by antibiotics (otitis media) or by surgical intervention such as replacing the ossified stapes in the oval window.

Sensorineural Hearing Loss

Hearing loss due to problems within the cochlea or in higher neural centers is known as sensorineural impairment. An auditory nerve problem is usually caused by tumors. The more common form of sensorineural hearing loss is that found in the cochlea. Infections, drugs, and trauma can cause cochlear hearing loss. Sometimes sensorineural loss is congenital.

The most sensitive parts of the cochlea, the hair cells and the stria vascularis, are likely to be involved in cochlear impairments. Although sensorineural loss is the most common type of impairment, treatment with hearing aids can be beneficial. However, you should note that the hearing aid does not restore normal hearing like eyeglasses restore 20/20 vision. The loss of the outer or inner hair cells is critical. These cells cannot be replaced if they are damaged. There are some interesting and promising studies that show that birds (chickens) can regenerate damaged hair cells (Travis, 1992). Whether or not scientists are able to induce regeneration within the human cochlea, however, is still to be determined. For the time being, it is wiser to rely on hearing protection than it is to hope that you can regenerate damaged hair cells.

Noise-Induced Hearing Loss

Noise-induced hearing loss (NIHL) is actually a subset of the sensorineural hearing loss category. I have, because of the importance of environmental noise pollution, taken the liberty to discuss NIHL as a separate class of dysfunction.

There are two types of NIHL. The first one is known as a temporary threshold shift. The decrease in sensitivity, an increase in threshold, occurs when you are exposed to a long duration sound that has a level greater than about 80 dB SPL. Most everyone has experienced a temporary loss of hearing. After you have incurred a temporary threshold shift, by attending a rock concert or listening to the radio or tapes on earphones at intense levels, an interesting phenomenon often accompanies the shift in threshold. When you leave the concert or take off the earphones and go to the "silent" normal world, your ears "ring." The ringing is the result of the overstimulation of the hair cells.

The second kind of NIHL is the more serious kind. It is a permanent threshold shift. In this situation, the individual becomes permanently hearing impaired because of the noise-induced destruction of the hair cells or the stria vascularis. The benefits of hearing aids may be beneficial, but, once again, the hearing never returns to normal. The permanent threshold shift, in conjunction with the normal hearing loss of aging, can be a devastating condition. The permanent threshold shift was, when it was first diagnosed, known as "boilermaker's ear" because individuals who worked in boiler manufacturing factories a few decades ago nearly always became deaf as a result of the exposure to the intense sounds during the workday. Today, in industries where high noise levels exist in the workplace, federal regulations require hearing protection if employees are exposed to noise levels greater than 85 dB SPL for 8 hours or longer.

An easily recognized sign of the beginning of permanent threshold shift due to noise exposure is the **4-kHz notch** in a hearing test. Noise trauma begins its insidious attack on hearing by destroying the most sensitive region of hearing first. It is insidious because it destroys the hearing without warning. NIHL, if it is not caused by an intense explosive blast such as gunfire or dynamite, is not painful. Consequently, the permanent threshold shift simply creeps up on you without warning. After a few years in a high-noise environment, you are permanently hearing impaired.

One other type of hearing deficit should be mentioned before we close this section. It is presbycusis. This is cochlear hearing loss that occurs because of normal aging. It was mentioned in the previous paragraph as an added consequence of NIHL. Presbycusis begins with a loss in the high frequencies and slowly expands in the low-frequency range. Although it is thought to be the result of the normal attrition of hair cells as a function of growing older, some scientists believe presbycusis is merely a symptom of our noisy industrial age. Whether that is the case or not, it is true that the cochlea did not evolve to handle the intense sounds now found in our society.

Summary

This chapter has introduced the auditory system from the cochlea to the cortex. The cochlea is the initial auditory portion of the inner ear. The normal movement of the tympanic membrane by external environmental sounds results in the movement of the ossicular chain and the initiation of the traveling wave within the cochlea. The cochlea, in turn, is an active system of receptors, supporting cells, and fluid that, together, produce a relatively finely tuned analysis of the impinging sound waveform. The transduction to neural action potentials is accomplished by the inner hair cells with fine-tuning provided by the outer hair cells. An excellent perspective of the neural aspects of hearing is provided by Geisler (1998).

The sensitivity of the auditory mechanism is one of the most acute sensory systems. An amazing aspect of the cochlea is its ability to generate the neural auditory code used to interpret music, language, noise, and the infinite kinds of sounds in our environment. The cochlea does this with only 15,500 receptors in each ear. This sparse number of receptors, in view of the organism's evolutionary necessity to perceive environmental sounds, is even more amazing. As a contrast, consider the human eye. There are within a single eye over 126 million receptors. The loss of 31,000 receptors in one eye is scarcely noticed. The loss of 31,000 auditory receptors, 15,500 from each ear, places you in a permanently silent world. The loss of our receptors by noise is a commonly encountered deficit.

Sound localization begins with the interaural processing of intensity and temporal cues in the superior olive. The inferior colliculus continues to process the localization information as well as initiate reflexes for head movement and visual search. The auditory cortex receives the majority of its inputs from the contralateral ear. The cortex is partitioned into primary and secondary areas. The cortex is further partitioned into the planum temporale (Wernicke's area) and Heschl's gyrus. The former area is assumed to be associated with speech perception and the latter with musical ability.

Suggested Readings

Borg, E., & Counter, S. A. (1989, August). The middle-ear muscles. *Scientific American*, pp. 74-80.

Geisler, C. D. (1998). *From sound to synapse.* New York: Oxford University Press.

Heffner, H. E., & Masterton, R. B. (1990). Sound localization in mammals: Brain stem mechanisms. In M. Berkley and W. Stebbins (Eds.), *Comparative perception, vol. 1: Discrimination.* New York: John Wiley.

Konishi, M. (1993, April). Listening with two ears. *Scientific American*, pp. 66-73.

Loeb, G. E. (1985, February). The functional replacement of the ear. *Scientific American*, 104-111.

Moore, B. C. J. (1997). *An introduction to the psychology of hearing.* New York: Academic Press.

CHAPTER 10

Vision

The Visual Stimulus

This chapter introduces the processes that provide us with visual images, colors, patterns, motion, and depth derived from the environmental stimuli. Given this goal, it is appropriate to begin with the energy in the universe. The energy striking the earth comes from the sun and beyond. It is in the form of radiation and travels at 186,000 miles per second (speed of light because it is light) and has the properties of waves and particles. The particles are called photons. Figure 10.1 shows a diagram of the range of electromagnetic radiation. The figure also reflects the very restricted range of the spectrum used by the human visual sense. As can be seen, the electromagnetic spectrum consists of very short wavelengths (gamma waves) and the much longer waves (radio and television). Near the middle is the narrow band of waves called the **visible spectrum.** This narrow band of wavelengths, often simply referred to as light, generates our visual sensations. The energy within the visible spectrum is at a level at which living organisms and their nuclear bonds are not destroyed. Too much energy (as in gamma waves) destroys or disrupts nuclear bonds. The longer wavelengths, on the other hand, lack enough energy to adequately stimulate receptors. Hence, the visible spectrum contains the necessary energy and electromagnetic waves (photons) to create our visual world. The blanket of ozone surrounding the earth helps protect us from the higher-level damaging radiation. The electromagnetic radiation shown in Figure 10.1 has wavelengths that are so short they are often measured in angstroms (gamma waves). The longer waves (radio and TV) are so long that they can be measured in meters. The usual metric for radiation is, however, the nanometer (nm) that is one billionth of a meter. You often find the measurement specified as millimicron (mμ). It makes no difference which verbal description of wavelength is used. *One nanometer* and *one millimicron* are just different words for the same quantity.

It probably comes as no surprise to learn that different creatures have different visible spectrums. Some hawks, for example, use ultraviolet radiation to detect their prey (and their eyes are structured differently too). Snakes use the infrared waves. The human visual system cannot process either the ultraviolet or the infrared. The visible spectrum does provide wavelengths used to produce our color perception. The colors we see are indicated in Figure 10.1 by the color nomenclature associated with the wavelengths in the visible spectrum.

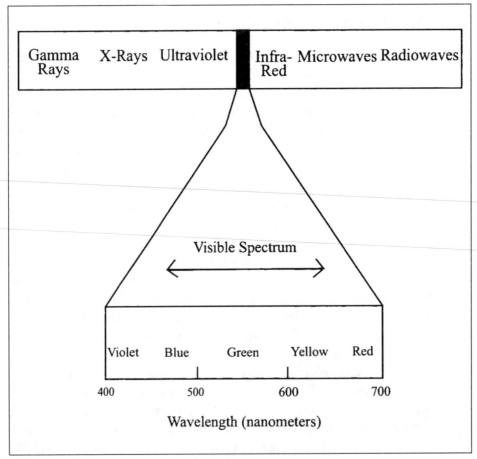

Figure 10.1. The Electromagnetic Spectrum

Before we continue with a discussion of the structure of the eye, there is one more important idea that must be noted. Only foolish individuals look directly at the sun. That is not the concept to remember because everyone knows that (or should). The important rule to understand is that the universe we see is based nearly entirely on reflected wavelengths. When light strikes an object in the environment, the object absorbs and reflects the wavelengths and photons selectively. If an object absorbs all the energy in the visible spectrum, it reflects nothing and the object, if seen at all, is perceived as black. On the other hand, if an object reflects all the wavelengths in the visible spectrum, the object is, if it is perceived, white. The point of this discussion is simple. The vast majority of our visual sensations are dependent on wavelengths reflected by the tangible objects in the environment. Of course, some things emit light. We see those objects if we focus on them (for example light bulbs, fire, and fireflies).

The Structure of the Eye

Figure 10.2 shows a cross section of the human eye. Our discussion begins with the **sclera.** The sclera surrounds the entire eye and is the membrane that provides structure to maintain the eyeball in a relatively round shape. The largest portion of the sclera appears white and surrounds most of the eye. In the front is an additional important feature. The sclera bulges out and is transparent, and light passes through it to reach the receptors inside the eye. The transparent portion of the sclera is the **cornea.** The function of the cornea with its transparency is to diffract or bend light radiation as it enters the eye. The cornea accounts for a little over two thirds of the diffraction that occurs (the lens accomplishes the remaining one third). Immediately behind the cornea is the anterior chamber formed by the cornea in the front and the iris in the back. The chamber is filled with a fluid, **aqueous humor,** that is continually produced and circulated. The aqueous humor bathes the cornea and iris and provides the oxygen and nutrients necessary for these structures.

When you look at your friend's eyes, the iris usually gets your attention. The iris provides the color of the eyes. Because of an individual's genetic endowment, the iris, like other objects in the world, is pigmented and absorbs some wavelengths and reflects others. The reflected wavelengths determine the eye color as perceived by others (or yourself if you look in a mirror). Because the iris is a muscle (actually two muscles), it can contract or relax. The contraction and relaxation affects the size of a hole in the center of the iris. This hole is the **pupil.** The iris automatically and reflexively controls the

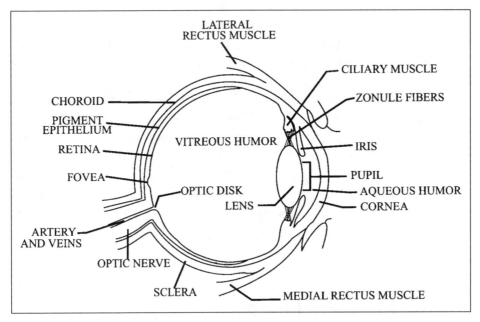

Figure 10.2. *Cross Section of the Human Eye*

amount of light entering the posterior chamber to reach the receptors. When the reflex occurs it changes the size of the pupil. When the light is dim, the iris relaxes and the pupil enlarges. When the light becomes too intense, vision becomes impaired and the iris contracts to make the pupil smaller. The restriction of the pupil reduces the amount of light entering the eye and improves the visual image.

Directly behind the iris is the **lens.** The lens is a remarkable structure; it is transparent and assumes different shapes. The shape of the lens is determined by a set of ciliary muscles acting in conjunction with many **zonule fibers.** The interaction between the **ciliary muscle** and zonule fibers determines the thickness of the lens.

First, it should be noted that the zonule fibers place a constant tension on the lens when the ciliary muscles are relaxed. When the zonule tension reduces, the lens becomes thicker. One end of the ciliary muscle is connected to the inner wall of the eye near one boundary of the zonule fibers. The other end of the ciliary muscle is attached to the sclera. The ends of the zonule fibers are attached, in turn, to the lens and the inner wall of the eye. This muscle and fiber configuration provides the means of changing the thickness of the lens. When the ciliary muscle contracts, the tension on the zonule fibers decreases. The decrease in fiber tension reduces, in turn, the tension on the lens. The result is that the lens, because of its elasticity, assumes its preferred configuration, relatively round. The contraction of the ciliary muscle reduces tension on the fibers and the lens changes its shape to become more spherical. This configuration allows one to clearly view objects in close proximity. This is near vision. Conversely, the relaxation of the ciliary muscle allows the zonule fibers to increase their tension on the lens. The increase in tension by the fibers pulls the lens in a thinner and flatter contour and reduces the diffraction of the light entering the eye. This configuration is used for distance viewing. The change in the lens shape and the subsequent focusing of the environmental image on the back of the eye provides us with our acuity and clear vision. The focusing is accomplished by the lens and is called **accommodation.** The accommodation by the lens results in our clear crisp image of the world. The spherical or round shape of the lens is produced when our eyes focus on objects closer than approximately 20 feet. As you read this sentence, your ciliary muscles are contracted just enough to allow the lens to refract (bend) the reflected light (remember, you are looking at reflected wavelengths) so you can see the words on the page. In short, the contraction or relaxation of the ciliary muscles affects the tension of the zonule fibers to provide the correct accommodation for a clear image.

Inside the eye, in the **vitreous chamber,** is a clear jellylike substance called the **vitreous humor.** The vitreous humor aids the sclera in its task of maintaining the eyeball in a relatively round configuration. In addition, it has a phagocytic (cell-eating) action that removes "floaters" from the eye. Floaters are blood cells or other cells that have broken away from the inner portions of the eye and drifted aimlessly through the vitreous humor. They can cause some distraction and impairment in the clarity of vision. Floaters, by analogy, could be called "eye dandruff." The debris floating in the vitreous humor can be seen if it crosses the field of view.

Surrounding the inside of the posterior chamber is the **retina.** The retina consists of the neurons and receptors that produce the activity used for visual sensation. Before we discuss the retina in detail, it is important to note two other layers of cells that lie just posterior and next to the retina. The cells that maintain a healthy and functional eye are the **ciliary** and **pigment epithelium.** The pigment epithelium lays next to the retina and in conjunction with the ciliary, supplies nutrients for the receptors while simultaneously removing debris (discarded receptor disks and membranes) that are constantly produced and discarded by the active receptors. In fact, a special glial cell conducts the debris cleanup. This is not surprising because there are specialized glial cells (astrocytes) in the central nervous system that remove unwanted debris. In humans, the pigment epithelium contains black melanin granules that absorb the stray light not captured by photoreceptors. The absorption of the stray light prevents a distortion of the visual image. In nocturnal animals, on the other hand, the epithelium differs significantly in its composition. In most nocturnal animals, the pigment epithelium, called the tapetum, is reflective in nature. The tapetum acts to reflect light rather than absorb it. The reflected light that is not absorbed by the receptors is captured as it rebounds from the back of the eye. The very weak light that is available at night is not wasted by such a system. The effects of the tapetum can be observed easily when car headlights strike the eyes of such animals (e.g., deer and rodents). Their eyes are "caught in the headlights" and we see the reflected light and their tapetum in action.

The Retina

The retina is the place where the brain first encounters the visible spectrum. This statement means that the neural elements within the eye are extensions of brain development. The neural elements become specialized to transduce electromagnetic radiation and generate action potentials. By looking through the pupil into the eye with a special instrument (an opthalmoscope), you can actually see the retina. It is composed of six different kinds of cells. Two of the cell types are true receptors: **rods** and **cones.** The other four are neurons. The neurons are the **bipolar, amacrine, horizontal,** and **ganglion** cells and are physically located in front of the receptors next to the vitreous humor. This means that light, as it enters the eye, must travel through the neural elements to reach the photosensitive receptors. Even more interesting is that the photosensitive portion of the receptor is oriented toward the rear of the eye so the light must pass through the receptor cell body to reach the photosensitive outer segment. This arrangement, however, causes no problem in visual sensation for two reasons. First, the cells are quite transparent and light passes through them readily. Second, the neurons are conveniently shunted to the side at a point called the **fovea** (see Figure 10.2). This means that light reaching the fovea falls exclusively on the receptors. An arrangement of the retinal cells not located in the fovea is shown diagrammatically in Figure 10.3.

Phototransduction

The transduction of light by the rods and cones is an interesting phenomenon. A single photon of light can energize and activate the transduction pro-

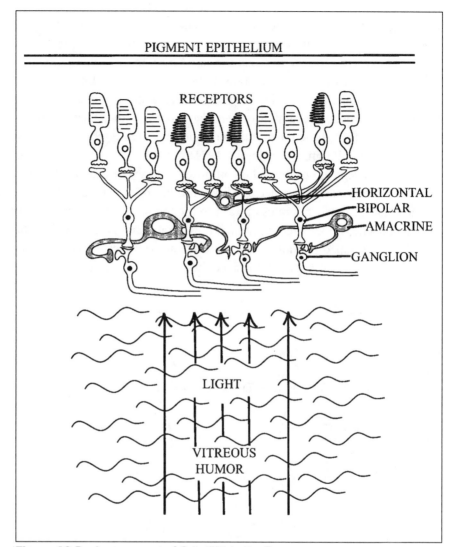

Figure 10.3. Arrangement of Cells Within the Eye

cess in a single receptor. More interesting still is that the transduction in the rods and cones are the same except for a single protein: opsin. The protein is, as we learn, quite important in the initiation of the action potentials. Before we begin discussing the process of transduction, it is necessary to briefly outline the structures of the rods and cones. They differ not so much in function as they do in structure. First, both of these receptors consist of two distinct segments. The first segment is at the end of the cell and initiates the transduction process—the **outer segment**. The second part of the cell—the inner segment—is similar to the soma of a neuron because it contains the nucleus and produces the necessary ingredients to maintain the cell. The inner segment has the synaptic terminal at the base. Given this overview, shown in Figure 10.4 with a diagram of the transduction operation, we can proceed to the photochemical process. The rod is used as a model to describe the transduction process of changing one energy form to another. Significant differences between the function of rods and cones are noted as we proceed (Yau, 1994; Yoshikami, Robinson, & Hagins, 1974).

The outer segment of the rod is composed of layers of disks enclosed in the outer membrane of the cell. Each disk is produced at the base of the outer segment, and it slowly migrates upward to the top of the stack. Once it has reached the end of the outer segment, it degenerates and is absorbed by the glial cells mentioned previously. All the disks are connected to each other through a narrow hairlike segment called the cilium. The cilium provides the

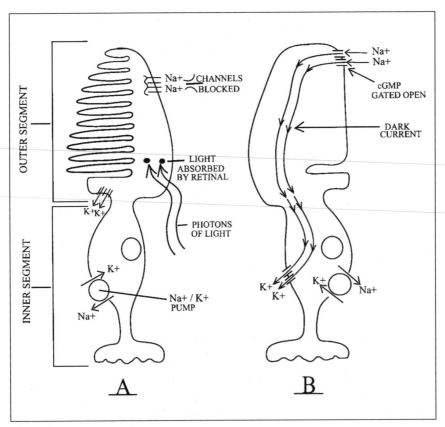

Figure 10.4. Diagrammatic Representation of Receptor Cell Transduction

bridge or passageway for the movement of the ions within the cell during transduction. The degeneration of the disks is continuous, and new outer segments are produced about every 8 days.

The disks within the outer segments are where the photons of light are absorbed. The chemical molecules that absorb the light initiate the process of visual sensation. Each rod contains possibly 1,000 to 2,000 disks with approximately 3 billion photon-absorbing molecules within each disk. The molecule that is involved in light absorption is **rhodopsin.** Rhodopsin is composed of two parts: retinal and opsin. Retinal is a molecule in its own right. It is long and straight when not coupled with opsin. In this straight form, it is called *all-trans* retinal. When the straight all-trans retinal joins forces with the protein opsin, it must bend to accommodate and hold the opsin. The all-trans retinal, when bent, becomes a form called *11-cis.* You can remember this easily if you just visualize the 11-cis retinal bent in a 90° angle to hold on to the protein opsin.

When the retinal portion of the rhodopsin absorbs a photon of light, the retinal molecule releases the opsin and reverts to its preferred configuration: a straight all-trans molecule. The straightening of the retinal molecule because of the absorption of a photon of light initiates the second step of the transduction process (the first was the absorption of the photon by retinal). The release of the opsin, the second step, initiates a cascade of events that changes the status of the receptor and "stops" the release of the neurotransmitter glutamate at the receptor synaptic terminal. Glutamate is constantly released in the absence of light. Complete darkness results in the release of more glutamate than does twilight or evening shadows. The absorption of light by retinal breaks the bond with the opsin protein and initiates the chemical events that terminate the release of the neurotransmitter. Unlike all the other receptors we have discussed, the rods and cones do not release a neurotransmitter when the adequate stimulus occurs. Instead, the receptor stops the release of glutamate and hyperpolarizes. The receptors are partially depolarized in the dark or dim light, and they hyperpolarize and stop releasing the neurotransmitter when a photon of light is absorbed by the retinal. A close look at the chemical events and membrane channels in the outer segment of the cell clarifies this situation.

Dark Current and Hyperpolarization

The story begins in the dark with the rods and cones depolarized with an internal potential between about −10 and −30 mv. As just noted, the receptors are depolarized above their resting potential when not stimulated by an adequate stimulus. The depolarization in the rods and cones in the dark is associated with a dark current flowing through the cell. The current is generated by Na^+ ions entering the outer segment of the cell through the outer membrane while K^+ ions steadily leave the cell from the inner segment. A question probably comes to mind at this point. If the Na^+ continues to influx and the K^+ continues to efflux, it appears that the cell soon becomes devoid of K^+ and filled with Na^+. This, of course, does not occur. The reason it does not happen is the familiar active transport system called the sodium-potassium pump. The pump maintains the ion balance and the cell continues to have a dark current while in the dark, and the Na^+/K^+ pump actively responds to the influx and efflux. The dark current maintains the depolarization and the synaptic membrane of the cell continually releases the neurotransmitter. Thus, in the dark, rods and cones have active synapses. The synapses are releasing their vesicles full of glutamate onto the postsynaptic dendrite of the bipolar and horizontal neurons.

How the Na^+ influx enters the outer segment of the receptor is answered by examining the effects of a molecule called cyclic guanosine monophosophate (cGMP). The cGMP maintains the open Na^+ channels in the outer segment and permits the passive influx of Na^+ into the cell (Fesenko, Kolesnikov, & Lyubarsky, 1985; Haynes & Yau, 1985). The cGMP is synthesized from guanosine triphosphate (GTP is an energy packet) by guanylate cyclase (GC) present in the outer segment. The K^+ channels in the inner segment are always open for the K^+ ions to efflux so there is a continuous dark current of Na^+ influx and K^+ efflux. The dark current, of course, declines if some of the Na^+ channels were too close. Any decline in the dark current, in turn, reduces the amount of neurotransmitter released by the vesicles. The way to hyperpolarize the rod (and the cone) and reduce the dark current is to close the Na^+ channels. It should not be surprising at this point in the discussion to note that the Na^+ channels close when a photon of light is absorbed. Our next task is to examine how the absorption of light closes the Na^+ channels.

Light Absorption and the Na^+ Channels

As we know, when the retinal molecule absorbs a photon of light, the molecule straightens (is isomerized) to the all-trans shape and frees the protein opsin. When the freed and unstable opsin breaks the bonds with the retinal, it activates a G-protein called **transducin.** *G-protein* is shorthand for a special binding protein named guanosine triphosphate. The "binding" aspect of the G-protein usually refers to the linking of a neurotransmitter molecule with the G-protein. In vision, however, it is the absorption of the light and the release of opsin that activates the transducin. The transducin, in turn, activates an enzyme called **phosphodiesterase (PDE)**. An enzyme is another protein that facilitates a chemical interaction but does not specifically enter the reaction. The enzyme PDE then begins to inactivate (hydrolyze) the cGMP to change it to GMP. The result is an ineffective molecule (GMP) that cannot keep the channels open for Na^+. The channels close and prevent Na^+ from entering the cell while K^+ continues to leave. The consequence is a hyperpolarized receptor with an internal voltage approaching the equilibrium potential for K^+, near -70 mv. This sequence of events is very fast. One photon can release hundreds of transducins to activate thousands of PDE enzymes. The PDE, in turn, causes the hydrolysis of 10^5 molecules of cGMP. The chemical events initiated by the photon take 1 second. The outcome is a reduction in the neurotransmitter release at the synapse with the bipolar cell. One last comment before we move on: After this chain of events gets started, why does it stop? The reason it stops is because the photon of light absorption lasts only a fraction of a second and the transducin activated by opsin is deactivated by another protein—opsin kinase. The deactivating protein, opsin kinase, breaks a nucleotide bond and stops the transducin activity. The chemical reaction comes to a rapid stop. The chain of events that occurs when a photon of light is absorbed is summarized below and shown in Figure 10.4:

1. Light is absorbed by retinal and isomerized to all-trans configuration.
2. Opsin becomes unstable because retinal breaks the bond.
3. Opsin activates the G-protein transducin.
4. Transducin activates phosphodiesterase (PDE).
5. PDE hydrolyzes (inactivates) cGMP to GMP.
6. Na^+ channels are no longer held open by cGMP and close.
7. Na^+ channels close, and K^+ channels remain open so the receptor hyperpolarizes.
8. The hyperpolarized receptor decreases the neurotransmitter release.
9. Opsin kinase terminates the light response.

Functional Differences Between Rods and Cones

The two receptors differ from each other in several ways. Rods and cones differ in structure, photochemical molecules, sensitivity, retinal distribution, synaptic connections, and function. The structural contrasts are evident and are shown in Figure 10.4. Briefly, the two types of receptors differ in their size and their disk morphology. The outer segment of rods contains approximately 1,000 to 2,000 identical disks. The disks in rods contain more photopigment (rhodopsin) and consequently capture more photons of light than cones. There is also a higher amplification in the rods than in the cones. This means that, in rods, more cGMP gets hydrolized for each absorbed photon of light. This amplification (more hydrolization) leads to a longer integration and a more sensitive cell. In other words, the rod responds longer and easily with a few photons of light. The high amplification and long integration leads to high sensitivity to scattered light (weak and not directly falling on any one rod). The high sensitivity is the reason that rods are effective in weak light (moonlight, starlight, and dark movie theaters). In contrast, the cones do not have individual disks to hold the photochemicals used in the transduction process. The photochemicals in cones are in the outer membrane of the cell and the shape of the cone is determined by the folding of the outer membrane. The folding of the membrane in the outer segment increases the surface area and provides more membrane exposure for light absorption. The amplification, sensitivity, and integration, however, are not equivalent to the rods. The cones require more light because they have fewer photochemicals and less amplification. The superiority of the cone to detect fine detail, however, is apparent with direct (not scattered) axial rays of daylight. The direct and precise convergence of nonscattered light on the fovea provides us with our excellent acuity during the day. The cones are activated.

The opsin molecules in the photochemical differ in the two receptors. All rods have the same opsin molecule. Because the opsin molecule determines the particular wavelength that can be absorbed most readily by the retinal, all the rods are similar in their response to light. The rods have an absorption peak near 500 nm. Each cone, on the other hand, has one of three different opsin molecules. The cone opsin molecules are also referred to as iodopsin (Wald, Brown, & Smith, 1955). The wavelength absorption characteristic of each cone depends on which opsin is bound to the retinal in the 11-cis configuration. The opsin determines the cone-wavelength absorption sensitivity (Marks, Dobelle, & MacNichol, (1964). This means that cones differ from each other as well as from the rods in their absorption characteristics. The opsin in some cones allows the retinal to best absorb a wavelength near 420 nm, whereas the other two cones have peak absorption near 530 and 560 nm. The different absorption spectra for the three cones provide the first step in color perception. The three different receptors are referred to as the short, medium, and long wavelength cones because their adequate stimulus is the short, medium, and long wavelengths in the visible spectrum. It should come as no surprise at this point to note that color vision only occurs when there is sufficient light in the surrounding world. Rods function well in dim light—cones do not.

The distribution of the rods and cones in the retina differs significantly. The optical center of the eye is called the macula. This area of the retina is approximately 5 to 6 mm in diameter and is filled with an abundance of cones and a few rods. In the center of the macula is the small indentation shown in Figure 10.2. This indentation is the fovea. It is about 1 mm in diameter and it contains only cones (the fovea is greatly exaggerated in size in Figure 10.2). Although no one has counted every cone, there are approximately 34,000 to 35,000 cones in the fovea and 5 to 6 million cones in all. The fovea, therefore, has a relatively small fraction of the total number of cones. However, the synaptic organization within the fovea makes this area of the retina probably the most important within the eye (Kolb, Linberg, & Fisher, 1992; Kuffler, 1953; Wässle & Boycott, 1991). Although cones are distributed throughout the retina, the majority (approximately 90%) are within the macula and fovea. The distribution of rods is relatively straightforward. The approximately 100 to 120 million rods are found in the peripheral areas of the retina, not in the fovea. The majority of the rods are located approximately 20° from the center of the macula. There are no receptors—rods or cones—at the optic disk where the ganglion cell axons that form the optic nerve exit the eye and blood enters (central artery) and leaves (central vein). Finally, there are a significantly greater number of cones and rods than there are neural fibers that form the optic nerve. This implies, quite correctly, that there is a convergence of 125 million receptors on 1 million ganglion cells. The convergence is important in producing the visual sensations we experience.

The synaptic connections between receptors—bipolar, horizontal, amacrine—and ganglion cells are complex, and a basic understanding of their organization is important to understanding visual processing. Because of this complexity, the discussion of convergence and synaptic connections is partitioned in two sections. First in the discussion is the convergence of receptor output to the neural cells and an examination of their response characteristics. The second discussion topic is the lateral organization of the horizontal and amacrine cells. During these discussions, the synaptic and neural processing that provide the foundation for visual sensations such as brightness, acuity, contrast, movement, and color are presented.

Convergence and Receptive Fields

Before we continue, we need to recall that a neurotransmitter can elicit both an excitatory and inhibitory response in different cells. An excitatory or inhibitory response by the same neurotransmitter is due to the neurotransmitter binding to different receptor membranes on the postsynaptic side of the synapse. In one case, the docking of the neurotransmitter with the membrane receptor results in an inhibitory graded potential. On a different cell, the same neurotransmitter can produce an excitatory response. This idea is important because the bipolar cell receives only one neurotransmitter, glutamate, from the receptor and the bipolar cell has either excitatory receptors for glutamate or inhibitory receptors. The bipolar cell is either inhibitory or excitatory, depending on its postsynaptic response to glutamate. In addition, the bipolar cells do not conduct action potentials. All the bipolar activity occurs with fast-conducting graded potentials. In fact, only two cells in the retina conduct action potentials—the amacrine and the ganglion cells. With these ideas in mind, the topics of convergence and **receptive fields** become easier to understand.

Figure 10.5 illustrates the convergence process and introduces the idea of a receptive field in vision. A receptive field can be defined as a circumscribed area on the retina that provides the input to a ganglion cell. The receptive field, of course, begins with the activation of receptors. The simplest possible receptive field is shown in Figure 10.5 by Cone A. The convergence shown by Cone A is indeed simple: no convergence. The cone, labeled A, has a direct path to a single bipolar cell and the subsequent ganglion cell. Any light absorbed by the cone affects the bipolar and the ganglion cell directly. There are no lateral connections from other cells in this diagram. Keep in mind that in this example the bipolar cell is assumed to be excitatory. This means that the bipolar cell depolarizes when the cone releases neurotransmitter and hyperpolarizes when the amount of neurotransmitter declines. Consequently, an excitatory bipolar cell hyperpolarizes when the cone absorbs light. The hyperpolarized bipolar cell then reduces the glutamate it releases to the ganglion cell. This sequence of events leads to a reduction in the number of action potentials generated by the ganglion cell. This sequence is important so the four steps are repeated here. First, when a spot of light falls on an area of the

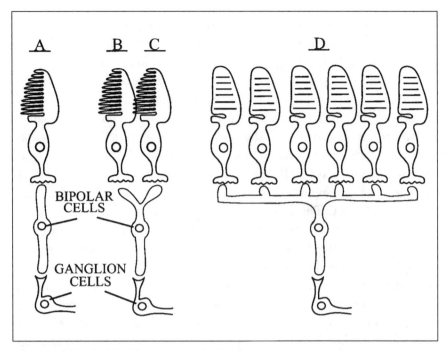

Figure 10.5. Cellular Convergence in the Retina

retina, in this case, on a single cone, it reduces the dark current and the cone hyperpolarizes. Second, the cone hyperpolarization decreases the amount of glutamate released at the synapse with the bipolar cell. Third, the reduction in the neurotransmitter removes the excitation of the bipolar cell, and the bipolar cell hyperpolarizes. Fourth, the hyperpolarized bipolar cell reduces the amount of neurotransmitter that is released at the synapse with the ganglion cell. The ganglion cell, in turn, produces fewer action potentials. The ganglion cell and the bipolar cell, in this situation, are both said to have an "off-center" receptive field. Light falling directly on the area of the retina served by the receptor turns off the activity sent to higher neural locations. Given this off-center situation, you may wonder if there is an "on-center" response, and if so how it occurs. The answer is that the inhibitory bipolar cell produces the on-center response when a light falls on the retina. The spot of light absorbed by the cone once again reduces the neurotransmitter release. However, with an inhibitory bipolar cell, the reduction in the neurotransmitter is equivalent to removing an inhibition. The reduction in neurotransmitter removes the inhibition, and the bipolar cell depolarizes. The depolarization increases the bipolar response at its synapse with the ganglion cell. The ganglion cell then depolarizes, and action potentials are sent to the higher centers. This sequence of events leads to the on-center receptive field. This direct signal pathway—cone to bipolar to ganglion cell—occurs only in the fovea.

Also shown in Figure 10.5 is a situation in which the convergence is more complex. In the discussion to follow, we assume that the bipolar cell is an inhibitory one. That is, if a light falls on the retina and the cones are stimulated, the bipolar cell depolarizes and the ganglion cell is activated to send action potentials. There are two cones, B and C, to be considered. The two cones converge on a single bipolar cell. This convergence means that a perception of two spots of light is impossible if one light falls only on Cone B and the other light only on Cone C. This is because the two cones converge on the same bipolar cell. The nervous system has no way to determine whether there are two lights—one illuminating Cone B and the other illuminating Cone C—or one spot of light illuminating both cones. The same bipolar and ganglion cell is involved regardless of the configuration of the lights. If, on the other hand, Cone A and Cone C each absorbed a photon of light you may distinguish the two lights as separate. There are different paths activated and different ganglion cells. There are, in short, two separate receptive fields activated and two sets of information are sent to the higher centers. Cones A and C each had their on-center receptive fields stimulated. The idea important here is that convergence leads to a lack of acuity. The more receptor outputs converge, the less you are able to differentiate between small separate objects in the environment. You may have noted that the receptors we just discussed were cones. The example assumes that the cones were all located within the fovea. The rule to remember is that cones have relatively little convergence so they provide us with sharp acuity.

Let us consider a different scenario by using Figure 10.5 again. Assume, in this example, that bipolar cells require six units of synaptic activity at their synapse with the receptors before they can activate the ganglion cell. We also assume, for this example, that to achieve the required six units at the synapse, Cone A must absorb six photons. Cones B and C together must absorb six photons to reach the threshold of activity for their shared bipolar cell. The scene is now set. Could you see a spot of light if the photons fell on Cone A but only five were absorbed? The answer is no, there was not enough light to generate the required response in the bipolar cell. What could you see if two photons were absorbed by Cone B and four photons were absorbed by Cone C at the same instant in time? You see a spot of light because of the convergence (recall "spatial summation"). The bipolar cell summates the input and receives enough activity to pass the information on to the ganglion cell. The sum of the activity from the two cones is sufficient. The bipolar cell activates the ganglion cell, and you see a spot of light. Note that neither Cone B nor Cone C, by itself, could accomplish the task. It required the summation of simultaneous activity from each receptor. The rule in this case is that convergence reduces acuity but increases sensitivity. A weak stimulus can activate several receptors just a little bit (for example, one photon for each of six receptors), and the convergence can summate to produce neural activity. Consider, for example, the rods labeled D in Figure 10.5. If a weak spot of light fell on the retina with just enough energy (one photon per rod) to activate the group of six rods, there would be a summation at the bipolar cell and a spot of light could be detected. The same weak light could not generate ganglion cell activity if it were absorbed by just one receptor. Sensitivity, then, increases when many converge on few. One last point before we move on. The receptive fields for bipolar cells (and ganglions) are larger when convergence occurs. This can be seen easily in Figure 10.5. The receptive field for the bipolar and ganglion cell associated with Cones B and C is larger than the receptive field of the bipolar cell receiving inputs from Cone A. Why? The answer is simple. Cones B and C cannot exist in the same space. They exist side by side and take up a greater space. The receptive field on the retina has to be larger. In fact, the on-center and off-center receptive fields vary in their size and are circular in their shape. More is said about the on-center and off-center receptive fields a little later in our discussion.

In summary, Figure 10.5 shows an extremely simplified retinal configuration. In this diagram, there are several rods and three cones. The rods, of course, represent the peripheral portion of the retina where rods are plentiful and cones are few. The point to note is the different amount of convergence for the rods and cones. The rods converge on a single ganglion cell while the cones converge less (in A, not at all). What this tells us is that the rods have poor acuity and very good sensitivity and the cones have good acuity and poor sensitivity. In fact, the rod sensitivity permits us to see in the dim light at night. The rods are more sensitive to the available light and generate the appropriate responses for vision. The details of the environment (and color) are not available. They are left to the high acuity cones that are not active in weak light.

Before we move on to a discussion of the horizontal cells, a brief summary may be useful concerning the straight-through neural flow from receptor to bipolar cell to ganglion cell.

First, rods are more sensitive and have lower thresholds than the cones. The rods, therefore, require less light to become active and are the primary visual receptors in very dim lighting conditions. There are many rods in the periphery of the retina, and their convergence on ganglion cells results in large circular receptive fields and relatively poor acuity. The rods have only one type of opsin and therefore do not provide any color information. The cones, in contrast, require more light, are less sensitive, have higher thresholds, provide us with color vision, have smaller circular receptive fields, and give us good acuity. There are more cones in the fovea, so color and acuity is best in this region of the eye.

Second, the bipolar cells are both excitatory and inhibitory and synapse directly on the ganglion cell. They do not conduct action potentials; rather they operate exclusively on the graded potentials. The inhibitory and excitatory aspect of the bipolar cells produces the on-center and off-center activity at the ganglion cell.

Lateral Processing by Horizontal Cells

The circular on-center and off-center receptive fields provide only part of the story for our visual sensations. The situation becomes more complex when horizontal cells become involved. The lateral processing modifies the receptive field (Peichl & Wässle, 1983). Our prior discussion pointed out that each ganglion cell (and bipolar cell) had a circular receptive field that was classified as either on-center or off-center. When horizontal cell activity is considered, the receptive field changes in size and response. The receptive field for each ganglion cell actually has a circular center and an antagonistic area that surrounds it (called an antagonistic surround). *Antagonistic* simply means that however the circular center responds, the circular surround responds in the opposite way. Assume, for example, that a ganglion cell sends action potentials when photons of light fall in the center of its receptive field. This ganglion cell has an on-center. If a light falls on the antagonistic surround instead of the center, however, the ganglion cell is turned off. This ganglion cell has a receptive field called an on-center off-surround. Horizontal-cell lateral activity makes this ganglion cell have these response characteristics (on-center off-surround). A light falling only on the on-center of the receptive field activates the ganglion cell (turns it on), whereas a light falling only on the off-surround inactivates the ganglion cell (turns it off) because of the horizontal-cell activity. The surround is antagonistic to the center. It probably comes as no surprise that if a ganglion cell has an off-center rather than an on-center, a light in the antagonistic surround activates the ganglion cell (turns it on) rather than inactivates it. Ganglion cells can have one or the other kind of receptive field. It is either an on-center off-surround or an off-center on-surround. These two types of ganglion cells provide parallel paths to the higher neural centers, and the combination of these two types of receptive fields provide us with our perception of edges and object contrast.

Figure 10.6 shows a simplified (very simplified) diagram of cells making up the two different kinds of ganglion receptive fields (Peichl, 1991). One is an off-center on-surround, and the other is an on-center off-surround. For simplicity, the figure shows only two receptors and one horizontal, bipolar, and ganglion cell for each neural system. Lateral processing by the horizontal cell is simple to understand. First, the horizontal cells are excitatory when glutamate is released by the receptors in the surround. Second, the horizontal cells make synaptic contact with receptors in the center of the receptive field, not with bipolar cells. Third, the horizontal-cell synaptic contact with the receptors is inhibitory. When the horizontal cell is active, it releases an inhibitory neurotransmitter and hyperpolarizes the receptor. When this inhibition is removed (by a decrease in the inhibitory neurotransmitter), the receptor depolarizes.

Given these conditions, consider what occurs if a light falls only on the surround of an on-center off-surround receptive field (the left side of Figure 10.6). The photons of light are absorbed and the receptor in the surround hyperpolarizes. The hyperpolarization decreases the release of glutamate at the synapse with the horizontal cell. The horizontal cell becomes hyperpolarized and stops releasing the inhibitory neurotransmitter to the receptor in the center of the receptive field. The receptor in the center of the field becomes more depolarized because of the decline in horizontal-cell inhibition. The depolarized receptor releases more glutamate to the bipolar cell. Remember, this is an on-center off-surround receptive field so the bipolar cell is an inhibitory one (inhibited by glutamate). Therefore, when the glutamate is increased at the receptor-bipolar synapse, the bipolar cell becomes more inhibited and reduces its activity at the ganglion-cell synapse. The consequence is that the ganglion-cell activity decreases. The light on the surround has done exactly what the name of the receptive field implies. When a light falls on the off-surround, the ganglion cell is inhibited (turned off) and the number of action potentials sent to higher centers declines. The antagonistic surround has done its job. The on-center bipolar and ganglion-cell pathway is turned off. This reduction in the ganglion-cell activity is shown in Figure 10.6(a). There is a decrease in action potentials when the surround is illuminated. The ganglion-cell response, when only the on-center is illuminated,

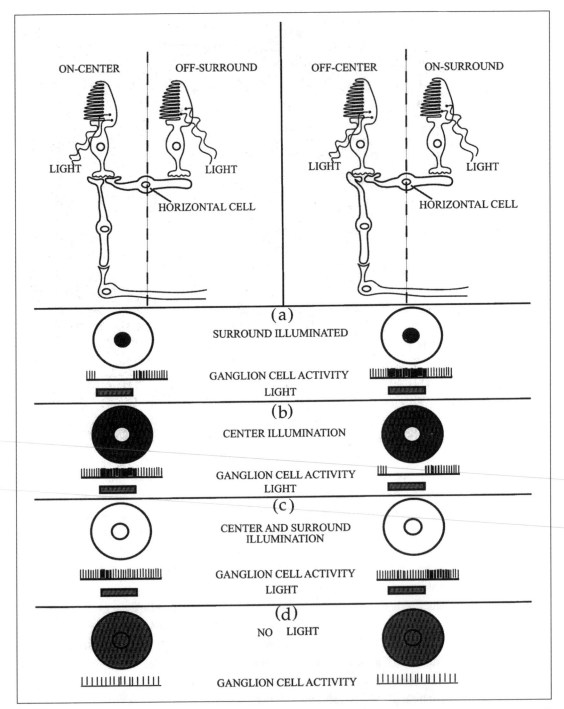

Figure 10.6. Ganglion Cell Response as a Function of Light Stimulation on the Center or Surround of the Receptive Field

NOTE: The on-center off-surround receptive field is on the left, the off-center on-surround is on the right. (a) The surround is illuminated, (b) the center is illuminated, (c) the center and surround are illuminated, and (d) no light on either the center or surround.

results in ganglion-cell activity (Figure 10.6[b]). When both the center and surround are illuminated, as shown in Figure 10.6(c), there is a constant but low output from the ganglion cell when the light is constant. Figure 10.6(c) also shows the usual response to a change in the stimulus, an on-response and an off-response. With no light falling on the receptive field, the ganglion cell responds randomly and spontaneously (Figure 10.6[d]).

The other pathway to the higher neural centers, the off-center and on-surround, is shown on the right in Figure 10.6. This path employs the same horizontal-cell activity as the on-center off-surround just discussed. The difference between the two parallel paths and their receptive fields is the type of bipolar cell in the system. The bipolar cell is excitatory in the off-center on-surround receptive field (it is inhibitory in the on-center off-surround). Thus, when the horizontal cell is inhibited and depolarizes the receptor cell, the bipolar cell becomes depolarized and activates the ganglion cell. The on-surround once again does its job. The on-surround is antagonistic to the off-center. Figure 10.6 shows, below the off-center on-surround neural diagram, the resulting neural activity of the ganglion cell with different configurations of light on the receptive fields. The ganglion-cell activity for four different lighting conditions is shown with the light falling only on the surround (a), only on the center (b), on both the center and surround simultaneously (c), and no light (d). The ganglion-cell output varies directly with the characteristics of the light pattern. The patterns of light in the present example are all circular and neatly fit the receptive field of the cell. This leads to the obvious question. Our world is not circular, so how do these circular receptive fields generate our perception of noncircular objects? The answer lies in the parallel processing by the two types of ganglion cells and their center-surround antagonistic organization.

One of the most important things our visual system does is differentiate objects in the environment. It does this is by contrasting the edges of the objects. For example, as you read this sentence and look at the words, there is an automatic contrast made between the dark letters and the white paper. The edges of the letters contrast with the background (the white paper). This is required if you are to see the letters. All you need to do is consider what you could see if the letters on the page suddenly became the same (no edges) as the white paper. An example of what you would see is the next line.

That is right. You see nothing. There are no edges and no contrast between the background (white paper) and the foreground (black type). So, you see nothing. Edges are straight, round, curved, and half-curved and provide the change in contrast between different objects. Letters of the alphabet are the objects in this example. The point here is that the receptive-field responses provide these edges by sending, in parallel, many signals about the environment. Where one receptive field (off-center) responds one way, another receptive field (on-center) responds in a completely different way. When many photoreceptors and ganglion cells are involved, the result is an edge. A simple way to demonstrate the manner in which this processing occurs is to consider Figure 10.7.

Note the left side of Figure 10.7. The figure shows a gray vertical bar with 10 receptive fields differentially located along the right edge. There are five off-center on-surround receptive fields (top five) and five on-center off-surround receptive fields (bottom five). Located to the right of each receptive field is a diagram showing the ganglion-cell activity as a function of the light impinging on the field. The important points to note are labeled A' and B' for the off-center on-surround and A and B for the on-center off-surround. First, contrast the ganglion-cell activity of A' and A. The ganglion-cell activity for these two receptive fields is significantly different. One receptive field (A') shows a strong response whereas the other receptive field (A) is inhibited. These two responses, keep in mind, are both sent to the higher neural centers at the same time. They both are significant responses. No response (A) is information just like a strong response (A'). The ganglion outputs noted at B' and B in the diagram are equally important although the activity is opposite of A' and A.

The message you should get from looking at Figure 10.7 is that when many receptive fields are activated along an edge, a clear message is sent to the higher centers about the environmental change (edge) where one object stops and another one begins. To see objects we depend on our ability to detect edges and contrast (where one object stops and another begins). The edges and the perceptual contrast between the objects are what permit us to navigate our world without bumping our heads or walking into some object in front of us.

Although our ability to detect edges by automatically contrasting differences in luminance is critical to our visual process, contrasts and edges can also provide interesting illusions. One such illusion is shown on the right in Figure 10.7. As you look at the diagram of the three bars, you no doubt see the center gray bar as varying in brightness. It appears dark gray at the top and lighter at the bottom. In contrast, the two bars on the sides are lighter at the top and darker at the bottom. Look at the center bar carefully. It surely varies in brightness. It is not a uniform gray, is it? The answer is, yes it is. It is a uniform

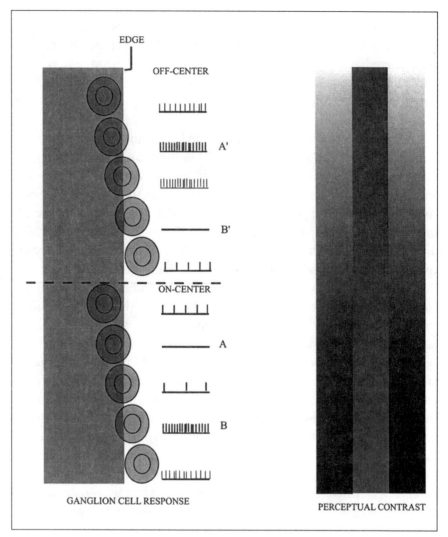

Figure 10.7. *Ganglion Cell Response to Edges and an Illusion of Brightness*

gray and is equally bright from the top to the bottom. You do not see it this way because of the contrast between the center bar and the two sidebars. What you see is an illusion, a false perception. To prove this to yourself, take two pieces of paper and cover the sidebars so you only see the center. What happened? The world changed. The center bar is now uniformly bright. This demonstrates the idea that the parallel paths and the ganglion-cell activity from the receptive fields provide a neural code about luminance contrasts (edges) in our environment. Without the luminance contrasts (edges), we are quite helpless. We are continually comparing and contrasting the background luminance with the object in the foreground. The center-surround antagonistic receptive fields provide us with this information. Occasionally we misperceive.

Introduction to Color Vision

Although more is said about color vision later in the chapter, it is appropriate to provide a background and begin at the beginning. The beginning, in this case, is the responses that occur within the retina when different wavelengths of light are transduced and processed. We already know that each cone contains one of three different opsins. The different opsins allow the retinal within the cone to absorb one wavelength more readily than another. The different absorption characteristics result in three types of cones. There are cones that absorb short wavelengths (420 nm), medium wavelengths (530 nm), and long wavelengths (560 nm). The fact that there are three different kinds of cones suggests that ganglion cells must also be involved in differentiating wavelengths because cones communicate with ganglion cells. In fact, ganglion cells associated with cones have unique receptive fields.

In the previous discussions, when a light was used to demonstrate the antagonistic center-surround characteristics of a receptive field, there was no mention of the particular wavelengths involved. Most likely, you assumed that a white spot of light was shined in the eye to stimulate the retina and the receptive field associated with the ganglion cell. This is often a correct assumption. You may ask, however, about what occurs if different wavelengths were used to obtain a ganglion-cell center-surround receptive field. By using different wavelengths, you can investigate the effects on ganglion-cell activity as a function of wavelength. When this is done, the results are quite interesting. Ganglion cells connected to cones not only have an antagonistic center-surround receptive field, many have a center-surround that is wavelength specific.

Four different receptive fields display antagonistic center-surrounds for particular wavelengths. There are ganglion cells that have an inhibitory surround and an excitatory center (–G/+R). Figure 10.8 shows the receptive field. There are also ganglion cells that have the opposite receptive fields. This type of ganglion cell receptive field is shown in Figure 10.8 with the +G and –R designation. The other two types of receptive fields are antagonistic for yellow and blue. They are, specifically, the –Y/+B and the +Y/–B shown in Figure 10.8. The designation of these receptive fields with the letters G, R, B, and Y comes from the perceptual response we get when short (blue), medium

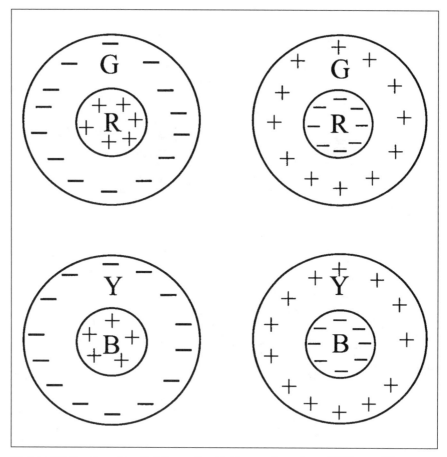

Figure 10.8. Ganglion Cell Receptive Fields as a Function of Different Wavelength Stimulation on the Center and Surround

(green), and long (red) wavelengths are presented. Our perception of yellow (Y) occurs when the cones that transduce medium and long wavelengths are stimulated equally. In other words, our perception of yellow is derived from the combined output of cones that connect to the −Y/+B and +Y/−B ganglion cells.

It would be helpful, at this point, if color processing in the retina were put in a simple model. Such a model is provided in Figure 10.9. The visible spectrum is shown at the top. The bipolar cells and the lateral processing by neural cells are not displayed in the figure. This model displays the three types of cones and their connections to three ganglion cells. For simplicity, only two of the four different wavelength antagonistic ganglion cells are shown (+R/−G and +Y/−B). The third ganglion cell is not wavelength specific and has a

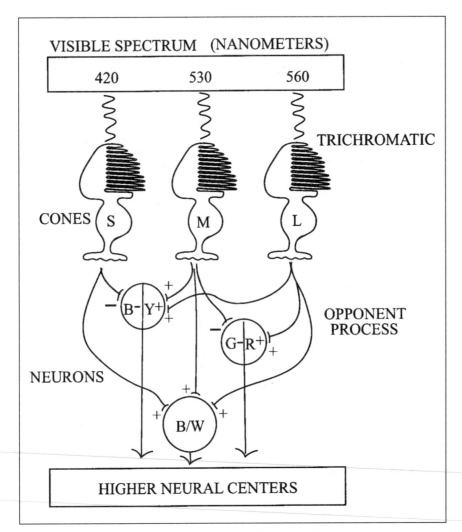

Figure 10.9. Model of the Trichromatic and Opponent Process Theories of Color Vision

center-surround that receives input from all three cones (B/W). The output from the three ganglion cells is sent to higher neural centers for additional processing.

In this first example, assume that a long wavelength stimulus (560 nm) is absorbed by Cone L. There are no other wavelengths in the stimulus. For ease of understanding, pretend that there are 20 units (photons) absorbed. The output of the Cone L is connected to three ganglion cells. It is connected to the +R half of the +R/–G ganglion cell and the +Y half of the +Y/–B ganglion. It is also connected to the third ganglion cell that is not wavelength specific—B/W. The question at this point is, what pattern of neural activity is sent to the higher neural centers? We begin with the +Y/–B ganglion cell. What happens at the +Y/–B cell? The answer is nothing. This is because the +Y needs simultaneous inputs from the L and M to become active and send a message to the higher neural centers. On the other hand, the +R/–G ganglion cell responds with excitatory output (+R). In this example, the output of the ganglion cell is assumed to be the same as the number of photons absorbed by the cone. So, 20 units of activity are sent to the higher centers from the +R/–G ganglion cell. In addition, the B/W ganglion cell forwards its output (20 units). The perception from the pattern of neural inputs is red with a particular brightness provided by the B/W cell.

As a second example, assume that two wavelengths are present in the stimulus, 530 and 560. Each wavelength has the same energy (20 photons). Cones L and M absorb their respective 20 units of light and send their output to the three ganglion cells, +R/–G, +Y/–B, and B/W. The result is the perception of a bright yellow light. This occurs because Cone L has absorbed 20 units and sent 20 units to the +R portion of the +R/–G, and to the +Y portion of the +Y/–B ganglion cells. It also sends 20 units to the B/W neural element. Cone M absorbs its 20 units and sends an identical amount of activity on to the –G (of the +R/–G ganglion cell), the +Y(of the +Y/–B ganglion), and the B/W ganglion. The result is that the 20 units of –G cancel the 20 units of +R so there is no output from the +R/–G ganglion cell. The +Y portion of the +Y/–B cell, on the other hand, receives what it needs to become active. The +Y requires simultaneous inputs from Cones L and M to initiate neural activity. This is exactly what it has. The result is 40 units of excitatory output from the +Y portion of the +Y/–B cell. Finally, the B/W cell sends 40 units of activity to the higher neural centers. This pattern of activity produces the perception of a bright yellow.

Given this model, it should be clear that a white light is perceived if Cones L and M each absorb 20 photons and Cone S absorbs 40. In this situation, both the +R/–G and +Y/–B ganglion cells have no output (the + and – cancel each other) and the B/W neural elements have 80 units of brightness (20 from L, 20 from M, and 40 from S). The result is the perception of white light (no color).

Before we move on to the higher neural centers and the pathways of the visual system, it is useful to take a moment and briefly discuss two guiding theories that have led to the discovery of the physiological mechanisms underlying color vision. The first theory is the **trichromatic theory of color vision.** Although this theory, like the next one to be discussed, has a long history, perhaps as far back as the 1600s, we consider the more recent times (the last 150 years or so). The trichromatic theory is solidly associated with two individuals. The first was an Englishman named Thomas Young and the other was a German named Hermann von Helmholtz (who provided us with the place theory of pitch discussed in Chapter 9). The theory was first espoused by Thomas Young and was based on his ideas and studies with color matching. His approach to color perception and his investigations led him to theorize that there were three receptors (or pigments) necessary for normal color vision. All the colors we perceive could be obtained by assuming that the eye captured light using three "pigments." The three pigments were assumed to absorb wavelengths that composed the primary colors: red, green, and blue. These three pigments absorbed light in the visible spectrum and could produce all the colors the human eye could detect. Thomas Young's ideas were recognized and championed by von Helmholtz. The theory came to be called, and still is today, the Young-Helmholtz trichromatic theory of color vision. What makes the theory so profound and interesting is that in the 1800s there were no physiological data available to support the theory. The theory came into being because of the psychophysical-matching investigations of Young and the acceptance and support of von Helmholtz, an eminent scientist. Supporting physiological data for the theory did not appear until the mid-20th century when technology had advanced to the point where individual cones could be subjected to precisely controlled wavelengths of light using a technique called microspectrophotometry (Brown & Wald, 1964). The name for the technique emphasizes the precision and control necessary to accomplish the task of measuring the absorption spectra for cones. The result was, as you know, the discovery of the S, M, and L absorption spectra associated with the three different opsins. The trichromatic theory was firmly established after years of debate.

As is often the case in science, there is seldom just one theory or scholarly position regarding important problems. Color perception was no different. The trichromatic theory of color vision had a rival. A German physician, Ewald Hering, proposed the other approach to the investigation of color vision. Hering's theory was initially based on his idea that there were not three pigments in the eye, there were four. Hering's approach was quite simple. For example, he asked his participants in his experiments to name the primary colors. They always said red, green, blue, and yellow. Yellow was clearly a primary color to his participants. Yellow is unlike any other color. The perception of yellow clearly is not a mixed or tinted composite of other colors. Orange and purple clearly are not primary colors because they are mixtures of other colors. This suggested to Hering that there were four, not three, pigments in the eye. In addition, Hering pointed out to his critics, and those who supported the other theory, that these four primary colors were not independent. Rather, red and green were perceptually paired and opposed each other. In addition, yellow and blue fit the same kind of opposition. Simple perceptual experiments supported this opponent idea. One of the experiments he asked his participants to perform was to report what they saw after they had studied a constant and stable image composed of one of the four primary colors. The participants always reported a visual afterimage in the complementary color. A visual afterimage occurs when you stare at one of the two opposing colors. For example (you may wish to try this), if you stare at an image of a red star for approximately 30 to 45 seconds and then shift your focus to an "X" on a sheet of white paper, a green star appears on the paper. If you reverse the process and stare at a green star after 30 to 45 seconds, you will see the red star on the white paper. The two colors, red and green, are opposing and complementary. The same kind of afterimages will occur for yellow and blue opposing pairs. A black-white afterimage can be seen by examining Figure 10.10. In short, Hering had psychophysical support for his "four pigments" theory. Like Young and Helmholtz, however, Hering had no physiological support for his ideas. The technology was not yet available. In the 1960s, the same time that investigators were using new technology to discover the three cones supporting the trichromatic theory, other scientists were zeroing in on neural recordings. Although the **opponent process theory of color vision,** as Hering's theory came to be called, did not find support for four pigments and four receptors, investigators did find strong evidence for the neural opponent cells. They found the same kind of antagonistic mechanisms we have already discussed. The opponent process theory is correct, but it applies to neurons (ganglion cells and other cells more central) and not to receptors (Hurvich & Jameson, 1957; Wiesel & Hubel, 1966). As you suspect by now, the two theories, when combined, produce an elegant story of how our visual system operates. Figure 10.9 is based on the combination.

Central Pathways

Our discussion begins with the **visual field.** The visual field is the world we see. Figure 10.11 diagrammatically shows the right and left visual fields and the central pathways to the cortex. In the figure, each eye has to receive a different perspective of the world. This is simply because the right eye is spatially to the right of the left eye and vice versa. The two eyes get different views of the same environment (the binocular area). Each eye is, however, blind to parts of the environment as noted by the right and left monocular areas. The nose prevents the left eye from seeing the right monocular field. Likewise, the right eye cannot see the left monocular area for the same reason. This is easy to check

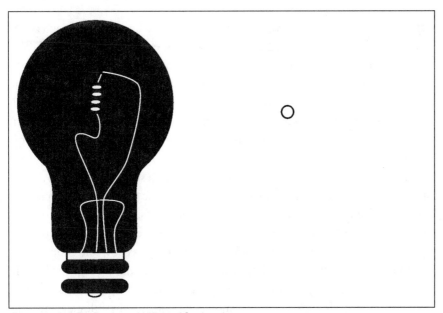

Figure 10.10. Back and White Afterimage

Focus on the black light bulb for 30 to 45 seconds and then stare at the spot to the right. Watch the light come on!

by closing one eye and noticing what part of your world disappears. Even though each eye receives a slightly different view of the world, we usually see a single perceptual image. The merging of the two images from the binocular area, one from each eye, is called **binocular fusion.** When an image from the right and left visual fields stimulates the same retinal area in each eye, there is no problem to overcome. The image is the same in each eye. This occurs when we fixate on an object in the environment (the "X" in Figure 10.11). All the objects that fall on an imaginary line passing through the fixation point stimulate the same retinal points in each eye. There is no disparity. This imaginary line is the dashed line in the visual field shown in Figure 10.11. The imaginary line is called the **horopter.**

Figure 10.11 shows the square and circle falling on the horopter and consequently stimulating each eye in the same retinal location because the relationships are the same. However, if the image from each eye is not on the horopter then each image stimulates a different retinal area. By following the solid line from the solid circle to the retina in Figure 10.11, you see that different points, relative to other objects, are stimulated in each eye. The image in each eye is, therefore, disparate. The slight difference between the two images is known as **binocular disparity.** Any object in the environment that does not lie on the imaginary horopter produces binocular disparity. The main point

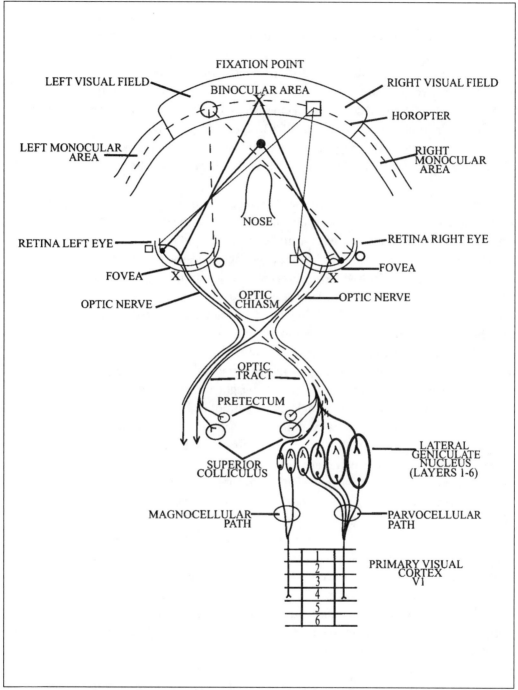

Figure 10.11. The Visual System From the Visual Field to the Cortex

NOTE: (a) orientation columns and (b) hypercolumns showing the combination of orientation columns with ocular dominance columns and the color components called blobs.

of this discussion is that when the visual system combines two disparate images in a single percept, we gain a strong cue for depth perception. Any object not on the horopter, too far away or too close, provides us with binocular disparity. The automatic calculation of distance is not unique to us. Predatory animals (lions, wolves, monkeys, and humans) have their eyes located in the front of their head to provide the depth cues necessary to capture their prey and find their food (Hubel & Wiesel, 1970). The "prey" (rabbits, rodents, deer) have their eyes located on each side of their head to encompass a greater field of view (larger visual field) to more easily see and escape from their predators.

The phenomenon of binocular disparity can be demonstrated easily. You simply close your left eye and then point to an object in the distance using your right eye. Then open your left eye and close your right eye. You see the environment shift noticeably. Your image has changed because each eye has a slightly different view. The right eye views the world from the right and the left eye sees it from the left. This difference is, once again, binocular disparity. There is, of course, always the possibility that the two images are so disparate that the visual system cannot put them together to produce a fused perception. When this occurs the visual system is "confused" and the perception alternates back and forth between the two different images. This alternation between one image and then the other, left eye then right eye, occurs because the two images are so disparate that a single image cannot be formed. This phenomenon is called **binocular rivalry.** Binocular rivalry occurs when the two eyes fail to focus on the same object (Blake & Camisa, 1978; Wiesenfelder & Blake, 1991). Because the two eyes are focused on different objects, there are two different images: one image in the left eye and a different one in the right eye. The two eyes must move and operate together to have normal binocular vision.

It is also interesting to ask, while we are on the topic of rivalry, a question concerning the inversion of our visual field in both eyes. This does not cause rivalry. This is because each eye receives the same inverted input. If glasses that invert the world are worn and not removed, the obvious occurs. The world is initially upside down, and you may be nauseated. If you keep the glasses on for a long period of time (a few days), your visual perception of the world changes. The world once again becomes upright and normal. This phenomenon illustrates the concept of plasticity: The brain changes to accommodate the sensory input. After a few days of wearing glasses that invert your world, your perception changes and becomes upright. You could walk around the environment very easily and even ride bicycles, locate objects, and probably even drive a car. The next question is, what happens when you remove the glasses that invert the visual field? The world once again is upside down. However, it only remains inverted for a short period (minutes). The visual system almost immediately can reverse itself and use the previous neural processes to synthesize the visual perceptions. The brain is indeed unique (Rossetti, Koga, & Mano, 1993; Sugita, 1996).

It is time to follow the visual path from the retina to the cortex. This is done easily using Figure 10.11. The figure shows the left and right visual fields when the eyes are focused on the "X." For this discussion, we focus on the dashed lines originating at the circle in the left visual field. When you follow the dashed lines, you see that the retina of the right eye is stimulated on the right side (temporal retinal field) and the retina of the left eye receives the same image near the nose (nasal retinal field). When you follow the dashed line leaving the left eye, you see it cross the midline at the optic chiasm (visual crossing) and join the dashed line coming from the right eye. The ganglion-cell axons from each eye form the optic tract and ascend to the **lateral geniculate nucleus** of the thalamus. Before the lateral geniculate, a branch of fibers leaves the optic tracts to synapse on cells in the pretectum and superior colliculus. The output of the lateral geniculate nucleus continues to the final destination via the optic radiations. The optic radiations consist of both the magnocellular and parvocellular paths that leave the six layers of the thalamus. These radiations are the neural input to the V1 area of the primary visual cortex in the occipital lobe. A final point regarding the pathway from the retina to the cortex is that the perception of objects in the left visual field (the circle in this example) has as its final destination in the right hemisphere. Likewise, the right visual field is projected to the left hemisphere. Although the pathways seem simple, the simplicity hides some elegant functions. We examine these in the next few pages.

The Thalamus and Other Neural Centers

There are two small but important deviations in the main pathway to the cortex. The first diversion is to the pretectum. Some of the axons from the retinal ganglion cells that form the optic tract synapse in the pretectum to provide information regarding the brightness of the light entering the eye. The output of the pretectum actives the muscles of the iris. A bright light, therefore, initiates a reflex controlled by the pretectum. A bright light falling on the retina causes a pupil constriction and a reduction in the amount of light entering the eye. A dim light produces pupil dilation. The reflex is initiated by the activity of retinal ganglion cells in the eye and controlled by the pretectum.

The second diversion, as seen in Figure 10.11, is to the superior colliculus. The auditory system provides information to the superior colliculus so the source of sounds could be visually located. The superior colliculus has an important role to play in our everyday activities. It controls our voluntary **saccadic eye movements.** Saccadic eye movement is the rapid eye movement we make as we shift our gaze from one portion of the visual field to another. The saccadic movements allow you to read this sentence. Your eyes jump from place to place as you process the information. The superior colliculus also integrates head movement with eye movement and body posture so we may focus directly on the object of interest while moving around in our environment.

The next neural center in the pathway to the cortex is the lateral geniculate nucleus of the thalamus. As Figure 10.11 indicates, there are six distinct layers within the geniculate. The input to these six layers is very specific and organized. The incoming ganglion fibers are sorted according to three criteria.

First, the ipsilateral (same side) inputs synapse only in Layers 2, 3, and 5. In Figure 10.11, the dashed lines from the temporal portion of the retina of the right eye form the ipsilateral path to Layers 2, 3, and 5. The contralateral (opposite side) inputs have their synapses in Layers 1, 4, and 6. The contralateral fibers in Figure 10.11 begin as the dashed lines originating in the left nasal retina. The dashed line changes to a solid line as they enter the thalamus and synapse on Layers 1, 4, and 6. Each layer of the lateral geniculate nucleus is associated with only one eye.

The second sorting characteristic of the input to the thalamus is the **retinotopic** locations found in each layer. Retinotopic means that each location in the retina has a specific place within each layer of the lateral geniculate. In other words, the retina is completely represented within each layer. Each point in the retina has a specific position in each layer of the lateral geniculate nucleus. If, for example, an electrode is inserted into the lateral geniculate, perpendicular to the surface, the recorded neural activity is all associated with the same spot in the retina. If the electrode is moved and the experiment repeated, the cells in the six layers are all active when a different part of the retina is stimulated.

The last sorting criterion is the size of the neural cells found within the layers. Layers 1 and 2 are composed of relatively large neurons. The output from these two layers is labeled magnocellular (large cells) in Figure 10.11. If recordings are taken from neurons located in Layers 1 and 2, the receptive fields are circular and have opposing center-surrounds like those found in the periphery of the retina. They do not respond to specific wavelengths. The magnocellular neurons respond best to movements in a particular direction. Like the ganglion cells, the neural cells in the lateral geniculate, Layers 1 and 2, are movement selective. They respond to a movement in one direction but not the other. The response of these cells strongly supports the thesis that they receive their input from the rods and their associated ganglion cells. Layers 3, 4, 5, and 6 are composed of small neurons and receive their input from the cones. These parvocellular (small cell) neurons are responsive to color, acuity, shape, and depth. The receptive fields you obtain when recording from neurons in each of the four parvocellular layers are similar to those of ganglion cells because they are circular in shape and have wavelength antagonistic center-surrounds (+R/–G, –R/+G, +Y/–B, –Y/+B). There are also cells within the parvocellular areas that also respond to motion.

There are two important points to emphasize before we go on to the next higher level. First, the parvocellular Layers 3 through 6 receive their input from the macular region of the retina. The increase in the amount of neural tissue in these four layers of lateral geniculate nucleus relative to the size of the macula and fovea reintroduces the idea of magnification. The increase in amount of neural tissue at the higher centers suggests, correctly, that the most important aspects of a sensory system are provided with more neurons to accomplish the more important tasks. In the case of vision, the most important tasks are acuity, depth, color, movement, and edges of objects processed by the cones and ganglion cells of the macula and the fovea. This does not mean, of course, that the more peripheral portions of the retina are immaterial and not considered important. The peripheral portion of the retina and the magnocellular layers are intimately related to our perception of peripheral movement in the visual field and extremely important when the light is dim.

The second point to note is the model presented representing color processing shown in Figure 10.9. This model is also applicable when it is applied to the processing found in the lateral geniculate nucleus. The neural elements in the model are simply shifted from the ganglion cells to the cells within the lateral geniculate nucleus. There are opponent process neurons in the lateral geniculate nucleus that perform the color-perception task in the same manner as the ganglion cells within the fovea (DeValois, Abramov, & Jacobs, 1966). In addition, because color perception is important, more neural tissue is provided for the task (magnification).

The afferent output of the lateral geniculate nucleus is sent to the primary visual cortex denoted as V1. The parvocellular and magnocellular paths leave the thalamus and form the optic radiations to the cortex. The final destination of the optic radiations is Layer 4 of the visual cortex. As is suggested by Figure 10.11, the visual cortex is organized in six layers with vertical columns. The organization of these columns and their significance is the next step in the story.

The Visual Cortex

We begin by briefly reviewing the procedures used to study the cortex. As we know, the neurons of the cortex can have their activity recorded by the insertion of a microelectrode. The insertion of electrodes into the primary visual cortex in the occipital lobe has provided us with the following information. First, the cortex, like the lateral geniculate, is retinotopic. This means that the retina is completely represented in the V1 region of the cortex. The neural activity and transduction that occurs at a particular location on the retina produces neural activity at particular location in V1 area of the cortex. If the stimulating light is shifted slightly to an adjacent retinal location, the cortical response also shifts. In short, by stimulating different areas of the retina, one can plot the entire retina in the cortex. Second, there are neurons in the cortex that respond specifically to bars of light oriented in particular directions. Some cortical cells respond best to horizontal bars of light, others prefer a different orientation. Unlike the lateral geniculate and ganglion cells, the receptive fields of these cortical cells respond best if the bar of light is elongated and is at a particular orientation on the retina. Third, there are cortical cells that respond best if the bar of light is at a particular orientation and moves in a specific direction. Fourth, there are cells in the cortex that respond best to angles (two bars of light form an angle). Fifth, there are vertical columns throughout the V1 area of the visual cortex that respond best to one eye rather than the other. The columns are vertical in the sense that if a microelectrode is inserted perpendicular to the surface of the cortex, the cellular responses are dominated by one eye—*ocular dominance columns*. This does not mean that there are no cells responding to binocular inputs. The estimate is that approximately 80% of the cortical cells are binocular and respond to activity from either eye. There are the binocular cells that respond specifically to the disparity between the two retinal images. The columns are, however, preferential for one eye over the other. These ocular dominance columns alternate (left, right, left, right) across the cortex. Finally, there are neural cells within the V1 area of the cortex that are color specific. These areas are called **blobs** because of the way they absorb chemicals and how they look when viewed with a microscope (Wong-Riley, 1979; Wong-Riley et al.,

1993). With this brief introduction, we begin examining the cortex more closely.

Neurons and Orientation Columns

There are three types of cortical cells that are of specific interest. They were discussed briefly in the previous paragraph. I expand on their function by considering the results of investigations that led to Nobel Prizes in physiology and medicine in 1981 for David Hubel and Torsten Wiesel. When Hubel and Wiesel inserted a microelectrode perpendicular to the surface of the cortex, they discovered neural cells that responded to bars of light that had a particular orientation. They named these cells **simple cells** (Hubel & Wiesel, 1959). Some simple cells respond to horizontal bars of light and other cells respond to bars at different orientations, for example, 60° or 90°. Each column contains cells that respond in the same orientation. Because there are multiple columns, all possible orientations, from 0° to 180°, are found. In short, the orientations vary systematically across columns, and all orientations are available for every location on the retina. The discovery of these adjacent columns led to the descriptive term **orientation columns.**

In addition to the simple cells in the orientation columns, there are two other cells within the columns that respond in a more complex manner. The first type of cell is the **complex cell** (Hubel & Wiesel, 1962). The complex cells not only require the bar of light to be in a particular orientation but also require that the bar of light be moving in a particular direction. So, within each orientation column there are simple and complex cells. The simple cell responds when the bar of light on the retina is in the correct orientation, and the complex cell responds when the bar of light moves and is also in the correct orientation.

The third cell in the story is the **end-stopped cell** (Hubel & Wiesel, 1965). This cell, in addition to the requirements that the bar of light be moving and at the right orientation, has further requirements before it responds. The moving of the bar of light must be bent (at a particular angle) and cannot be too long. The bar of light is also restricted in its length (end stopped). The orientation columns containing these cells are depicted in Figure 10.12.

Figure 10.12(a) shows a series of columns that contain cells that systematically change their preferred orientation (0° to 180°). Each complete sequence of orientation columns shown in Figure 10.12(a) represents the same location on the retina. The cortex has retinotopic maps like the lateral geniculate. That is, the retina is "mapped" on the cortex, and each retinal

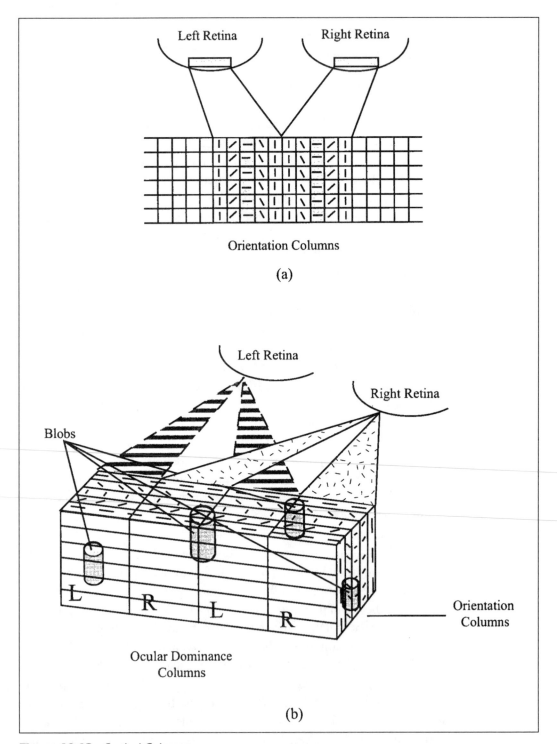

Figure 10.12. Cortical Columns.

NOTE: (a) orientation columns, (b) hypercolumns showing the combination of orientation columns with ocular dominance columns and the color components called **blobs**.

location has many orientation columns associated with each location. Each column is composed of neurons that have different orientations and functions. This means that there are multiple columns of cortical cells that process afferent activity from every location on the retina. Regardless of retinal location, there are columns that contain cells that respond to the perceptually important aspects of the visual field. These important aspects are, of course, orientation, movement, length, shape (angle), and color. The color blobs, of course, are found only in those columns that respond to the parvocellular layers of the thalamus and the macula of the retina.

Ocular Dominance Columns and Blobs

Perhaps the simplest way to understand ocular dominance and blobs is to consider Figure 10.12(b). This figure shows an expanded configuration of the orientation columns. This configuration, probably because it is a little more complex, is called a **hypercolumn.** Each hypercolumn consists of three components: orientation columns, ocular dominance columns, and blobs (Hubel & Wiesel, 1968, 1974a, 1974b; Michael, 1979, 1981; Ts'o & Gilbert, 1988). The orientation columns within each hypercolumn are the same as previously discussed. What is different when a hypercolumn is formed is the configuration. The hypercolumn is a three-dimensional configuration with alternating ocular dominance columns combined with the orientation columns. The two hypercolumns depicted in Figure 10.12(b) are shown as three-dimensional cubes with a complete set of orientation columns (from 0° to 180°) for each ocular dominance column. As noted previously, the hypercolumns that receive inputs from the macula (cones) contain cells specifically responsive to different wavelengths. Because blobs are associated with color vision, they do not occur in all hypercolumns. The blobs are noted in Figure 10.12(b) by the small shaded columns within the hypercolumns. Aside from refining our sense of color, the cells within the blobs are unique in another way as well. Their receptive field is circular and often has a **double color-opponent receptive field** configuration. This means, for example, that the cell could have a −R/+G center and a +R/−G surround. This particular configuration yields a very active cell if, for example, the cell were simultaneously stimulated with a medium wavelength in the center and a long wavelength in the surround.

Retinotopic organization is achieved when groups of hypercolumns represent different retinal locations. It needs to be emphasized that each hypercolumn encompasses less than 0.2 mm of cortical surface, and there are a significantly large number of hypercolumns dedicated to the macula.

A representation of the retinotopic organization and cortical magnification is shown in Figure 10.13. The most important area of the retina—the macula and fovea—are provided with a significantly larger portion of the visual cortex. This is seen in the figure by noting that the area in the visual field representing the macula (numbered 1, 2, 3, and 4) is assigned a significantly large portion of the visual cortex. The cortical magnification is a continuation of the neural magnification that occurred in the lateral geniculate where the four parvocellular layers of the thalamus were dedicated to the macular region of the retina.

A final and important topic requires consideration before we move on. We refer here to **stereopsis** or binocular depth perception. The cortical neurons that respond to binocular inputs also provide us with our stereopsis. These cells, often referred to as disparity selective cells, respond to the differences between the two retinal fields. The size of the disparity between the retinal images determines the response by the disparity-selective neurons. Some cells respond to small disparities and others respond to slightly greater disparity. If the disparity is too large, however, there is no stereopsis because the disparity-selective cells fail to respond.

Ventral and Dorsal Paths

The flow of afferent sensory information does not stop at the occipital lobe and the V1 primary cortex. Other paths and other areas of the brain make significant contributions. More than 30 different anatomical areas provide visual processing. We do not attempt to discuss them all; rather, we examine two parallel paths and some of their neural centers as they flow through the cortex. These two paths—the ventral and dorsal—and their interactions provide a strong endorsement regarding the complexity of our visual system (Callaway & Wiser, 1996; Livingstone & Hubel, 1987; Merigan & Maunsell, 1993; Ungerleider & Mishkin, 1982).

The two parallel paths begin at the retina and are followed by afferent inputs to the lateral geniculate. The parvocellular and magnocellular layers, in turn, provide the major inputs to the ventral and dorsal cortical paths. Figure 10.14 provides an overview of the cortical areas and a schematic diagram of the flow of information through the ventral and dorsal pathways. Figure 10.14(a) shows the locations of specific areas in each pathway. Figure 10.14(b) is a diagrammatic representation of each pathway. The solid lines in this latter diagram indicate the afferent flow of information through each pathway. The dashed lines indicate that there is a significant amount of

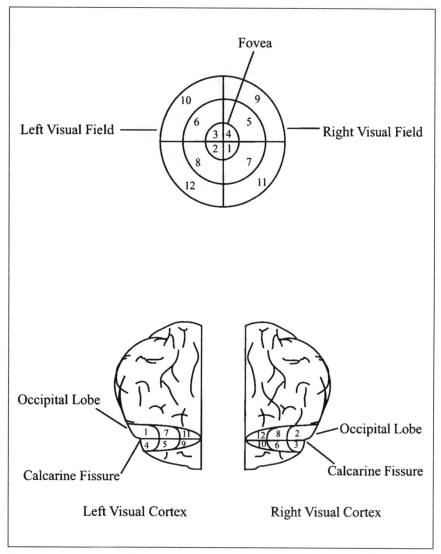

Figure 10.13. Cortical Magnification of the Visual Field on the Occipital Lobe

interaction between the two paths and among the different areas of the cortex. The position of the individual areas within each path is labeled but you must keep in mind that they do not function independently. The complexity of the system defies a complete understanding of all the functions and interactions. This, however, does not deter us. As we examine these higher cortical functions, we make some speculations and conjectures about how our perception of the world occurs.

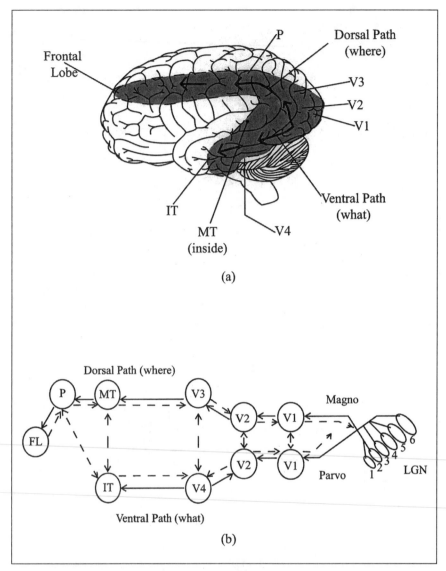

Figure 10.14. The Cortical Paths Within the Cortex and the Dorsal and Ventral Paths

NOTE: (a) overview and (b) a diagram showing the flow of activity through the ventral and dorsal pathways.

The starting points are the parallel paths into the V1 area of the cortex. The parvocellular and magnocellular layers of the thalamus synapse on different layers within the V1 cortex. This implies that there may be functional differences between the two pathways. The neural processing of movement may be under the control of one path and color, orientation, and disparity in the other. To an extent, this is correct.

Looking at the ventral pathway first, we note that afferent input comes from the parvocellular path and there are wavelength sensitive cells within the V4 area. This suggests that color processing occurs within the ventral path and specifically in the region of V4 (Spitzer, Desimone, & Moran, 1988). The V4 area is not, however, restricted to a single perceptual task. There are important orientation cells that very likely provide pattern recognition and the depth perception necessary to clearly perceive objects in the world (Merigan, 1996; Merigan & Pham, 1998; Tanaka, 1966). The output of the V4 continues to an area in the temporal cortex labeled inferior temporal (IT). The inferior temporal area is involved with color, shape, edges, and very likely depth perception (Desimone, Schein, Moran, & Ungerleider, 1998). In fact, there are some cells within the inferior temporal region that are selective for extremely complex pattern recognition: faces of other monkeys. The probability is that the human species processes faces in the same manner. The objects in the world have to be identified, and the ventral pathway is intimately associated with this task. What is it? Have I seen this face before? Is this milk the right color? We return to this topic later.

When the dorsal pathway is considered, it is clear that the magnocellular path is providing the bulk of the input. This suggests that the magnocellular pathway very likely supplies the inputs to areas associated with peripheral movement in the visual field. The medial temporal area (MT) that is buried on the medial side of the temporal lobe has a large number of cells that are movement reactive (Zeki, 1974). The cells, not surprisingly, are similar to the complex cells that require movement in a particular direction and are orientation dependent as well (Rodman & Albright, 1989). Although the medial temporal area of the cortex is within the dorsal pathway (Figure 10.14[b]), it also plays a role in the ventral pathway. This is logical. Movement and motion in the visual field are very important and moving objects, once they are detected, need to be identified (what is it?). The dorsal path from the medial temporal area continues on to the posterior portion of the parietal lobe (Lomber, Payne, Cornwell, & Long, 1996; P in Figure 10.14[a]). The parietal lobe is associated with the "where" aspect of our world. This part of the brain searches for objects in the visual field. The cognitive word associated with this task is *attention*. The parietal lobe directs the eye movement to the objects in the visual field and controls the voluntary guided visual movement (Colby, Duhamel, & Goldberg, 1995; Lynch, Mountcastle, Talbot, & Yin, 1977; Thier & Erickson, 1992). The dorsal pathway, in general, appears directly related to attention and planned motor tasks (see it, reach for it). This idea fits the "where" aspect of the dorsal pathway: Where is it? I'll get it. These two short sentences, "Where is it?" and "I'll get it" are processed in the dorsal pathway. The parietal lobe (P) searches (where is it) and controls the movement of the body (I'll get it). The "decision" about the identification of the object, however, is a ventral pathway function. Clearly, the two paths are not independent. The ventral-stream neural mechanisms identify and answer the question "what" while the dorsal streams operates "where." Once the identification is formed and the "where" is confirmed, the dorsal pathway can initiate motor activity. For the ventral path to make decisions and identifications, it clearly has to have inputs from memory and emotions. This is certainly the case. The ventral path has direct contact with the limbic system as well as the frontal lobes. There are, then, cognitive and noncognitive elements involved in our visual search and understanding of the world. For us (or monkeys) to "know" and recognize a face, that face must be stored in memory before it can be retrieved (Perrett, Rolls, & Caan, 1982). On the other hand, the automatic (noncognitive) responses we make to environmental events are clearly only dorsal pathway functions. For example, when your pal unexpectedly decides to share her lunch by tossing you something from across the room, you quickly move your hands and catch the morsel of candy. The dorsal pathway automatically takes care of the visual tracking (where) while simultaneously providing the motor movement for you to catch it. You may even recognize the brand of candy (what) as it flies through the air to your waiting hands (Barlow, 1997). The final message to remember is that depth, color, movement, memory, noncognitive responses, and object images all occur interactively with the two "separate" streams of cortical processing. It is easy to remember that one parallel path provides you with the "where" information while the other gives you the knowledge to recognize "what" it is. It is easy, but it is not complete. The two parallel paths converse with each other. When parts and areas within these streams, from retina to cortex, have problems interacting or functioning, visual malfunctions can readily occur.

A final question may occur to you at this point. As you read these words, which visual path is most active? Clearly, the dorsal is involved so you know "where" to look. However, perhaps more important, the ventral path in the left hemisphere (if you are right handed) is intimately involved in figuring out "what" you are reading. The visual system is sending information to the auditory system and Wernicke's area for cognitive interpretation of the words and what they mean. If you are like many students you are also taking notes on "what" you are reading, while simultaneously you need to know "where" your hand, pen, and paper are located. You do not even think about what your sensory system is doing when it operates correctly. So, life may be complex, but your brain smooths out the rough edges when it can.

Dysfunctions

Visual problems come in a variety of forms and under several different conditions. The individual may be born with a difficulty or the loss of vision may occur as a function of aging or disease. In addition, there are always the unfortunate problems that can occur because of damage caused by accidents. The following paragraphs provide an overview of some of the possible problems that can occur. You should keep in mind as these problems are discussed that some of them are correctable, but not all of them.

Myopia, Hyperopia, and Presbyopia

Nearly the first thing that you encounter when asked about problems in vision is a statement that refers to the problems of **myopia, hyperopia,** or **presbyopia.** These are problems in refraction. The light is not bent correctly so the image you wish to see fails to be focused directly on the retina. The image is blurred. These conditions are usually corrected with the use of glasses or contact lenses.

Myopia is the word used to describe when an individual can see nearby items but has difficulty seeing objects in the distance. Myopia is nearsightedness and is caused by a change in the shape of the eyeball. The eyeball has become too long. The change in length, from the front to the back, affects the optics of the eye so distant objects cannot be focused correctly on the retina. The image always falls too close to the lens and not on the retina. Even when the ciliary muscles of the eye relax, as they do when accommodating for distance viewing, the normal lens flattens its shape and contour so distant objects may be precisely focused on the retina. However, with myopia the lens accommodation cannot correct the problem. Even when the lens is as flat as it can become, the image still cannot be focused on the retina because the retina is too far away. Because the eyeball is too long, the correction for myopia is usually a pair of glasses (or contact lenses) that have a concave shape to correct for the long eyeball and the inability of the lens to accommodate sufficiently.

Hyperopia is, basically, the opposite of myopia. You are unable to see nearby objects. You can see faraway mountains and the beautiful ships on the ocean but cannot read the newspaper. The accommodation by the lens, once again, is of no help. When the ciliary muscles contract to allow the lens to change to its more circular or round shape and attempt to focus the image directly on the retina, it cannot do the task and refract the light enough to have the image fall on the retina. In contrast to myopia, the focused image with hyperopia occurs behind the retina. The shape of the eye has become too short so the correction, once again, is a lens in front of the eye (glasses or contact lenses) to correct the optics. The lens in this case is convex or rounded so the light is bent as it enters the eye and the image falls on the retina clearly. The eye is focused, and the book can be read.

The word *presybopia* is loosely translated as "old vision." This kind of refractive problem results in farsightedness and the inability to accommodate and bring close objects in focus. The reason for this problem, however, is not a short eyeball. The problem is in the lens. The lens is unique because it continues to add layers and lose its elasticity as we age. These changes make the lens less capable of changing shape so when the ciliary muscles contract, the lens, because it has hardened, cannot become spherical enough to bring the nearby objects in focus. The correction for presbyopia is the same as it is for hyperopia: A convex lens in front of the eye offsets an inadequate lens in the eye. Reading glasses become a common part of the apparel of the elderly.

Glaucoma

Glaucoma is a progressive disease caused by the failure of aqueous humor to be drained from the anterior chamber of the eye. Should the drainage of the aqueous humor become blocked, the pressure within the chamber increases, and permanent blindness can occur. This blockage and the buildup of the pressure is **glaucoma.** The loss of vision occurs because the pressure within the anterior chamber builds to such a level that the vitreous humor behind the lens is forced back against the optic disk. The optic disk is where the blood enters the eye and the axons of the ganglion cells exit. As the pressure builds within the eye, vision is permanently damaged because the neurons of the optic nerve are damaged and die. Fortunately, this disaster can be avoided by the use of drugs to open the closed outlets for the aqueous humor or by laser surgery to provide new exits. Glaucoma is a very common cause of permanent blindness when it is not treated. The first symptoms observed are slow and gradual loss of vision in the periphery of the visual field. This is because the first ganglion cells that are affected are those coming from the peripheral portion of the eye.

Age-Related Macular Degeneration

Age-related macular degeneration (AMD) is cruel and incurable. The symptoms begin, as you can guess, with the loss of sharp central vision. In the most severe form of the disease, there is a significant and finally permanent failure of the visual system to provide color, perception of fine print, faces of loved ones, and clear images of the world. The ability to drive down the street in a car is totally out of the question. As you probably surmise from this brief description, this form of the disease is devastating to the individual. The less severe of the two forms is called "dry" AMD. This form accounts for the majority of the cases. In this condition, the macula is raised from its retinal moorings by an accumulation of deposits under the macula. This form progresses slowly and is often not diagnosed for over a year and usually does not result in a complete loss of vision. One reason the dry form is often not noticed is that it is painless and may only occur in one eye. When this occurs, the unaffected eye compensates for the loss of vision. When the dry form changes to the "wet" form there is, unfortunately, an eventual permanent loss of central vision. About 10 to 15% of the dry form of AMD develops into the wet form. The wet AMD is caused by the development and leakage of new blood vessels in the eye. The blood vessels form around the macula and eventually cause the blindness. Sometimes the wet form develops very rapidly with little notice and no warning. Once one eye is affected, the other eye very likely succumbs. The only treatments available do not replace the lost vision. In a few select cases, the treatment can stop or slow the progression. However, it does not work in most cases. This treatment is a laser zap to the bleeding blood vessels. This usually stops the bleeding, but it simultaneously creates a permanent scar on the macula. A relatively new procedure still under investigation and being examined is called photodynamic therapy. This procedure entails the injection of a drug that accumulates in the damaged blood vesicles of the eye. The drug is then used as a target for a light that is directed in the eye. The drug is extremely light sensitive and becomes active when the light appears. The activity destroys the blood vesicles that contain the drug without causing damage to the neural elements in the eye. This procedure shows promise, but it is not a cure. The outlook for this disease is bleak.

Strabismus Ambylopia

The child is born with two eyes. The problem is they do not move together or focus on the same object. This problem is **strabismus ambylopia.** It is also called "lazy eye" because one eye just appears to lag behind and fails to focus on the object of interest. If this problem is not corrected before the child is about 6 years of age, the lazy eye is permanently "turned off." This means that there is a "critical period" in the child's development. The eyes must be fused and operational before the critical period is over. If the brain tries for years (5 or 6) and is unsuccessful in obtaining a consistent fused image from the two eyes, the result is one nonfunctional eye. The individual becomes permanently monocular. The correction for the problem is surgery on the lazy eye to correct the erroneous wandering and lack of a fused image. This is accomplished by detaching one or more of the muscles of the lazy wandering eye and reattaching it in such a way that the eyes move together and form a single image. The surgery is usually successful.

Damage to or Diseases of the Optic Nerve and Tract

It is easy to imagine the visual deficit that occurs when the optic nerve from one eye is destroyed or damaged. The entire visual field from the affected eye is lost. Although this is not a likely event, it can occur if there is a tumor or injury that either puts pressure on the nerve or severs it entirely. If, on the other hand, a tumor or growth destroys or puts pressure on the optic chiasm, the visual effects are different. In this case, the individual has tunnel vision. This occurs because the nasal retinal fibers from each eye cross the optic chiasm, and these are the cells that receive information from the right and left visual fields. The central portion of the visual field remains unaffected. This kind of occurrence is not a fantasy. The pituitary gland lies directly beneath the optic chiasm. When the pituitary is tumorous, the pressure on the chiasm is a common occurrence. The physicians even have a name for this situation: bitemporal hemianopia.

When tumors, stokes, and other unfortunate occurrences affect the optic tract, the result is often a scotoma (blank spots in the visual field). The particular location of the scotoma is used to determine the source of the problem. The scotoma also occurs in both eyes because the optic radiations carry information from both retinas.

Ventral Stream Disruption

When the ventral stream of inputs occurs because of a stroke, the brain has significant interruptions in normal functioning. The patient (usually a patient because the problem is so serious) often cannot recognize objects in the environment. This is serious because the objects that are not recognized are often formerly familiar objects such as faces (wife, husband, friend). This disturbing situation occurs when the strokes occur in the right hemisphere. Although the patient does not recognize the face, the patient knows that it is a face. These kinds of visual deficits have a clinical name: prosopagnosia, the inability to recognize faces. The loss of object recognition is often not restricted to a single class of objects such as faces. It can often extend to other classifications and different objects. The individual may identify an animal as a dog but is unable to identify it as his or her own and fails to recall the dog's name. When these patients are subjected to a brain scan, as they often are as a means of diagnosis, it is interesting to note that the emotional centers within the limbic system are often involved with the visual recognition. The appearance of a formerly familiar face often initiates an emotional response in the amygdala of the limbic system, possibly indicating recognition, but there is no overt statement to confirm the familiarity.

Summary

This chapter had the task of summarizing and presenting a complex, possibly the most complex, sensory system. It began with a presentation of the environmental stimulus and the visual spectrum. The small section of the electromagnetic spectrum that is used for vision is rather unique in its effects on our "brain." The brain in this case is the retina of the eye. The retina consists of only six different kinds of cells, but they provide the basic inputs for the entire visual process and initiate the standards for movement, color, shape, and depth. Like the auditory system, the visual periphery is extremely complex. The different transduction by the rods and cones lays the groundwork for color, acuity, stereopsis, and motion. The wavelength absorption characteristics of the rods and cones are dependent on the opsin within the cells. The cones are predominantly found in the macula and fovea and are responsible for acuity, color vision, and depth perception. The dark current and the hyperpolarization of the receptors are unique to the visual system. The expectation that all receptors operate on a depolarization concept to initiate sensory activity is incorrect. Rather than the usual depolarization when the adequate stimulus occurs, the receptors hyperpolarize and the neurotransmitter release is terminated to initiate the visual activity begun by the absorption of the photons of light. The Nobel Prize-winning work that produced the physiological foundation for the trichromatic theory and opponent process theory of color vision were significant steps in understanding color vision. The immediate neural molding of receptor output by lateral neural processes play a significant role in the parallel pathways to higher neural centers. The parallel paths created within the retina and sent to the thalamus continues to the cortex in the parvocellular and magnocellular optic radiations to the cortex. In the visual cortex, the orientation and ocular dominance columns were merged to form hypercolumns. The neural responses of the simple, complex, end-stopped cells within the hypercolumns continued to form and refine the perception of shape, movement, and depth perception. The blobs within the hypercolumns expanded the color processing with cells that had double-color opponent receptive fields. The parallel afferent paths leaving the V1, V2, V3, and V4 areas of the cortex formed the dorsal and ventral pathways and further provide ingredients to "where" and "what" is in our visual field. The visual sense has been discussed and written about by many investigators. For further interesting and lucid presentations of the visual sense consult Cornsweet (1970), Gegenfurtner & Sharpe (1999), Held (1989), and Zeki (1993).

Suggested Readings

Cornsweet, T. N. (1970). *Visual perception.* New York: Academic Press.

Gegenfurtner, K. R., & Sharpe, L. T. (Eds.). (1999). *Color vision: From genes to perception.* New York: Cambridge University Press.

Held, R. (1989). *Readings from the encyclopedia of neuroscience: Sensory systems, vol. 1: Vision and visual systems.* Boston: Birkhäuser.

Perrett, D. I., Rolls, E. T., & Caan, W. (1982). Visual neurons responsive to faces in the monkey temporal cortex. *Experimental Brain Research, 47,* 329-342.

Ungerleider, I. G., & Mishkin, M. (1982). Two cortical visual systems. In D. Ingle, M. A. Goodale, & R. J. W. Mansfield (Eds.), *Analysis of visual behavior.* Cambridge: MIT Press.

Zeki, S. (1993). *A vision of the brain.* Cambridge, MA: Blackwell Scientific Publications.

Glossary

absolute refractory period The period of time required for an action potential to reach its maximum depolarized level, approximately 1 msec, is the absolute refractory period.

accommodation The focusing of the lens accomplished by changes in the ciliary muscles and the zonule fibers.

acetylcholine (Ach) A neurotransmitter found in the nerve-skeletal muscle junctions, cortex, and basal nucleus. It is intimately involved in Alzheimer's disease.

acoustic neurinoma This is a central cause of dizziness caused by a tumor in the internal auditory meatus. The pressure on the nerve causes false signals to be sent to the brain. The tumor usually occurs in Schwann cells in the vestibular nerve. Hearing can be affected.

action potential The terms *spike, impulse,* and *neural impulse* are used interchangeably with the term *action potential.* An action potential is the electrical-chemical ion exchange across the axon membrane that is the basis of nervous system function.

active transport The movement of ions by cellular metabolic processes is active transport.

acuity The ability to discriminate fine detail that is directly related to small receptive fields.

acupuncture A form of pain relief that may occur when needles are inserted into areas of the body and electrically stimulated.

adaptation A decrease, and in some cases a complete cessation, of a receptor's response to a constant unchanging stimulus.

A-delta A large myelinated sensory axon.

adenosine monophosphate (cAMP) A second messenger in olfaction, cyclic adenosine monophosphate.

adenosine triphosphate (ATP) An energy packet found in cells that allows them to be active. When activated by adenylyl cyclase, it is converted into the second messenger cAMP.

adenylyl cyclase An enzyme in the cilia membrane that, when activated by an olfactory stimulus, converts ATP into a second messenger cAMP.

adequate stimulus The stimulus that most readily causes a change in neural or receptor activity: an increase (excitation) or decrease (inhibition).

afferent Refers to the direction of impulse flow in the nervous system. The afferent flow refers to the sensory flow into the central nervous system.

age-related macular degeneration (AMD) The degeneration of the macula within the retina that causes permanent visual impairment in the elderly.

ageusia No sense of taste.

agonist A chemical compound that elicits a distinct and measurable change in the biological organism by mimicking another chemical, usually a neurotransmitter.

Alzheimer's disease A terminal disease that causes dementia and is intimately associated with the degeneration of neurons that produce the neurotransmitter acetylcholine.

amacrine neurons Neurons in the retina that are involved with lateral processing.

amines A class of organic compounds found within the body that are related to pain perception.

amplitude Refers to the magnitude or size of a stimulus in terms of energy. In general, the greater the amplitude or size of a stimulus the greater the perceptual response. The amplitude of an auditory stimulus is measured in decibels (dB).

ampulla The enlargement in the semicircular canal where it joins the utricle. Receptors for vestibular sensory transduction of angular motion are located within the ampulla.

amygdala A part of the limbic system that is intimately associated with aggression.

analgesia Relief from pain without a loss of consciousness.

angular rate of acceleration   The tilt of the body or head, or movement of the head, that activates the ampulla in the semicircular canals; refers to angular acceleration or angular velocity.

antagonist   A chemical compound that prevents or reverses the effect of a neurotransmitter or agonist.

anterior commissure   A lateral band of fiber that extends from one olfactory bulb to the other. In this particular case, the anterior commissure has axons from the mitral and tufted cells that extend to areas in the contralateral olfactory bulb homotopic to the sending ipsilateral bulb.

anterior insula-operculum   An area of the cortex that forms the floor of the lateral sulcus. The insula is within the fissure and overlying the insula is the operculum. A region of cortex that is associated with taste.

anterorgrade degeneration   *See* orthograde degeneration.

antihelix   One of two ridges around the superior portion of the pinna. The helix begins at the top of the pinna and runs around the outer edge. The antihelix makes an approximate half-circle below the helix.

aqueous humor   Fills the anterior chamber and is continually produced and circulated. It bathes the cornea and iris and provides oxygen and nutrients for these structures.

arborizations   Refers to the branching of axons and dendrites at their distal extremity. The arborization permits more synaptic contact with other neurons or physiological elements.

arch (or tunnel) of Corti   The structural marker that partitions the inner and outer rows of hair cells within the cochlea.

ATP   adenosine triphosphate is an energy packet in the olfactory receptor that, when activated by adenylyl cyclase, is converted into the second messenger cAMP.

audiogram   A measure of the absolute threshold of human hearing. A common hearing test.

auricle   The pinna is sometimes referred to as the auricle.

axoaxonic   The synaptic designation used when one axon synapses upon another axon.

axodendritic   When an axon makes a synaptic connection with a dendrite, it is an axodendritic synapse.

axon   The conducting fiber of a neuron.

axon hillock   The area on the soma where the axon is produced and leaves the soma. It is also known as the initial segment.

axoplasm   The internal supporting fluid or plasma within an axon.

axosomatic   When an axon synapses on the cell body or soma of another neuron, it is an axosomatic synapse.

axotomy   When an axon is cut, it is called an axotomy.

bandpass noise   The band of frequencies that pass through a filter after the elimination of high and low frequencies.

basal cells   The basal cell is located in the olfactory epithelium, divides by mitosis, and replaces olfactory receptors.

Bell-Magendie law   A statement that refers to the division of a spinal nerve into afferent and efferent portions (roots)—one dorsal and one ventral. The sensory (afferent) root enters the dorsal horn and the motor (efferent) root leaves the ventral horn.

best frequency   The frequency with the lowest intensity that produces an increase in neural activity.

binocular disparity   When an object in the environment is not on the imaginary horopter, the image in each eye is different (disparate). The slight difference in the image of each eye is binocular disparity.

binocular fusion   The single perceptual image formed by the merging (fusing) images from two eyes.

binocular rivalry   When a continual alternation of a single image occurs because the images to the two eyes are so disparate that binocular fusion cannot occur; the continual perceptual alternation of the image is binocular rivalry.

bipolar neurons   Bipolar neurons are in the retina and synapse directly with true receptors.

blobs   The neural cells within the V1 area of the cortex that are color specific.

bony labyrinth   The vestibular and cochlear labyrinth formed within the temporal bone that contains the membranes, cells, and fluids of the peripheral organs.

Bowman's gland   The gland that produce the mucus within the nasal passages.

Broca's area   Broca's area is located in the frontal lobe adjacent to the motor cortex and is directly associated with speech phonation, articulation, and facial expression.

caloric test   Because of the proximity of the horizontal semicircular canal and the external auditory meatus, when warm or cool water (or air) enters the external auditory canal a temperature change will occur in fluids of the canal. This exchange of heat produces predictable nystagmus and provides a means of examining the vestibular system.

capture   When there is a discrepancy between different sensory modalities, one of the two senses will usually predominate over the other and capture the perception.

case of the missing fundamental   The perception of the fundamental frequency in a harmonic complex when the fundamental does not physically exist. It is an illusion.

cation   An ion that has a positive charge.

cell body   The cell body is the main protoplasmic mass of a cell that produces the internal metabolic means of cell survival. The cell body is also called a soma or perikaryon.

Centigrade   A metric scale used to quantify temperature. Zero degrees Centigrade is equivalent to 32 degrees on the Fahrenheit scale. To change Centigrade to Fahrenheit, multiple the degrees Centigrade by 9, divide the product by 5, and then add 32 degrees.

central fissure   A deep sulcus (fissure) that partitions the cerebral cortex from front to rear. The frontal lobe is anterior to the central fissure and the parietal lobe is directly posterior to the central fissure. The central fissure is also known as the fissure of Rolando.

central nervous system (CNS)   Consists of the brain and spinal cord.

cerebrovascular accident (CVA)   Commonly known as a stroke. The CVA can occur because the vessels become closed, occlusive CVA, or because the vessels burst, hemorrhagic CVA.

cerumen   The "ear wax" within the external auditory meatus. The cerumen provides protection and moisture for the tissues within the ear canal.

C-fibers   Small unmyelinated sensory fibers usually associated with protopathic pain.

cGMP   A second messenger in the transduction process of olfaction: cyclic guanosine monophosophate.

channel blockage   If a chemical stimulus blocks an ion channel in a taste receptor membrane, the process is called channel blockage.

characteristic frequency (CF)   The frequency with the lowest intensity that will increase the firing rate of a neuron.

chemical sensitive   This refers to the membrane of a neuron that changes state (becomes excited or inhibited) because of a chemical contact.

chorda tympani   A branch of the facial nerve that serves the anterior two thirds of the tongue.

ciliary epithelium   Cells behind the retina that help maintain a healthy and functional eye by supplying nutrients for receptors and removing the continually produced debris of rods and cones.

ciliary muscles   Muscles that provide accommodation by changing the shape of the lens.

ciliated cells   The olfactory ciliated cells move mucus through the nasal passages toward the nasopharynx to help maintain a passageway for inspired air and to provide better receptor and airborne chemical interaction.

circumvallate   A type of papillae found on the posterior portion of the tongue.

CNS   Central Nervous System. Consists of the brain and spinal cord.

cochlea   The cochlea is the auditory portion of the inner ear carved into the temporal bone. It is snail-shaped and has a notable coiled appearance. It makes about $2\frac{3}{4}$ turns as it spirals from its base, near the oval and round windows, to its apex.

compensatory movements   Eye movements that compensate for head movements.

complex cell   A cortical cell that requires the bar of light to be in a particular orientation and moving in a particular direction.

complex waveform   A waveform that has more than one frequency. The most complex is noise.

concentration gradient   The inequality in ion concentrations on each side of a neural membrane results in a potential difference across the membrane. The potential difference is the result of unequal ionic concentrations.

concha   The relatively deep depression at the opening of the external auditory meatus.

conductive hearing loss   Hearing loss associated with the failure of sound to be conducted through the external and middle ear.

cones   One of two types of true receptors in the eye (rods are the other true receptor). The cones are responsible for color vision and visual acuity.

conjugate movement   Voluntary eye movement. This type of eye movement is controlled by the frontal eye field in the motor cortex and is occurring now as you read this sentence.

cornea   The transparent portion of the sclera located in the front of the eye. It accounts for approximately two thirds of the bending or diffraction of entering light.

corpus callosum   The band of fibers that connects the left and right hemispheres of the cerebral cortex.

cortical magnification   The most important features of a sensory system require, and receive, the largest portion of the cortex. An example in the somatosensory system is the area of cortex devoted to the fingers and thumb.

cranial nerves   The 12 nerves found within the skull.

cribriform plate   Also known as the ethmoid bone, it lies below the olfactory bulbs and above the nasal cavity. The fila olfactoria pass through the cribriform plate to enter the olfactory bulb.

crista   The supporting structure holding the hair cells receptors in the ampulla of the vestibular system.

cross-adaptation   The failure to taste a chemical stimulus after having been adapted by a previous stimulus is cross adaptation.

cupula   The gelatinous mass that lays over the vestibular hair cells and extends from the crista to the roof of the ampulla.

CVA   *See* cerebrovascular accident (a stroke).

cyclic adenosine monophosphate (cAMP)   A second messenger in olfaction.

cyclic guanosine monophosophate (cGMP)   A second messenger in the transduction process of olfaction.

dark current   The continual influx of Na^+ and efflux of K^+ when the rod or cone is in the dark. The dark current depolarizes the receptor.

decibel (dB)   The unit of measurement of a sound amplitude, intensity, or perception. Named after Alexander Graham Bell.

Deiter cells   A group of supporting cells within the cochlea that helps form the organ of Corti.

depolarized   If a cell is depolarized, the internal potential is more positive than the resting value.

dermatome   The body surface that is innervated by the dorsal root of a spinal nerve.

direct entry   When ions from a chemical stimulus enter a receptor directly to initiate action potentials in the gustatory sense.

direct gating   When a chemical stimulus changes the configuration of a taste receptor membrane and opens cation gates to initiate a depolarization.

doctrine of specific nerve energies   The theory postulating that sensory perception depends on a specific and direct line to a particular cortical location.

dopamine   A neurotransmitter involved in motor behavior and schizophrenia. Loss of dopamine leads to Parkinson's disease; excess dopamine causes schizophrenia.

dorsal column   A major afferent path within the dorsal horn of the spinal cord.

dorsal horn   The back portion of the spinal column where afferent fibers enter the central nervous system.

dorsal root   The sensory portion of a spinal nerve.

double color-opponent receptive field   When the center and surround of a neuron's receptive field each responds to two opponent wavelengths, the neuron has a double color-opponent receptive field. An example is when a neuron has a −R/+G center and a +R/−G surround.

dysgeusia   A distortion of the perception of taste. It can be an hallucination or an unpleasant taste that occurs when a pleasant morsel is presented.

efferent   Refers to the direction of impulse flow in the nervous system. The efferent flow refers to the motor or outward flow of impulses from the central nervous system.

efflux   The exit of ions from a cell.

electrical gradient   When a difference in electrical charge exists between two locations, an electrical inequality exists. The difference in electrical charge is an electrical gradient.

electrotonic   The term can refer to (a) a slow graded potential that occurs post-synaptically as a function of the amount of neurotransmitter released or (b) electrotonic transmission. Electrotonic transmission is the conduction of action potentials between neurons without chemical neurotransmitters.

end bouton   The initial part of the synapse is a structure called the end bouton. The end bouton is located at the distal end of the axon.

endogenous   Produced from within. The cell produces the neurotransmitter endogenously.

endolymph   The fluid that fills the scala media within the auditory system and the membranous labyrinth of the vestibular system.

endolymphatic potential   The +80 mv endolymphatic potential, produced by the stria vascularis, provides the medium for hair-cell modulation in the auditory and vestibular modalities.

endorphins   Neurotransmitters that mimic opiates and bind to receptors that alleviate pain.

end-stopped cell   A neural cortical cell that responds to a bent moving bar of light that is also restricted in length (end stopped).

enkephalins   Neurotransmitters that mimic opiates and bind to receptors that alleviate pain.

entorhinal cortex   A portion of the limbic system associated with olfactory emotional responses.

epicritic   The initial rush of action potentials that causes a sharp, piercing pain is called an epicritic pain.

EPSP   *See* excitatory postsynaptic potential.

ethmoid bone   Also known as the cribriform plate. It is the bone that lies below the olfactory bulbs and the frontal lobe.

eustachian tube   A narrow tube that leads from the middle ear to the throat that functions to equalize pressure across the tympanic membrane.

evoked otoacoustic emissions   An evoked otoacoustic emission is generated within the cochlea by outer hair cells and is recorded within the ear canal. It is produced (evoked) when an acoustic signal is presented to the ear.

excitation   Excitation is associated with the depolarization of the neuron. When the internal voltages is increased above the resting potential and a spike is generated, the cell is in a state of excitation.

excitatory postsynaptic potential (EPSP)   When the postsynaptic membrane is depolarized by a neurotransmitter, the result is an excitatory postsynaptic potential.

external auditory meatus   The ear canal. It is sealed at the end by the tympanic membrane, the eardrum.

external ear   The portion of the auditory system that includes the pinna, external auditory meatus, and tympanic membrane.

extrapyramidal tract   A section of the spinal cord that when viewed in cross-section appears similar in shape to another pyramidal area of the spinal cord; hence, it is another or "extra" pyramidal pathway.

Fahrenheit   A metric scale used to quantify temperature. Thirty-two degrees Fahrenheit is equivalent to 0 degrees on the Centigrade scale. To change Fahrenheit to Centigrade subtract 32 degrees from the Fahrenheit then multiple the result by 5 and divide the product by 9.

fast adaptation   One of the two classes of mechanoreceptors (slow adaptation is the other). Receptors that adapt rapidly (stop responding) when the stimulus is non-changing and constant is a fast adapting receptor.

fila olfactoria   A bundle of unmyelinated olfactory receptor axons that pass through the cribriform plate and enter the olfactory bulb forms the fila olfactoria.

first messenger   The first chemical to bond with the receptor membrane.

foliate   A type of papillae that is found on the sides of the tongue.

Fourier analysis   A mathematical method used to analyze a complex waveform into its separate components.

4-kHz notch   The initial loss in hearing that occurs as a result of noise pollution. The loss is first seen in an audiogram at 4,000 Hz.

fovea   The region of the macula of the eye where acute color vision and fine detail is transduced by cones.

free nerve endings   Neural elements with no receptor at the distal portion.

frequency   Refers to the number of complete cycles or oscillations that occur in a one second interval of time. It is measured in Hertz (Hz).

frequency-intensity principle   When the environmental stimulus increases in strength, the nervous system increases the number of action potentials generated. This is the frequency-intensity principle.

frequency tuning curve (FTC)   The FTC is obtained by manipulating the frequency and intensity of an auditory stimulus while recording the activity of an afferent fiber coming from the cochlea. The response of the neuron reflects the cell's frequency selectivity.

frontal eye field   Located in the motor cortex and controls voluntary saccadic eye movement.

frontal lobe   A region of the cerebral cortex anterior to the central fissure and the parietal lobe.

fundamental frequency   The lowest frequency in a complex waveform.

fungiform   A type of papillae found on the anterior two thirds of the tongue. The majority of the fungiform papillae are on the tip. One half of these papillae have no taste buds and therefore no taste receptors.

gamma-amino butyric acid (GABA)   A neurotransmitter found within the central nervous system that is nearly always inhibitory in its effects.

ganglion   A gathering of neural cell bodies.

ganglion neuron   The primary sensory neuron of the visual system. It directly conducts action potentials to the higher neural centers.

gap junctions   The structural connection between neurons where action potentials can be conducted without a synapse from one neuron to another is a gap junction.

generator potential   A small local variation in cellular potential that can change cellular response. The generator potential is a local graded potential.

glabrous   Hairless skin such as the finger tips.

glaucoma   The loss of vision due to increased pressure within the anterior chamber that destroys ganglion axons as they exit the eyeball.

glia   A classification of supportive cells within the nervous system. Astrocytes, microglia, oligodendrocytes, and Schwann cells are some of the different classifications of glia cells.

glial scar   The proliferation of astrocytes and microglia due to trauma or injury can produce a glial scar that has been associated with the inability of damaged neural elements to repair themselves.

glomeruli   The axons of olfactory receptors enter the olfactory bulb and infiltrate a complex of glomeruli (*glomeruli* is plural for *glomerulus*). A glial sheath is formed around each glomerulus to separate it from the other neural elements.

glossopharyngeal nerve   The IX cranial nerve serving the posterior foliate papillae and the circumvallate papillae within the gustatory sense.

glutamate A major neurotransmitter in the brain that is most often excitatory in nature. A principle transmitter in the visual system.

glycine A neurotransmitter found in the spinal cord and brain that is nearly always inhibitory in effect.

graded potential A change in potential within a postsynaptic neuron as a function of the amount of neurotransmitter released by the presynaptic neuron. The potential is graded and not an all-or-none response (like an action potential). It varies in size (excitatory or inhibitory) as a function of the amount of neurotransmitter released at the synapse.

granule cells Cells that make contact with the mitral cells in the olfactory bulb and send their axons laterally in a manner similar to that of the periglomerular cells.

gyrus A normal convolution or enlargement that is defined by fissures in the cortex.

hair cell A true receptor within the auditory and vestibular systems.

hallucination The perception of a nonexisting stimulus.

harmonic An exact multiple of the lowest frequency in a complex waveform.

helicotrema The hole at the apex of the basilar membrane connecting the scala tympani and the scala vestibule.

helix One of two ridges around the superior portion of the pinna. The helix begins at the top of the pinna and runs around the outer edge.

Henson cells A group of supporting cells within the cochlea that helps form the organ of Corti.

heroin A highly addictive opiate derived from the poppy.

high-pass noise The high frequencies that pass through a filter after the low frequencies have been removed.

hippocampus A part of the limbic system associated with emotions and intimately related to short-term memory processing.

histamine A widely distributed amine found in the human body. Can be involved with pain when injuries occur.

homunculus A distorted neural representation or map of one half the body in the cortex is called a somatosensory homunculus. *Homunculus* is Latin for "little man."

horizontal neurons Neurons in the retina intimately associated with receptive fields and lateral processing.

horopter   All objects in a visual field that fall on an imaginary line (the horopter) that passes through the fixation point stimulate the same retinal points in each eye. Objects falling on the horopter produce no retinal disparity.

horseradish peroxidase (HRP)   A substance used to stain and delineate the neural elements of a cell.

hydrophilic   Water-soluble taste stimuli.

hypercolumn   Consists of three components: orientation columns, ocular dominance columns, and blobs.

hyperopia   Farsightedness that occurs because the eyeball has become too short.

hyperpolarize   If a neuron is hyperpolarized, it is more negative than the resting potential.

hypothalamus   A part of the limbic system that lies immediately ventral to the thalamus.

iatrogenic   A disorder that is caused by a physician.

illusion   A false perception of a sensory event. The existing stimuli are misinterpreted.

impedance mismatch   A loss of energy caused by the difference in impedance (resistance) when there is a interface between two different mediums such as air and fluid.

impulse   *See* action potential.

incus   The middle bone in the ossicular chain.

indirect gating   Indirect gating occurs when the initiating event in taste reception indirectly opens channels for ionic exchange by using a second messenger.

influx   The movement of ions into the interior of the cell is referred to as an influx.

inhibition   A cell that is hyperpolarized (below its resting level) is in a state of inhibition.

inhibitory postsynaptic potential (IPSP)   An inhibitory postsynaptic potential occurs at a postsynaptic membrane when a neuortransmitter produces a decrease in the voltage across the postsynaptic membrane. The membrane is hyperpolarized and locally inhibited.

initial segment   The area on the soma where the axon is produced and leaves the soma. It is also known as the axon hillock.

inner ear   Composed of the peripheral mechanisms of the vestibular and auditory systems. The inner ear consists of the semicircular canals, ampulla, utricle, saccule, and the cochlea.

inner hair cell   One of the two true receptors located within the scala media of the cochlea.

inner segment   The function of the inner segment of a rod or cone is similar to that of a neuron. It contains the cell nucleus and produces necessary ingredients to maintain the cell.

intensity   The magnitude or size of a stimulus. In audition, it is measured in decibels.

intensity level (IL)   A stimulus measured in watt/cm^2 with a reference value of 10^{-16} watt/cm^2, is expressed as intensity level, IL.

internal auditory meatus   The passageway in the petrous bone used by the VIII cranial nerve to enter the brainstem.

interneurons   A dense group of neurons within the laminae (layers) of the spinal cord that communicate and interact with each other and process incoming (afferent) and outgoing (efferent) impulses.

ion   Atom that has gained or lost an electrons.

ionic channels   The channel or pore within neural membrane that permits the passage of ions.

ionic flow   The movement of ions is ionic flow. It is from the Greek verb that means "to move."

ipsilateral   Ipsilateral means the same (ipsi) side (lateral).

kinocilium   A single large cilium on the vestibular hair cell receptor.

Krause end bulb   A modified neuron that acts as a somatosensory receptor and responds to tactile pressures and light touch.

labyrinth   Refers to the inner ear where both the vestibular and auditory peripheral mechanisms are found. It is sculpted within the temporal bone and has the chambers, fluids, membranes, receptors, and structures necessary for auditory and vestibular function.

laminae   A layer of neural cells, interneurons, within the spinal cord.

lateral fissure   Separates the parietal and temporal lobes and is also known as the Sylvian sulcus.

lateral geniculate nucleus (LGN)   The ganglion cell axons ascend to the lateral geniculate nucleus of the thalamus. This portion of the thalamus is associated with vision.

lateral spinothalamic tract   The lateral spinothalamic tract is located laterally, to the side, of the spinal cord and conducts information from the spinal cord to an area within the brain called the thalamus, hence the name lateral spinothalamic tract.

lens   A transparent structure at the anterior portion of the eye that changes shape, diffracts light, and provides accommodation and a clear image on the retina.

limbic system   A neural system in the brain stem associated with emotions. It includes the following neural elements: amygdala, hypothalamus, hippocampus, and entorhinal cortex.

line spectrum   The display of the amplitude of a waveform plotted on a vertical axis and frequency that is represented on the horizontal axis.

linear acceleration   An abrupt and rapid straight-line movement.

Lissauer's tract   A short neural pathway that connects closely aligned laminar layers within the spinal cord.

lobule   Part of the pinna, usually referred to as the earlobe.

local graded potential   A postsynaptic potential that varies in size (is graded) as a function of the amount of neurotransmitter released and is restricted to the synaptic area (is local).

longitudinal fissure   The longitudinal fissure divides the left and right hemispheres.

low-pass noise   The low frequencies that pass through an electronic filter after the high frequencies have been removed.

macula   The macula is the spot where the receptors are located. From the Latin *macula,* meaning "spot."

malleus   The first bone in the sequence forming the ossicular chain. The malleus is attached to the tympanic membrane and the incus.

McClintock effect   The synchronization of menstrual cycles in women who live together.

mechanoreceptor   A receptor that responds to pressure, movement of hairs, and depression of the skin.

medial lemniscus   A neural path in the brain stem that receives fibers from the spinothalamic tract associated with pain.

medulla   A group of neurons that form a nucleus or aggregate of cells within the brainstem. The medulla is the first destination of afferent neurons from the dorsal column of the spinal cord.

Meissner's corpuscle A modified neuron that acts as a somatosensory receptor. Responds to light tactile pressures.

membranous labyrinth The membranous labyrinth is within the bony labyrinth of the petrous bone. It contains fluid, specialized receptors, supporting cells, membranes, and structures for the vestibular sense.

Merkel's cells (Merkel's disc) A modified neuron that acts as a somatosensory receptor. It responds to light touch (skin deformation and light pressure).

middle ear The medial portion of the peripheral auditory system, which includes the ossicles, eustachian tube, stapedius and tensor tympani muscles, and the round and oval windows.

mitral cells Shaped like a Bishop's headdress, they are found in the olfactory bulb, receive inputs from the receptors, and send axons centrally to form the lateral olfactory tract.

modified neuron A modified neuron has modifications that permit it to change environmental stimuli into neural impulses. Unlike a true receptor, it does not produce a generator potential.

modiolus The location where nerve fibers enter and exit the cochlea.

morphine An opiate substance derived from the poppy and named after Morpheus, the Greek god of dreams.

morphological axis of polarity Refers to the systematic organization and orientation of the cilia on the hair cells. When cilia are bent or displaced in one direction, the hair cell depolarizes; when the cilia are bent in the opposite direction, the hair cell hyperpolarizes. The direction in which the cilia are moved determines the receptor response.

myelin The glial sheath that wraps an axon. The glia is either an oligodendrocyte (in the CNS) or a Schwann cell (in the PNS).

myopia Nearsightedness caused by a long eyeball.

naloxone An antagonist for morphine and heroin overdose.

nares The two entrances to the nasal cavity separated by the nasal septum.

nasal septum The dividing cartilage that separates the two nasal chambers.

nerve An afferent or efferent gathering of neural axons that conduct impulses within the nervous system.

neural impulse *See* action potential.

neural plasticity Refers to the ability of the nervous system to change as a function of an environmental event such as an injury or learning.

neurogenic   A sensation that is perceived as painful because of an injury to the nervous system is referred to as neurogenic.

neuroglia   *See* glia.

neuroleptic   An antischizophrenic drug.

nociceptor   A pain receptor (fiber) that has the capability of responding to physiological insults or injuries. Chemicals released by damaged or diseased organs and tissues act as stimuli and instigate the action potentials necessary for the perception of pain.

nodes of Ranvier   The nodes of Ranvier are the separations or interruptions between myelin sheaths that wrap an axon.

noise   Any complex, nonperiodic, auditory stimulus.

noise-induced hearing loss   A form of sensorineural hearing loss that is the result of environmental factors such as impulsive or continuously loud noise.

nystagmus   Small and rapid uncontrollable horizontal movements of the eyes.

occipital lobe   A region of the cerebral cortex associated with visual processing, it lies posterior to the parietal lobe.

Ohm's acoustic law   Refers to the frequency analysis capabilities of the auditory system.

olfactory cilia   Are on the olfactory knob and are the place where olfactory transduction occurs.

olfactory epithelium   Lies on the lateral and medial wall of each nasal passageway and has embedded within it the receptors and supporting cells.

olfactory knob   Located at the distal end of the short dendritic process of the olfactory receptor and accommodates 10 to 12 cilia.

olfactory receptor   An unmyelinated bipolar neuron associated with the transduction of odors.

oligodendrocyte   Within the central nervous system myelin is formed by a glial cell known as the oligodendrocyte.

olivocochlear bundle   The olivocochlear bundle originates from the ipsilateral and contralateral superior olive and is the efferent path leading to the hair cells within the cochlea.

opponent process theory of color vision   A theory originally proposed as an alternative to the trichromatic theory. The theory suggests that color vision is also an opponent process: The perception of red-green and blue-yellow are neurological opponent processes.

optic radiations The afferent fibers that leave the lateral geniculate nucleus and ascend to the cortex. The radiations consist of magnocellular and parvocellular paths leaving the six layers of the thalamus.

orbitofrontal neocortex The final path of the olfactory system is thought to be from the thalamus to the orbitofrontal neocortex located in the ventral portion of the frontal lobe.

organ of Corti Consists of several different cells and tissues that together produce action potentials for the sense of hearing. These cells and tissues include the basilar membrane, tectorial membrane, outer and inner hair cells, arch of Corti, pillar cells, and supporting cells of Henson and Deiter.

orientation column A vertical column of cortical cells composed of simple and complex cells.

orthograde degeneration The degeneration of an axon in the direction of impulse flow, away from the cell body and toward the axon terminal, is orthograde degeneration. This is also known as anterograde degeneration and Wallerian degeneration.

osseous spiral lamina A bony shelf supporting the basilar membrane.

ossicles The three smallest bones in the human body—the malleus, incus, and stapes—located in the middle ear.

ossicular chain The three bones that compose the ossicles (the malleus, incus, and stapes) that are linked together.

otitis media An infection in the middle ear that causes conductive hearing loss.

otoacoustic emissions Weak signals transmitted from the inner ear, through the middle ear, to the tympanic membrane, and then into the ear canal. Once the sound reaches the ear canal, a sensitive speaker can be used to record it. There are two types of otoacoustic emissions—those spontaneously generated and those evoked by a stimulus.

otoconia These otolith stones (from the Greek *lithos,* for "stone"), made of calcium carbonate, provide the necessary mass to deform the hair cells in the vestibular system when the head or body is tilted.

otoliths The otolith organs, the utricle and saccule, that respond to gravitational forces.

otosclerosis   Ossification (bone growth) that restricts the movement of the stapes and the oval window. This causes conductive hearing loss.

outer hair cell (OHC)   One of the two true receptors found within the cochlea of the auditory system.

outer segment   The area at the distal end of the visual receptor that initiates the transduction process. One of two distinct areas of visual receptors.

oval window   The thin membrane that separates the middle and inner ear and has the stapes attached to it on the lateral side (in the middle ear). On the medial side of the oval window is the perilymph within the inner ear.

Pacinian corpuscle   A modified neuron that acts as a somatosensory and proprioceptive receptor. It responds to deep pressure, joint movement, and vibration.

papillae   Small bumps on the tongue. The fungiform, circumvallate, and foliate papillae contain taste buds.

paradoxical cold   A cold perception that occurs with a hot stimulus.

parietal lobe   A region of the cerebral cortex separated from the temporal lobe by the lateral fissure. The parietal lobe is posterior to the fissure of Rolando (lateral fissure) and has neural areas associated with somatosensory and visual systems.

Parkinson's disease   A neurological deficit that affects movement. The symptoms are motor rigidity, movement difficulty in arms and legs, and limb tremor. The cause is the depletion of dopamine due to the degeneration of neural cells in the brain that produce this neurotransmitter.

passive transport   The movement of ions across the cell membrane with no metabolic cell involvement is passive transport.

pattern theory   The theory that postulates that sensory organization and perception is the result of the pattern of neural activity arriving at higher neural centers.

Penfield, Wilder   A surgeon who, while performing neural surgery to cure epileptic seizures in patients, discovered the homunculus associated with the somatosensory system.

peptides (bradykinin)   A compound formed by amino acids joined by peptide bonds. Bradykinin is an example of a peptide released from plasma.

periglomerular cell   The cell that sends its axon laterally from one glomerulus to another within the olfactory bulb.

perikaryon   The cell body of a neuron.

perilymph   The fluid surrounding the membranous labyrinth in the vestibular system and the scala media in the auditory system. Perilymph is ionically similar to cerebrospinal fluid.

periodic waveform   Repeats itself and is periodically predictable. Here, *periodic* means that if you know the amplitude of a waveform of at any one point in time, you can know the amplitude of the wave at a future time.

periodicity pitch   The pitch that is perceived when a complex waveform is presented. It is also often referred to as residue pitch when the complex is without a fundamental frequency.

peripheral nervous system (PNS)   That part of the nervous system that is outside of the brain and spinal cord.

petrous   Refers to the temporal portion of the skull where the vestibular and auditory labyrinth are formed within the bone (from the Latin *petrosa,* for "stony").

phase   Every "pure tone frequency" can be partitioned into 360 degrees. Each degree in the cycle is referred to as a particular phase angle in degrees. A sinusoid has a starting phase of zero degrees.

phase locking   Used to indicate that bursts of activity from neural fibers "follow" the frequency of the stimulus by firing at the same point (e.g., at 90 degrees) in each cycle of the stimulus.

pheromone   A chemical produced by males and females for the purpose of sexual attraction.

phosphodiesterase (PDE)   An enzyme that rapidly inactivates the cAMP by changing the cAMP configuration to the noncyclic AMP. This stops the transduction within the olfactory cilia. Also inactivates cGMP in the visual system by changing it to GMP.

pigment epithelium   Lies next to the retina and, in conjunction with the ciliary, supplies nutrients for receptors and removes discarded receptor discs and membranes.

pillar cells   Forms the arch (or tunnel) of Corti.

pilomotor reflex   The reflexive shivering (goose pimples or chill bumps) that occurs when the body is chilled. It was handed down from our ancestral past as a method of generating body heat.

pinna   The ear. *Pinna* is Latin for "wing." It is part of the external auditory system and important in localization.

place theory of pitch   States that the perception of pitch is dependent on the displacement of the basilar membrane at a particular place. The place that is maximally displaced depends on the traveling wave and the frequency of the stimulus.

plexiform layer   The outer synaptic region of the olfactory bulb.

plexuses   The joining or merging of fibers from different spinal nerves into a plexus (braid) forms a peripheral nerve composed of fibers of several spinal nerves. From the Latin for "braid."

PNS   *See* peripheral nervous system.

polarized   When the voltage within a cell differs from the voltage outside the cell, the cell is polarized. The cell can be either depolarized or hyperpolarized.

postcentral gyrus   The bump (gyrus) or convulsions of neural cortex that form the anterior portion of the parietal lobe associated with the somatosensory system.

postsynaptic   Refers to the dendrite or soma portion (the receiving side) of a synapse.

postsynaptic potential   The ionic exchange at the postsynaptic membrane that occurs as a result of a neurotransmitter binding with specific molecular receptors in the membrane produces a voltage change at the membrane. The voltage change is a postsynaptic potential.

postural reflex   The ability to maintain an erect and upright position while moving about the environment depends on the postural reflex (also called the "neck reflex" and the "righting postural reflex").

potential-sensitive   Potential-sensitive means that the "pores" or gates that allow ions to pass through the cell membrane open or close as a function of the potential across the membrane.

power   A measure of physical energy with a reference of watts per centimeter squared in the auditory domain.

presbycusis   Sensorineural hearing loss that is assumed to be the result of age.

presbyopia   A visual refractive problem that results in farsightedness and the inability to accommodate and bring close objects into focus. Caused by a hardening of the lens.

presbyosmia   The loss of smell as a function of age.

presynaptic   Refers to the axon end bouton portion of the synapse.

primary sensory neuron (PSN)   The first afferent neuron in a sensory path. The neuron that is synaptically connected to the receptor.

proprioception   Sensory inputs from muscles, joints, and internal organs.

prostaglandin   A physiological compound that produces nociceptor activity and the perception of pain.

protein kinase   Protein kinase functions as a Na^+/K^+ channel inhibitor when not bound with cAMP. When bound with cAMP the protein kinase becomes active and opens channels for Na^+ and K^+ ions. Influx of these positively charged ions results in an olfactory receptor depolarization

protopathic   A continual barrage of neural activity that produces a ceaseless and perpetual pain is protopathic.

PSN   *See* primary sensory neuron.

pupil   The hole in the center of the iris that controls the amount of light entering the eye.

pyramidal tract   An efferent pathway within the ventral horn of the spinal cord.

pyriform cortex   A relatively small area of tissue lying at the end of the hippocampus and used in olfactory mechanisms.

quantum   Quantum is the term used to designate the entire package of neurotransmitter stored and released by a single vesicle in the presynaptic terminal of a synapse.

radioactive 14C-deoxyglucose   A radioactive substance used to experimentally delineate the neural elements of a cell.

receptive field   A peripheral area of a sensory system that, when stimulated by an adequate stimulus, elicits a response from a neural fiber.

receptive membrane   The postsynaptic portion of a synapse. The membrane that receives the neurotransmitter.

receptor   A specialized cell that transduces (changes) one energy form (environmental stimuli) into an energy that is used by the nervous system (action potentials) to produce sensory experiences.

receptor potential   A local graded potential produced by a true receptor when it responds to the occurrence of an environmental stimulus. The receptor potential generates the action potentials that occur in the PSN by causing the release of the neurotransmitter at the synapse with the PSN.

relative refractory period   The portion of the action potential that immediately follows the maximum depolarization is the relative refractory period.

residue pitch   *See* periodicity pitch.

resonance theory of pitch   A theory of hearing initially proposed by von Helmholtz. The resonance theory was later modified to become the place theory of pitch.

respiratory epithelium   Cleans and warms the air in the nasal cavities and provides a moist humidity using a rich supply of blood vessels and Bowman's glands.

resting potential   The potential within a cell when it is not conducting action potentials. It is inactive and at rest. The internal resting potential is approximately –70 mv relative to the outside.

retina   Is in the vitreous chamber of the eye and consists of the neurons and receptors necessary for visual sensation.

retinotopic   Means that the retina is completely mapped within the thalamus and the cortex. Each location on the retina has a specific place of neural activity in each layer of the lateral geniculate and visual cortex.

retrograde degeneration   Retrograde degeneration refers to the degeneration from the zone of trauma on the axon toward the cell body.

re-uptake   When the neurotransmitter returns to a presynaptic membrane it is often taken back into the neuron that generated it. The absorption of the neurotransmitter back into the sending neuron is re-uptake.

rhodopsin   The molecule involved in light absorption and consists of retinal and opsin.

rods   One of the two types of true receptors in the eye (the other type is the cones). The rods are very sensitive (low thresholds) and do not provide color vision.

round window   One of the two membranes separating the middle ear and inner ear. Functions to relieve the pressure during hydromechanical events within the cochlea.

Ruffini end organ   A modified neuron that acts as a kinesthetic and somatosensory receptor. Responds to pressure on skin, muscles, joints, and internal organs. It is also called a Ruffini ending.

saccadic eye movements   The voluntary eye movements involved with visual scanning of the environment.

saccule   One of the otolith organs that responds to linear acceleration.

saltatory conduction   When an axon is myelinated, the electrical impulses functionally leap from node-to-node along the axon. This functional leap is called saltatory conduction.

sapid   Refers to a stimulus that leads to gustatory sensory activity and a perceptual experience.

scala media   The cochlea is partitioned into three scala or canals (also called ducts). The inner scala is the scala media. It is filled with endolymph and contains auditory receptors.

scala tympani   One of the three scala or canals within the cochlea. The scala tympani lies below the scala media and the basilar membrane.

scala vestibuli   One of the three scala or canals within the cochlea. The scala vestibuli lies above Reissner's membrane.

Scarpa's vestibular ganglion   The location of the cell bodies for the primary sensory neurons of the vestibular sense.

schizophrenia   Entails all or some of the following phenomena: loss of contact with reality, emotional disorders, hallucinations, distortion of reality, indifference, paranoid ideas, delusions, incoherence, illogical thoughts, and grossly disorganized personality and behavior. Excess dopamine is intimately involved in this mental disorder.

Schwann cell   In the peripheral nervous system the myelin sheath is formed by a glial Schwann cell.

sclera   The membrane that provides the shape of the eyeball and appears white in appearance.

second messenger   A chemical sequence within a receptor that carries out the task of opening ionic channels after being activated by the first messenger in the sequence.

semicircular canals   The pairs of peripheral organs in the vestibular system (horizontal, superior, and posterior) that respond to three-dimensional angular rates of acceleration of the head or body.

sensorineural hearing loss   Hearing loss due to problems within the cochlea (hair-cell degeneration) or in higher neural centers (e.g., tumors).

sensory fibers   The afferent axons that conduct sensory impulses.

serotonin   A neurotransmitter that is intimately related to depression and aggression.

shingles   The reactivation of the geniculate herpes zoster virus (chicken pox) results in shingles. Shingles has been associated with taste dysfunctions, severe pain, axonal degeneration, and demyelination of the sensory ganglion nerve cells.

simple cells   Cortical cells that respond to bars of light that have a particular orientation are simple cells.

sinusoid   A single frequency that has its starting point at zero-degrees phase angle.

slow adaption (SA)   One of the two classes of mechanoreceptors (fast adaption is the other). The rate of time required for a mechanoreceptor to adapt or stop responding to a nonchanging constant stimulus is the functional feature dividing the mechanoreceptors into two different classes. Merkel's cells, Ruffini endings, and C-fibers are examples of slow-adapting receptors.

sodium-potassium pump   The active transport of Na^+ from inside the cell to the outside and the movement of K^+ into the cell is accomplished by a cellular metabolic process known as the sodium-potassium pump.

soma   *See* cell body.

sound pressure level (SPL)   A measure of sound pressure using 0.0002 dynes/cm^2 as the reference for the calculation of decibels.

sound shadow   A sound shadow reflects the fact that the high frequencies do not flow around the object in the environment, the head in this case. The sound in the sound shadow is less intense. The high frequencies are deflected and an intensity difference occurs. The object (head) will cause an intensity difference between the ears.

spatial summation   The algebraic summation of graded potentials that occur near each other (i.e., synapses that are spatially side by side).

spike   *See* action potential.

spinal nerves   Enter (efferent) and leave (afferent) the spinal cord.

spiral ligament   The basilar membrane is located between the outer walls of the scala media and is attached to the wall on one side by the spiral ligament and on the other side by the osseous spiral lamina.

spontaneous otoacoustic emission   A weak, spontaneously generated acoustic signal that is generated from within the cochlea and is produced by outer hair cells. The signal is recorded when it reaches the ear canal.

stapedius muscle   One of two muscles in the middle ear that act to protect the hearing mechanism when loud sounds occur. It is attached at one end to the bone within the middle ear and at the other end to the stapes.

Contraction causes the footplate of the stapes to be drawn into the middle ear.

stapes   The third bone in the ossicular chain from the tympanic membrane to the oval window. The stapes is connected to the incus and the oval window.

stereocilia   The 60 to 70 cilia (hairlike appendages on the top of the hair cell). The deformation or bending of the stereocilia is intimately related to hair-cell transduction.

stereopsis   Binocular depth perception.

strabismus ambylopia   The failure of the two eyes to move together and focus on the same object. The unsuccessful capability of obtaining a consistent fused image from the two eyes results in one eye becoming nonfunctional.

stria vascularis   Composed of secretory cells located on the outer wall of the scala media. The cells produce endolymph and the +80 millivolt endolymphatic potential.

substance P   A group of peptides that are major neurotransmitters in pain perception.

substantia gelatinosa (SG)   Interneurons in Laminae 1 and 2 of the spinal cord that are intimately related to the sensation of pain.

sulcus   A sulcus is a deep groove or fissure within the cerebral cortex.

superior olive   A group of cells that use time (phase) of arrival and intensity cues in sound localization.

superior petrosal   A branch of the VII cranial nerve that innervates the nonlingual taste receptors in the oral cavity (not the tongue).

synapse   The functional connection between neurons is called a synapse.

synaptic cleft   The gap between the presynaptic and postsynaptic portions of the synapse.

tardive dyskinesia   An iatrogenic disorder that includes involuntary movement of the mouth, tongue, arms, and legs.

taste buds   Small cuplike structures that contain taste receptors. The taste buds are, in turn, embedded within small bumps on the tongue called papillae.

taste receptors   The chemical receptors associated with the gustatory sensations.

T-cells Interneurons in the spinal cord that transmit pain impulses to the medulla through the spinothalamic tract.

temporal lobe One of the four lobes of the cerebral cortex. It lies below the parietal lobe and the lateral fissure and is anterior to the occipital lobe. It is intimately associated with audition and vision.

temporal summation The arrival of many action potentials at a synapse in a short interval of time is cumulative. This results in a large postsynaptic potential. The more rapid the arrival of the spikes, the larger the postsynaptic potential.

TENS *See* transcutaneous electrical nerve stimulation.

tensor tympani A muscle attached to the tympanic membrane. It works in conjunction with the stapedius muscle as a protective reflex for intense sounds. The tensor tympani draws the tympanic membrane inward making it taut.

thalamus A major aggregate of neurons within the brain that both acts as a relay station for afferent inputs as well as a major processing center for sensory systems. Functionally partitioned into separate nuclei for the different sensory systems.

thermoreceptor A neural fiber that is particularly sensitive to temperature variations of the skin is referred to as a "thermoreceptor"—a "cold receptor" or a "warm receptor."

tinnitus A continuous ringing or noise within the ear.

tip links Tip links are fine strands of connective tissue that attach the tip of one small stereocilium to the shaft of a large stereocilium in an adjacent row. They connect the stereocilia in the vestibular and auditory senses.

tonic Refers to steady or constant activity of a system such as the semicircular canals when it has adapted to a constant nonchanging situation.

tonotopic map A map of the basilar membrane activity in the frequency domain. The map refers to areas of the nervous system where activity is determined by the frequency of the stimulus.

tragus A little flap of tissue near the entrance to the concha, toward the anterior portion of the pinna.

transcutaneous electrical nerve stimulation (TENS) The placement of an electrical pulse generator near the spinal cord to relieve chronic pain.

transduce Used to specify what a sensory receptor accomplishes. The process of changing one energy form (environmental energy) into another form of energy (neural impulses) is to transduce (change) the energy.

transducin A G-protein activated by all-trans retinal when a photon of light is absorbed. Transducin activates an enzyme called phosphodiesterase (PDE).

traveling wave A hydromechanical movement within the inner ear that modulates the scala media and the internal fluids, cells, and structures to produce a maximum point of stimulation along the basilar membrane. The point of maximum stimulation is a function of frequency.

triangular fossa A small depression above the antihelix and below the superior portion of the helix of the pinna. *Fossa* is Latin for "ditch."

trichromatic theory of color vision Hypothesizes that color vision depends on receptors that respond best to three different wavelengths: short (420 nm), medium (530 nm), and long (560 nm). Initially proposed by Thomas Young and Hermann von Helmholtz.

true receptor A receptor that generates a receptor potential in response to an environmental stimulus. It has no axon and no dendrite and generates no action potentials.

tufted cell Neural cells within the olfactory bulb that receive input directly from the olfactory receptors and whose axons help form the lateral olfactory tract.

tympanic membrane Lies at the end of the external auditory meatus, commonly referred to as the eardrum.

umami A glutamate derived from seaweed. The term means savoriness. The chemical substance, commonly known as MSG (monosodium glutamate), is a candidate to become one of the primary tastes joining salty, sour, bitter, and sweet.

utricle One of the two otolith organs that responds to gravity and linear acceleration.

vagus The X cranial nerve.

vallate A short-hand version of the *circumvallate*. Refers to the circumvallate papillae.

ventral basal nucleus An area within the thalamus associated with the somatosensory system.

ventral column A major efferent pathway from the central nervous system that lies within the ventral horn of the spinal cord.

ventral horn The ventral (belly) portion of the spinal column where efferent fibers leave the central nervous system.

ventral root The efferent portion of a spinal nerve.

ventrobasal medial nucleus   An area within the thalamus associated with the gustatory system.

vertigo   The sensation of spinning or rapid dizziness where the surroundings appear to be spinning out of control. In such cases, once causes such as high blood pressure, heart rhythm, and visual disease are ruled out, it is usually found to be a problem with the vestibular system in the inner ear.

vesicle   A presynaptic container located within the end bouton at the synapse. It holds a single quanta of neurotransmitter.

vestibular ganglion   The cell bodies for the primary sensory neurons of the vestibular sense. Located in Scarpa's vestibular ganglion near the internal auditory meatus.

vestibular neuronitis   A vestibular disorder usually first experienced as a severe case of vertigo. The vertigo and loss of balance can continue for extended periods of time. The disorder is assumed to be a viral illness associated with an infected nerve.

vestibular nuclear complex   The destination of the primary sensory neurons of the vestibular system in the brain stem. After the complex has integrated the sensory information from the semicircular canals, utricle, and saccule, it is forwarded to nuclei associated with the vestibulo-ocular, vestibulo-spinal, and vestibulo-cerebellar systems.

vestibule   The middle portion of the labyrinth between the semicircular canals and the cochlea.

vestibulocochlear nerve   The VIII cranial nerve consists of primary afferent fibers from the vestibular and auditory modalities. It enters the brain stem through the internal auditory meatus.

vestibulo-ocular reflex (VR)   The smooth visual perception maintained because of compensatory eye movements is the result of the vestibulo-ocular reflex. As the head moves, the vestibular system and the ocular muscles are coordinated to maintain a stable visual percept.

VIII cranial nerve   The vestibulocochlear nerve that enters the brain stem through the internal auditory meatus.

visible spectrum   The narrow band of electromagnetic radiation that stimulates our visual system. The wavelengths that activate the visual modality range from approximately 400 to 700 nm.

visual field   The environment you perceive as the external world.

vitreous chamber   The posterior chamber of the eye containing vitreous humor.

vitreous humor   The clear fluid within vitreous chamber of the eye that provides nutrients and helps maintain the shape of the eye.

volley theory   Specifies low frequencies are perceived as a function of phase locking. The perceived pitch is a result of the number of neural impulses reaching higher centers rather than the pitch being determined by activity at a place on the basilar membrane.

voltage sensitive   Refers to the neuron's sensitivity to voltage variations across its membrane. The neuron's membrane changes configuration (opens/closes channels) as a function of voltage changes across the membrane. Hence, the neuron is voltage sensitive.

von Békésy, Georg   A Nobel prize winning investigator of the auditory system. Discovered the traveling wave.

von Helmholtz, H. L. F.   A scientist whose contributions rank him among the elite. His work encompassed physiology and physics. He was instrumental in forming the trichromatic theory of color vision and the resonance theory of hearing.

Wallerian degeneration   *See* orthograde degeneration.

watt/cm^2   A unit of power measured in watts per centimeter squared.

waveform   Refers to an acoustic stimulus. The waveform may be complex (more than one frequency) or simple (only a single frequency).

Wernicke's area   Wernicke's area lies in the left temporal lobe and has been associated with the comprehension and understanding of language.

Wever, Glenn   The originator of the volley theory of hearing.

white noise   The special name applied when a complex wave contains all the frequencies between 1 and 20,000 Hertz and each frequency has the same average amplitude.

zonule fibers   Fibers attached to the lens of the eye that work in conjunction with the ciliary muscles to change the shape of the lens and provide accommodation and clear vision.

References

Amoore, J. E. (1964). Current status of the steric theory of odor. *Annals of the New York Academy of Sciences, 116*, 457-476.

Amoore, J. E. (1982). Odor theory and odor classification. In F. Theimer (Ed.), *Fragrance chemistry: The science of the sense of smell* (pp. 27-76). New York: Academic Press.

Barber, H. O., & Sharpe, J. A. (1988). *Vestibular disorders.* Chicago: Year Book Medical Publishers.

Barlow, H. B. (1997). The knowledge used in vision and where it comes from. *Philosophical Transactions of the Royal Society of London, B, 352*, 1141-1147.

Barondes, S. (1994). Thinking about Prozac. *Science, 263*, pp. 102-113.

Bartoshuk, L. M. (1978). History of taste research. In E. C. Carterette & M. P. Friedman (Eds.), *Handbook of perception, vol. 6A: Tasting and smelling.* New York: Academic Press.

Batteau, D. W. (1967). The role of pinna in human localization. *Proceedings of the Royal Society of London, B, 168*, 158-180.

Beauchamp, G. K., & Bartoshuk, L. M. (Eds.). (1997). *Tasting and smelling, Handbook of perception and cognition* (2nd ed.). San Diego, CA: Academic Press.

Benson, T. E., Burd, G. D., Green, C. A., Pedersen, P. E. Landis, D. M. D., & Shepherd, G. M. (1985). High resolution 2-deoxyglucose autoradiography in quick-frozen slabs of neonatal rat olfactory bulb. *Brain Research, 339*, 67-78.

Blake, R., & Camisa, J. (1978). Is binocular vision always monocular? *Science, 200*, pp. 1497-1499.

Borg, E., & Counter, S. A. (1989, August). The middle-ear muscles. *Scientific American, 261*, pp. 74-80.

Brand, J., Teeter, J., Cagan, R., & Kare, M. (Eds.). (1989). *Chemical senses, vol. 1: Receptor events and transduction in taste and olfaction.* New York: Marcel Dekker.

Brodal, A. (1981). *Neurological anatomy in relation to clinical medicine* (3rd ed.). New York: Oxford University Press.

Brown, P. K., & Wald, G. (1964). Visual pigments in single rods and cones of the human retina. *Science, 144,* pp. 45-52.

Burgess, P. R., & Perl, E. R. (1973). Cutaneous mechanoreceptors and nociceptors. In A. Iggo (Ed.), *Handbook of sensory physiology, vol. 2: Somatosensory systems.* Heidelberg: Springer-Verlag.

Callaway, E. M., & Wiser, A. K. (1996). Contributions of individual layer 2-5 spiny neurons to local circuits in macaque primary visual cortex. *Visual Neuroscience, 13,* 907-922.

Colby, C. L., Duhamel, J. -R., & Goldberg, M. E. (1995). Oculocentric spatial representation in parietal cortex. *Cerebral Cortex, 5,* 470-481.

Cometto-Muniz, J. E., & Cain, W. S. (1990). Thresholds for odor and nasal pungency. *Physiology and Behavior, 48,* 719-725.

Cometto-Muniz, J. E., Cain, W. S., & Abraham, M. H. (1998). Nasal pungency and odor of homologous aldehydes and carboxylic acids. *Experimental Brain Research, 118,* 180-188.

Cornsweet, T. N. (1970). *Visual perception.* New York: Academic Press.

Dallos, P. (1992). The active cochlea. *Journal of Neuroscience, 12*(12), 4575-4585.

Dallos, P., & Harris, D. (1978). Properties of auditory nerve responses in absence of outer hair cells. *Journal of Neurophysiology, 41,* 365-383.

Davis, A. B. (1982, Sept./Oct.). The development of anesthesia. *American Scientist, 70,* pp. 522-528.

Desimone, R., Schein, S. J., Moran, J., & Ungerleider, L. G. (1998). Contour, color, and shape analysis beyond the striate cortex. *Vision Research, 25,* 441-452.

Deutsch, D. (1992, August). Paradoxes of musical pitch. *Scientific American,* pp. 88-95.

DeValois, R. I., Abramov, I., & Jacobs, G. H. (1966). Analysis of response patterns of the LGN cells. *Journal of Optical Society of America, 56,* 966-977.

Eccles, J. C. (1964). *The physiology of synapses.* New York: Academic Press.

Eccles, J. C. (1976). From electrical to chemical transmission in the central nervous system. The closing address of the sir henry dale centennial symposium. *Notes Recorded at the Royal Society of London, 30,* 219-230.

Evans, E. F. (1982). Basic physics and psychophysics of sound, In H. B. Barlow & J. D. Mollon (Eds.), *The senses.* New York: Cambridge University Press.

Fesenko, E. E., Kolesnikov, S. S., & Lyubarsky, A. L. (1985). Induction by cyclic GMP of cationic conductance in plasma membrane of retinal rod outer segment. *Nature, 313,* pp. 310-313.

Finger, T. F., Silver, W. L., & Restrepo, D. (2000). *The neurobiology of taste and smell* (2nd ed.). New York: Wiley-Liss.

Fischler, H., Frei, E., Spira, D., & Rubinstein, M. (1967). Dynamic response of middle ear structures. *Journal of the Acoustical Society of America, 41,* 1220-1231.

Gegenfurtner, K. R., & Sharpe, L. T. (Eds.). (1999). *Color vision: From genes to perception.* New York: Cambridge University Press.

Geisler, C. D. (1998). *From sound to synapse.* New York: Oxford University Press.

Gelfand, S. A. (1990). *Hearing: An introduction to psychological and physiological acoustics* (2nd ed.). New York: Marcel Dekker.

Getchell, T. V., Doty, R. L., Bartoshuk, L. M., & Snow, J. B., Jr. (Eds.). (1991). *Smell and taste in health and disease.* New York: Raven Press.

Gilbertson, T. A., Damak, S., & Margolskee, R. F. (2000). The molecular physiology of taste transduction. *Current Opinion in Neurobiology, 10,* 519-527.

Grigg, P., Cinerman, G. A., & Riley, L. H. (1973). Joint position sense after total hip replacement. *Journal of Bone and Joint Surgery, 55A,* 1016-1025.

Gulick, W. L., Gescheider, G. A., & Frisina, R. D. (1989). Hearing. New York: Oxford University Press.

Halpern, B. P. (1999). Taste. In R. A. Wilson & F. Keil (Eds.), *The MIT encyclopedia of the cognitive sciences.* Cambridge, UK: Bradford Books.

Halpern, M. (1987). The organization and function of vomeronasal system. *Annual Review of Neuroscience, 10,* 325-362.

Hamalainen, H., Vartiamen, M., Karvanen, L., & Jarvilehto, T. (1982). Paradoxical heat sensations during moderate cooling of the skin, *Brain Research, 251,* 77-81.

Hansson, P., & Ekblom, A. (1983). Transcutaneous electrical nerve stimulation (TENS) as compared to placebo TENS for the relief of acute orofacial pain. *Pain, 15,* 157-165.

Haynes, L. W., & Yau, K.-W. (1985). Cyclic GMP sensitive conductance in outer segment membranes of catfish cones. *Nature, 317,* pp. 61-64.

Heffner, H. E., & Masterton, R. B. (1990). Sound localization in mammals: Brain stem mechanisms. In M. Berkley & W. Stebbins (Eds.), *Comparative perception, vol. 1: Discrimination.* New York: Wiley.

Heimer, L. (1983). *The human brain and spinal cord: Functional neuroanatomy and dissection guide.* New York: Springer.

Held, R. (1989). *Readings from the encyclopedia of neuroscience: Sensory systems, vol. 1: Vision and visual systems.* Boston: Birkhäuser.

Herness, M. S., & Gilbertson, T. A. (1999). Cellular mechanisms of taste transduction. *Annual Review of Physiology, 61,* 873-890.

Hodgkin, A. L. (1964). *The conduction of the nervous impulse.* Springfield, IL: Charles C Thomas.

Hodgkin, A. L. (1992). *Chance and design: Reminiscences of science in peace and war.* Cambridge, UK: Cambridge University Press.

Holden, C. (1996). Sex and olfaction. *Science, 273,* pp. 313.

Hubel, D. H., & Wiesel, T. N. (1959). Receptive fields of single neurons in the cat's striate cortex. *Journal of Physiology, 148,* 574-591.

Hubel, D. H., & Wiesel, T. N. (1962). Receptive fields, binocular interaction and functional architecture in the cat's visual cortex. *Journal of Neurophysiology, 16,* 106-154.

Hubel, D. H., and Wiesel, T. N. (1965). Receptive fields and functional architecture in two non-striate visual areas (18 and 19) of the cat. *Journal of Neurophysiology, 28,* 229-289.

Hubel, D. H., & Wiesel, T. N. (1968). Receptive fields and functional architecture of monkey striate cortex. *Journal of Physiology, 195,* 215-243.

Hubel, D. H., & Wiesel, T. N. (1970). Stereoscopic vision in macaque monkey. *Nature, 225,* pp. 41-42.

Hubel, D. H., & Wiesel, T. N. (1974a). Sequence regularity and geometry of orientation columns in the monkey striate cortex. *Journal of Comparative Neurology, 158,* 267-294.

Hubel, D. H., & Wiesel, T. N. (1974b). Uniformity of monkey striate cortex: A parallel relationship between field size, scatter, and magnification factor. *Journal of Comparative Neurology, 158,* 295-306.

Hudspeth, A. J. (1982). Extracellular current flow and the site of transduction by vertebrate hair cells. *Journal of Neuroscience, 2,* 1-10.

Hudspeth, A. J. (1985). The cellular basis of hearing: The biophysics of hair cells. *Science, 230,* pp. 745-752.

Hudspeth, A. J. (1989). How the ear's works work. *Nature, 341,* pp. 397-404.

Hurvich, L. M., & Jameson, D. (1957). An opponent-process theory of color vision. *Psychological Review, 64,* 384-404.

Iggo, A., & Andres, K. H. (1982). Morphology of cutaneous receptors. *Annual Review Neuroscience, 5,* 1-31.

Jacobs, B. L. (1994, September-October). Serotonin, motor activity, and depression-related disorders. *American Scientist, 82,* pp. 456-463.

Johansson, R. S., & Vallbo, A. B. (1983). Tactile sensory coding in the glabrous skin of the human hand. *Trends in Neuroscience, 6,* 27-32.

Kaas, J. H., Merzenich, M. M., & Killackey, H. P. (1983). The reorganization of somatic sensory cortex following peripheral nerve damage in adult and developing mammals. *Annual Review of Neuroscience, 6,* 325-336.

Kaas, J. H., Nelson, R. J., Sur, M., & Merzenich, M. M. (1981). Organization of somatosensory cortex in primates. In F. O. Schmitt, F. G. Worden, G. Adelman, & S. G. Dennis (Eds.), *The organization of the cerbral cortex: Proceedings of a neurosciences research program colloquium.* Cambridge: MIT Press.

Kandel, E. R., Schwartz, J. H., & Jessell, T. M. (1995). *Essentials of neural science and behavior.* Norwalk, CT: Appleton & Lange.

Kemp, D. T. (1978). Stimulated acoustic emissions from within the human auditory system. *Journal of the Acoustical Society of America, 64,* 1386-1391.

Khanna, S. M., & Leonard, D. G. B. (1982). Basilar membrane tuning in the cat cochlea. *Science, 215,* pp. 303-304.

Kimelberg, H. K., & Norenberg, M. D. (1989, August). Astrocytes. *Scientific American,* pp. 88-95.

Kinnamon, S. C. (1988). Taste transduction: A diversity of mechanisms. *Trends in Neuroscience, 11,* 491-496.

Kinnamon, S. C., & Cummings, T. A. (1992). Chemosensory transduction mechanisms in taste. *Annual Review of Physiology, 54,* 715-731.

Kolb, H., Linberg, K. A., & Fisher, S. K. (1992). Neurons of the human retina: A Golgi study. *Journal of Comparative Neurology, 318,* 147-187.

Konishi, M. (1993, April). Listening with two ears. *Scientific American,* pp. 66-73.

Kuffler, S. W. (1953). Discharge patterns and functional organization of mammalian retina. *Journal of Neurophysiology, 16,* 37-68.

Lancet, D. (1986). Vertebrate olfactory reception. *Annual Review of Neuroscience, 9,* 329-355.

Le Guerer, A. (1994). *Scent: The essential and mysterious powers of smell.* New York: Kodansha America.

Licklider, J. C. R. (1954). Periodicity pitch and place pitch. *Journal of the Acoustical Society of America, 26,* 945 (A).

Licklider, J. C. R. (1956). Auditory frequency analysis. In C. Cherry (Ed.), *Information theory*. New York: Academic Press.

Livingstone, M. S., & Hubel, D. H. (1987). Psychophysical evidence for separate channels for the perception of form, color, movement, and depth. *Journal of Neuroscience, 7*, 3461-3468.

Lomber, S. G., Payne, B. R., Cornwell, P., & Long, K. D. (1996). Perceptual and cognitive visual functions of parietal temporal cortices in the cat. *Cerebral Cortex, 6*, 673-695.

Long, R. R. (1977). Sensitivity of cutaneous cold fibers to noxious heat: Paradoxical cold discharge. *Journal of Neurophysiology, 40*, 489-502.

Lynch, J. C., Mountcastle, V. B., Talbot, W. H., & Yin, T. C. T. (1977). Parietal lobe mechanisms for directed visual attention. *Journal of Neurophysiology, 40*, 362-389.

Marks, W. B., Dobelle, W. H., & MacNichol, E. F. (1964). Visual pigments of single primate cones. *Science, 143*, pp. 1181-1183.

Masterton, R. B. (1992). Role of the central auditory system in hearing: The new direction. *Trends in Neurosciences, 15*, 280-285.

McClintock, M. K. (1971). Menstrual synchrony and suppression. *Nature, 229*, pp. 244-245.

McLauglin, S., & Margolskee, R. F. (1994, November-December). The sense of taste. *American Scientist, 82*, pp. 538-545.

Melzack, R. (1992, April). Phantom limbs. *Scientific American*, pp. 120-126.

Melzack, R., & Wall, P. D. (1965). Pain mechanisms: A new theory. *Science, 150*, pp. 971-979.

Merigan, W. H. (1996). Basic visual capacities and shape discrimination after lesions of extrastriate area V4 in macaques. *Visual Neuroscience, 13*, 51-60.

Merigan, W. H., & Maunsell, J. H. R. (1993). How parallel are the primitive visual pathways? *Annual Review of Neuroscience, 16*, 369-402.

Merigan, W. H., & Pham, H. A. (1998). V4 lesions in macaques affect both single- and multiple-viewpoint shape discrimination. *Visual Neuroscience, 15*, 359-367.

Merskey, H., & Bogduk, N. (Eds.). (1994). *Classification of chronic pain* (2nd ed.), Seattle, WA: IAPS Press.

Meyer, J., Furness, D. N., Zenner, H.-P., Hackney, C. M., & Gummer, A. W. (1998). Evidence for opening of hair-cell transducer channels after tip-link loss. *Journal of Neuroscience, 18*, 6748-6756.

Michael, C. R. (1979). Color-sensitive hypercomplex cells in monkey striate cortex. *Neurophysiology, 42,* 726-744.

Michael, C. R. (1981). Columnar organization of color cells in monkey's striate cortex. *Journal of Neurophysiology, 46,* 587-604.

Miller, I. J., Jr. (1989, June). Variations in human taste bud density as a function of age from nutrition and the chemical senses in aging: Recent advances and current research needs. *Annals of the New York Academy of Sciences,* 307-319.

Moore, B. C. J. (1997). *An introduction to the psychology of hearing.* New York: Academic Press.

Mountcastle, V. B. (1980). Sensory receptors and neural encoding: Introduction to sensory processes. In V. B. Mountcastle (Ed.), *Medical physiology* (Vol. 1, 14th ed.). St. Louis, MO: Mosby.

Mozell, M. M., Smith, B. P., Smith, P. E., Sullivan, R. L., & Swender, P. (1969). Nasal chemoreception in flavor identification. *Archives of Otolaryngology, 90,* 367-373.

Narayan, S. S., Temchin, A. N., Reico, A., & Ruggero, M. A. (1998). Frequency tuning of basilar membrane and auditory nerve fibers in the same cochleae. *Science, 282,* pp. 1882-1884.

O'Connell, R. J., & Meredith, M. (1984). Effects of volatile and nonvolatile chemical signals on male sex behaviors mediated by the main and accessory olfactory system. *Behavioral Neuroscience, 98,* 1083-1093.

Paysan, J., & Breer, H. (2001). Molecular physiology of odor detection: Current views. *Pflugers Archives-European Journal of Physiology, 441*(5), 579-586.

Peichl, L. (1991). Alpha ganglion cells in mammalian retinae: Common properties, species differences, and some comments on other ganglion cells. *Visual Neuroscience, 7,* 155-169.

Peichl, L., & Wässle, H. (1983). The structural correlate of the receptive field centre of α ganglion cells in the cat retina. *Journal of Physiology, 341,* 309-324.

Penfield, W., & Rasmussen, T. (1950). *The cerebral cortex of man: A clinical study of localization of function.* New York: Macmillan.

Perrett, D. I., Rolls, E. T., & Caan, W. (1982). Visual neurons responsive to faces in the monkey temporal cortex. *Experimental Brain Research, 47,* 329-342.

Peters, A., Palay, S. L., & Webster, H. de F. (1991). *The fine structure of the nervous system: Neurons and their supporting cells* (3rd ed.). New York: Oxford University Press.

Pfaffmann, C. (1978a). Neurophysiological mechanisms of taste. *American Journal of Clinical Nutrition, 31*, 1058-1067.

Pfaffmann, C. (1978b). The vertebrate phylogeny, neural code, and integrative processes of taste. In E. C. Carterette & M. P. Friedman (Eds.), *Handbook of perception, vol. 6A: Tasting and smelling.* New York: Academic Press.

Phillips, M. (1992, July). Breath tests in medicine. *Scientific American,* pp. 74-79.

Pickles, J. O., Comis, S. D., & Osborne, M. P. (1984). Cross-links between stereocilia in the guinea pig organ of Corti, and their possible relation to sensory transduction. *Hearing Research, 15,* 103-112.

Pickles, J. O., & Corey, D. P. (1992). Mechanoelectrical transduction by hair cells. *Trends in Neuroscience, 15,* 254-259.

Pons, T. P., Garraghty, P. E., Friedman, D. P., & Mishkin, M. (1987). Physiological evidence for serial processing in somatosensory cortex. *Science, 237,* pp. 417-420.

Posner, M. I. (Ed.). (1989). *Foundations of cognitive science.* Cambridge: MIT Press.

Reed, R. R. (1990). How does the nose know? *Cell, 60,* 1-2.

Reger, S. N. (1960). Effect of middle ear muscle action on certain psychological measurements. *Annals of Otolaryngology, Rhinology, Laryngology, 69,* 1179-1198.

Rodin, J., Bartoshuk, L., Peterson, C., & Schank, D. (1990). Bulimia and taste: Possible interactions. *Journal of Abnormal Psychology, 99,* 32-39.

Rodman, H. R., & Albright, T. D. (1989). Single-unit analysis of pattern-motion selective properties in the middle temporal visual area (MT). *Experimental Brain Research, 75,* 53-64.

Roe, A. W., Pallas, S. L., Hahm, J.-O., & Sur, M. (1990). A map of visual space induced in primary auditory cortex. *Science, 250,* pp. 818-820.

Rossetti, Y., Koga, K., & Mano, T. (1993). Prismatic displacement of vision induces transient changes in the timing of eye-hand coordination. *Perception and Psychophysics, 54,* 355-364.

Rozin, P. (1990). Social and moral aspects of food and eating. In I. Rock (Ed.), *The legacy of Solomon Asch: Essays in cognition and social psychology.* Hillsdale, NJ: Erlbaum.

Rutherford, W. (1886). A new theory of hearing. *Journal of Anatomy and Physiology, 21,* 166-168.

Sato, T. (1980). Recent advances in the physiology of taste cells. *Progress in Neurobiology, 14,* 25-67.

Schnapf, J. L., & Baylor, D. A. (1987). How photoreceptor cells respond to light. *Scientific American, 256,* 40-47.

Schouten, J. F., Ritsma, R. J., & Cardozo, B. L. (1962). Pitch of the residue. *Journal of the Acoustical Society of America, 34,* 1418-1424.

Schwenk, K. (1994). Why snakes have forked tongues. *Science, 263,* pp. 1573-1577.

Shepherd, G. M. (1985). The olfactory system: the uses of neural space for nonspatial modality. *Progress in Clinical Biological Research, 176,* 99-114.

Snyder, S. H. (1986). *Drugs and the brain.* New York: Scientific American Library.

Spitzer, H., Desimone, R., & Moran, J. (1988). Increased attention enhances both behavioral and neuronal performance. *Science, 240,* pp. 338-340.

Stockwell, C. W. (1988). Conventional bithermal caloric tests. In H. O. Barber & J. A. Sharpe (Eds.), *Vestibular disorders.* Boca Raton, FL: Year Book Medical Publishers.

Stoddart, D. M. (1990). *The scented ape: The biology and culture of human odor.* New York: Cambridge University Press.

Sugita, Y. (1996). Global plasticity in adult visual cortex following reversal of visual input. *Nature, 380,* pp. 523-526.

Tanaka, K. (1996). Inferotemporal cortex and object vision. *Annual Review of Neuroscience, 19,* 109-138.

Thier, P., & Erickson, R. G. (1992). Responses of visual-tracking neurons from cortical area MST-I to visual, eye and head motion. *European Journal of Neuroscience, 4,* 539-553.

Travis, J. (1992). Can "hair cells" unlock deafness? *Science, 257,* pp. 1344-1345.

Ts'o, D. Y., & Gilbert, C. D. (1988). The organization of chromatic and spatial interactions in the primate striate cortex. *Journal of Neuroscience, 8,* 1712-1727.

Turk, D. (1994). Perspectives on chronic pain: The role of psychological factors. *Current Directions in Psychological Science, 3*(2), 45-48.

Ungerleider, I. G., & Mishkin, M. (1982). Two cortical visual systems. In D. Ingle, M. A. Goodale, & R. J. W. Mansfield (Eds.), *Analysis of visual behavior.* Cambridge: MIT Press.

von Békésy, G. (1947). The variation of phase along the basilar membrane with sinusoidal vibrations. *Journal of the Acoustical Society of America, 19*, 452-460.

von Békésy, G. (1960). *Experiments in hearing.* New York: McGraw-Hill.

von Bergeijk, W. A., Pierce, J. R., & David, E. E., Jr. (1960). *Waves and the ear.* Garden City, NY: Doubleday,

von Helmholtz, H. L. F. (1954). *Die lehre von den tonenpfindungen als physiologische grundlege für die theorie der musik* [On the sensations of tone as a physiological basis for the theory of music] (A. J. Ellis, Trans.). New York: Dover. (Original work published in 1863)

Wald, G., Brown, P. K., & Smith, P. H. (1955). Iodopsin. *Journal of General Physiology, 38*, 623-681.

Wall, P. D., & Melzack, R. (Eds.). (1994). *Textbook of pain* (3rd ed.). Edinburgh, Scotland: Churchill Livingstone.

Warfield, C. A., Stein, J. M., & Frank, H. A. (1985). The effect of transcutaneous electrical nerve stimulation on pain after thoracotomy. *Annals of Thoracic Surgery, 39*, 462-465.

Wässle, H., & Boycott, B. B. (1991). Functional architecture of the mammalian retina. *Physiological Review, 71*, 447-470.

Wever, E. G. (1949). *Theory of hearing.* New York: Wiley.

Wever, E. G., & Bray, C. W. (1937). The perception of low tones and the resonance-volley theory. *Journal of Psychology, 3*, 101-114.

Wever, E. G., & Lawrence, M. (1954). *Physiological acoustics.* Princeton, NJ: Princeton University Press.

Wiesel, T. N., & Hubel, D. H. (1966). Spatial and chromatic interactions in the lateral geniculate body of the rhesus monkey. *Journal of Neurophysiology, 29*, 1115-1156.

Wiesenfelder, H., & Blake, R. (1991). Apparent motion can survive binocular rivalry suppression. *Vision Research, 31*, 1589-1599.

Wightman, F. L., & Kistler, D. J. (1989). Headphone simulation of free field listening I: Stimulus synthesis. *Journal of the Acoustical Society of America, 85*, 858-867.

Wong-Riley, M. T. T. (1979). Changes in the visual system of monocularly sutured or enucleated cats demonstrable with cytochrome oxidase histochemistry. *Brain Research, 171*, 11-28.

Wong-Riley, M. T. T., Hevner, R. F., Cutlan, R., Earnest, M., Eagan, R., Frost, J., & Nguyen, T. (1993). Cytochrome oxidase in the human visual cortex: Distribution in the developing and adult brain. *Visual Neuroscience, 10*, 41-58.

Yau, K.-W. (1994). Phototransduction mechanism in retinal rods and cones. *Investigations in Ophthalmology & Visual Science, 35,* 9-32.

Yoshikami, S., Robinson, W. E., & Hagins, W. A. (1974). Topology of the outer segment membranes of retinal rods and cones revealed by fluorescent probe. *Science, 185,* pp. 1176-1179.

Zeki, S. (1974). Functional organization of a visual area in the posterior bank of the superior temporal sulcus of the rhesus monkey. *Journal of Physiology, 236,* 549-573.

Zeki, S. (1993). *A vision of the brain.* Cambridge, MA: Blackwell Scientific Publications.

Index

About the Author

David R. Soderquist is Professor of Psychology at the University of North Carolina at Greensboro, where he has been a member of the faculty since 1968. He was recruited in 1968 by the Department of Psychology to aid in the development of a nationally visible experimental doctoral program. He helped the department achieve this goal through his excellence in teaching and research. During this time, he served for over two decades as the faculty advisor for Psi Chi, the national honor society in psychology. He received numerous "certificates of appreciation" from his students for his dedication and commitment to Psi Chi and the advancement of undergraduate education. He has taught a wide spectrum of undergraduate psychology courses: Introductory Psychology (with a laboratory), Research Methods, Introduction to Statistics, Biological Psychology, Sensory Processes, Perception, Psychological Tests and Measurement, and undergraduate research honors courses. At the graduate level, he has taught Sensory Processes, Experimental Design, Graduate Statistics, and seminars in Animal Psychophysics and Auditory Perception. He has mentored not only doctoral students in his auditory psychophysics laboratory but also students in social, developmental, and clinical areas of psychology. His research has been supported by national foundations as well as university-sponsored grants.

Dr. Soderquist has presented numerous papers at professional meetings and published his research in many scientific journals: *Journal of the Acoustical Society of America, Journal of Auditory Research, Human Factors, Psychological Bulletin, Bulletin of the Psychonomic Society, Perception and Psychophysics, Current Psychological Research and Reviews, Educational and Psychological Measurement,* and *Journal of Experimental Child Psychology.*

He received his B.S. and M.S. degrees in psychology from Utah State University in 1961 and 1963. He then joined System Development Corporation as a Human Factors Specialist with the responsibility of training U.S. Air Force personnel in computerized air defense. He returned to academic psychology in 1965 and received his Ph.D. from Vanderbilt University in 1968 with an emphasis in statistics and auditory psychophysics.